CORONARY ARTERY DISEASE – NEW INSIGHTS AND NOVEL APPROACHES

Edited by **Angelo Squeri**

Coronary Artery Disease – New Insights and Novel Approaches
Edited by Angelo Squeri

Published by InTech
Janeza Trdine 9, 51000 Rijeka, Croatia

Publishing Process Manager Vedran Greblo

Technical Editor Teodora Smiljanic

Cover Designer InTech Design Team

Additional hard copies can be obtained from orders@intechopen.com

Coronary Artery Disease – New Insights and Novel Approaches, Edited by Angelo Squeri
p. cm.
ISBN 978-953-51-0344-8

For EU product safety concerns:
IN TECH d.o.o., Prolaz Marije Krucifikse Kozulić 3, 51000 Rijeka, Croatia,
info@intechopen.com or visit our website at intechopen.com.

Meet the editor

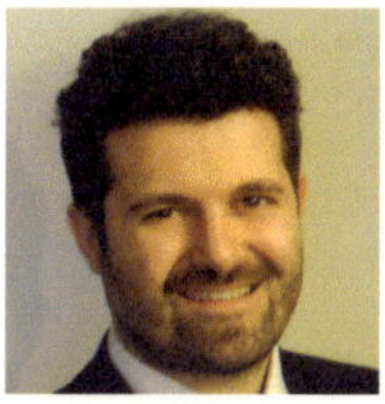

Angelo Squeri MD is a clinical cardiologist at Maria Cecilia Hospital, GVM Care & Research (Cotignola, Italy). He graduated in medicine in 2003 at the Università degli Studi di Parma where he also received his fellowship in Cardiology. He developed his interest in echocardiography especially in stress echocardiography with myocardial perfusion study, publishing several articles in the field of coronary artery disease. He also developed an expertise in valvular heart disease and three dimensional echocardiography, becoming a member of the "European Society of Cardiology Working group on valvular heart disease". He has also been an invited speaker at a number of international meetings and serves as reviewer for several journals.

Contents

Preface

Coronary Artery disease is one of the leading causes of death in industrialized countries and is responsible for one out of every six deaths in the United States. Remarkably, coronary artery disease is also largely preventable. The pathogenesis is complex and involves many different pathways that are only partially understood. Recently, the morbidity and mortality of ischaemic heart disease have substantially improved because of progress in therapeutic strategies, represented by the dramatic evolution of percutaneous coronary intervention. The biggest challenge in the next years is, however, to reduce the incidence of coronary artery disease worldwide.

A complete knowledge of the mechanisms responsible for the development of ischaemic heart disease is an essential prerequisite to a better management of this pathology improving prevention and therapy.

This monograph deals with the pathophysiology of atherosclerosis with emphasis on epigenetics, metabolomics, inflammation, molecular and cellular mechanisms involved in cardiovascular disease development.

This book has been written with the intention of providing new concepts about coronary artery disease pathogenesis that may link various aspects of the disease, going beyond the traditional risk factors.

Angelo Squeri, MD
Maria Cecilia Hospital – GVM Care & Research
Italy

Part 1

Pathogenesis

1

Gene Polymorphism and Coronary Heart Disease

Nduna Dzimiri
King Faisal Specialist Hospital and Research Centre
Saudi Arabia

1. Introduction

Like all other organs and tissues in a mammalian body, the heart muscle requires oxygen-rich blood in order to function, while oxygen-depleted blood needs to be transported away from organs. The first requirement is accomplished through the coronary artery networks which serve to furnish blood supply to the cardiac muscle, while the second is attained through a network of blood veins.

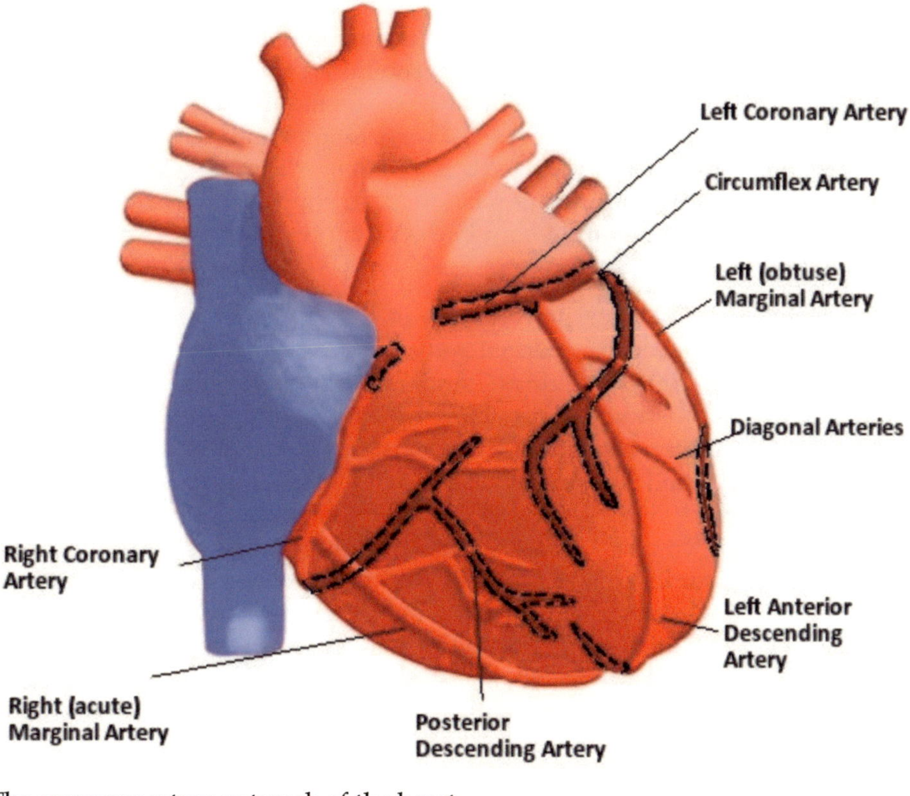

Fig. 1. The coronary artery network of the heart.

The coronary artery system consists of two main arteries, the left and right arteries, and their marginal arterial network. Anatomically, the left main coronary artery (LMCA) consists of the left anterior descending artery and the circumflex branch that supplies blood to the left ventricle and atrium (Figure 1). Additional arteries branching off the LMCA furnish the left heart side muscles with blood. These include the circumvent artery, which branches off the left coronary artery and encircles the muscle to supply blood to the lateral side and back of the heart, and the left anterior descending artery, which supplies the blood to the front of the left side of the heart. The right coronary artery, on the other hand, branches into the right posterior descending and acute marginal arteries to supply blood to the right ventricle, right atrium sinoatrial node (cluster of cells in the right atrial wall that regulate the heart's rhythmic rate) and the atrioventricular node. Other smaller branches of the coronary arteries include the acute marginal, posterior descending, obtuse marginal, septal perforator and the diagonals, which provide the surrounding network with blood supply.

2. What causes coronary artery disease?

Since coronary arteries deliver blood to the heart muscle, disease can have serious implications by reducing the flow of oxygen and nutrients to the heart, which in turn may lead to a heart attack and possibly death. Besides, the susceptibility and function of the vessel wall are dependent on the balance of several counteracting forces, i.e., vasoconstricting versus vasodilating, growth-promoting versus growth-inhibiting and proapoptotic versus antiapoptotic functions. While these factors are tightly balanced in a normal healthy vessel, under pathophysiologic conditions this balance is upset resulting in the development of vascular hypertrophy and the generation of proatherogenic vascular lesions, thereby triggering the initiation and progression of coronary artery disease (CAD) or atherosclerosis (as it is often called). CAD is a complex disorder, which culminates in the coronary bed system failing to furnish adequate blood supply to the heart. The disease has no clear etiology and manifests itself both in the young (early onset) as in familial cases as well as in adults (late onset).

One major culprit for CAD is a perturbation in lipid metabolism. A lipid is any fatty material or fat-like substance, e.g. normal body fat, cholesterol (i.e. high density and low density lipoproteins), other steroids, and substances containing fats, such as phospholipids, glycolipids and lipoproteins. Specifically, cholesterol (Chol) constitutes one of the most clinically important lipid substances, and alterations in the balance between its synthesis and the metabolism of its by-products is a major source of cardiovascular complications. Together with its metabolites, Chol plays a variety of essential roles in living systems. In fact, virtually all animal cells require Chol, which they acquire through synthesis or uptake, but only the liver can degrade it. Failure of metabolic pathways to break these substances down as required, or by the system to maintain the right balance, will lead to their increased levels, and therefore predispose an individual to acquiring CAD. Circulating lipoproteins are regulated at various levels, ranging from Chol synthesis, transport and metabolism. Chol biosynthesis comprises the condensation of acetyl-CoA and acetoacetyl-CoA into 3-hydroxy-3-methylglutaryl-coenzyme A (HMG-CoA), which in turn is reduced to mevalonate by the HMG-CoA reductase (HMGCR) followed by oxidoreduction and decarboxylation intermediate steps leading to the conversion of lanosterol to Chol. It is regulated through feedback inhibition by sterols and non-sterol metabolites derived from mevalonate. The HMGCR, an integral glycoprotein of endoplasmic reticulum membranes that remains in the endoplasmic reticulum after synthesis and glycosylation, is the rate-limiting enzyme in Chol biosynthesis in vertebrates.

The maintenance of Chol homeostasis encompasses diverse metabolic pathways linked to its transportation, metabolism and its metabolic by-products. Since Chol is insoluble in blood, it is transported in the circulatory system within a large range of lipoproteins in blood. Thereby, its transportation to peripheral tissues is accomplished by the lipoproteins, chylomicrons, very low density lipoproteins (VLDLs) and low density lipoproteins (LDLs), while high-density lipoprotein (HDL) particles transport it back to the liver for excretion. Functionally, LDL is a metabolic end-product of the triglyceride (TG)-rich lipoproteins (i.e. VDLDs). Lipoprotein metabolism constitutes a major component in the regulation of Chol homeostasis. Systems regulating Chol levels include the LDL receptor (LDLR) pathway and its ligand the apolipoprotein B100 (Apo B), which are involved in the maintenance of its homeostasis in the body by regulating the hepatic catabolism of LDL-Cholesterol (LDL-C), and the proprotein convertase subtilisin/kexin type 9 (PCSK9). The serine protease PCSK9 is a member of the proteinase K subfamily of subtilases that also affects plasma LDL-C levels by altering LDLR levels via a post-transcriptional mechanism[1], and cellular Chol metabolism by regulating both LDLR and circulating Apo B-containing lipoprotein levels in LDLR-dependent and -independent fashions[2-4]. It regulates LDL-C levels apparently both intracellularly and by behaving as a secreted protein that can be internalized by binding the LDLR. In the liver, it controls the plasma LDL-C level by post-transcriptionally downregulating the LDLR through binding to the epidermal growth factor-like repeat A (EGF-A) domain of the LDLR[5], independently of its catalytic activity. The LDLR regulates the plasma LDL-C concentration by internalizing Apo B and Apo E-containing lipoproteins via receptor-mediated endocytosis. Apo B is a large, amphipathic glycoprotein that plays a central role in human lipoprotein metabolism. Two forms of Apo B are produced from the *Apo B* gene through a unique posttranscriptional editing process: Apo B-48, which is required for chylomicron production in the small intestine, and Apo B required for VLDL production in the liver. In addition to being the essential structural component of VLDL, Apo B is the ligand for LDLR-mediated endocytosis of LDL particles. Lipoprotein (a) [Lp(a)] contains an LDL-like moiety, in which the Apo B component is covalently linked to the unique glycoprotein apolipoprotein(a) (Apo A). Apo A-I is essential for the formation of HDL particles. Apo A-I-containing HDL particles play a primary role in Chol efflux from membranes, at least partly, through interactions with the adenosine triphosphate-binding cassette transporter A1 (ABCA1). The ABCA1 regulates the rate-controlling step in the removal of cellular Chol, i.e. the efflux of cellular Chol and phospholipids to an apolipoprotein acceptor. Apo A is composed of repeated loop-shaped units called kringles, the sequences of which are highly similar to a kringle motif present in the fibrinolytic proenzyme plasminogen. Variability in the number of repeated kringle units in the Apo A molecule gives rise to different-sized Lp(a) isoforms in the population. Based on the similarity of Lp(a) to both LDL and plasminogen, its function is thought to represent a link between atherosclerosis and thrombosis. However, determination of the function of Lp(a) in vivo remains elusive. Mechanistically, elevated Lp(a) levels may either induce a prothrombotic/anti-fibrinolytic effect as Apo A resembles both plasminogen and plasmin but has no fibrinolytic activity, and/or may accelerate atherosclerosis because, like LDL, the Lp(a) particle is Chol-rich. Apolipoprotein E (apo E) is also a constituent of various lipoproteins and plays an important role in the transport of Chol and other lipids among cells of various tissues.

Apart from lipoproteins, circulating VLDLs serve as vehicles for transporting lipids to peripheral tissues for energy homeostasis. VLDLs are TG-rich particles synthesized in hepatocytes and secreted from the liver in a pathway that is tightly regulated by insulin. Hepatic VLDL production is stimulated in response to reduced insulin action, resulting in increased release of VLDL into the blood under fasting conditions, while it is suppressed in response to increased insulin release after meals. This effect is critical for preventing prolonged excursion of postprandial plasma lipid profiles in normal individuals. HDL particles are key players in the reverse Chol transport by shuttling it from peripheral cells (e.g. macrophages) to the liver or other tissues. This complex process is thought to represent the basis for the antiatherogenic properties of HDL particles. Accordingly, the particles mediate the uptake of peripheral Chol and return it to the liver for bile acid secretion through exchange of core lipids with other lipoproteins or selective uptake by specific receptors. These particles vary in size and density, mainly because of differences in the number of apolipoprotein (apo) particles and the amount of Chol ester in the core of HDL molecule.

The majority of lipoprotein disorders result from a combination of polygenic predisposition and poor lifestyle habits, including physical inactivity, increased visceral adipose tissue, increased caloric intake, and cigarette smoking. Plasma elevation of LDL-C, VLDL and Lp(a), as well as reduced HDL-C levels are predisposing factors for CAD. The amount of Chol transported is inversely correlated with the risk for CAD. Reduced circulating levels of HDL-C are a frequent lipoprotein disorder in CAD patients and can be caused by either genetic and/or environmental factors (sedentary lifestyle, diabetes mellitus, smoking, obesity or a diet enriched in carbohydrates. Lp(a) is a unique lipoprotein particle consisting of a moiety identical to LDL to which the glycoprotein Apo(a) that is homologous to plasminogen is covalently attached. These features have suggested that Lp(a) may contribute to both proatherogenic and prothrombotic/antifibrinolytic processes, which constitute a risk factor for premature cardiovascular disease. Among others, the association between elevated Lp(a) levels and increased CAD risk, indicates that elevated Lp(a), like elevated LDL-C, is causally related to premature CAD. However, although Lp(a) has been shown to accumulate in atherosclerotic lesions, its contribution to the development of atheromas is unclear. This uncertainty is related in part to the structural complexity of the Apo A component of Lp(a) (particularly apo A isoform size heterogeneity), which also poses a challenge for standardization of the measurement of Lp(a) in plasma. However, while LDL and Lp(a) are now believed to be atherogenic, the role of VLDL as an independent risk factor remains controversial. On the other hand, the HDL is the only lipoprotein that has been established as antiatherogenic, thought to reduce CAD risk by mediating Chol efflux from the periphery by way of transportation to the liver for excretion.

Hepatic lipase (HL), a member of the lipase superfamily, is a lipolytic enzyme that is produced primarily by hepatocytes, where it is secreted and bound to the hepatocyte surface and readily released by heparin. It is homologous to LPL and pancreatic lipase and hydrolyzes TGs and phospholipids in all lipoproteins, but is predominant in the conversion of IDL to LDL and the conversion of post-prandial TG-rich HDL into the post absorptive TG-poor HDL. Thus, the enzyme contributes to the regulation of plasma TG levels by facilitating its exudation from the VLDL pool, in a fashion that is governed by the composition and quality of HDL particles. It is thought that HL directly couples HDL lipid metabolism to tissue/cellular lipid metabolism[43]. Accordingly, hepatic lipase HDL regulates the release of HL from the liver and HDL, controls HL transport and activation in the circulation in a fashion that is regulated by factors that release it from the liver and activate it in the bloodstream. Therefore, alterations in HDL-apolipoprotein composition can disturb HL function by inhibiting the release and activation of the enzyme, thereby affecting plasma TG levels and CAD risk. It has been suggested that the HL pathway potentially provides the hepatocyte with a mechanism for the uptake of a subset of phospholipids enriched in unsaturated fatty acids and may allow the uptake of cholesteryl ester, free Chol, and phospholipid without catabolism of HDL apolipoproteins[43]. HL plays a secondary role in the clearance of chylomicron remnants by the liver[43]. Consistent with IDL being a substrate for HL, the human post-heparin HL activity is inversely correlated with IDL-C concentration only in subjects with a hyperlipidaemia involving VLDL. HDL-C has been reported to be inversely correlated to HL activity, leading to the suggestion that lowering HL would increase its levels. Common hormonal factors, such as estrogen, have also been shown to upregulate Apo A and HDL-C and lower HL. Hence this relationship may not be specific. However, an increase in HDL-C, Apo A, or HDL -triglycerides has been observed in severe deficiency of HL. Apart from heparin, HL also binds o the LDLR-related protein. This has led to the notion that enzymatically inactive HL may play a role in hepatic lipoprotein uptake, forming a bridge by binding to the lipoprotein and to the cell surface, raising the possibility that production and secretion of mutant inactive HL could promote clearance of VLDL remnants.

One of the important proteins involved in lipoprotein metabolism is the CETP. Plasma CETP facilitates the transfer of cholesteryl ester from HDL to Apo B-containing lipoproteins by catalyzing the transfer of insoluble esters in the reverse transport of Chol. Thus, CETP is involved in maintaining the balance between the LDL-C, ("bad" Chol) and HDL-C ("good" Chol), which is a risk factor for hyperlipidaemia. Since CETP regulates the plasma levels of HDL-C and the size of HDL particles, it is considered to be a key protein in reverse Chol transport, a protective system against atherosclerosis. In mediating the transfer of cholesteryl esters from antiatherogenic HDL to proatherogenic apolipoprotein apo-B-containing lipoprotein particles (including VLDL, VLDL remnants, IDL, and LDL), the CETP plays a critical role not only in the RCT pathway but also in the intravascular remodeling and recycling of HDL particles[6,7].

In mammalian cells, Chol homeostasis is controlled primarily by regulated cleavage of membrane-bound transcription factors, the sterol regulatory element binding proteins (SREBPs)[8-10] and their cleavage-activating protein (SCAP)[11,12]. The SREBPs activate specific genes involved in Chol synthesis, LDL endocytosis, fatty acid synthesis and glucose metabolism, providing a link between lipid and carbohydrate metabolism[13]. All three SREBP isoforms SREBP-1a, SREBP-1c and SREBP-2 (encoded by two genes) that are synthesized as 125 kDa precursor proteins localized to the endoplasmic reticulum[14], and play a central role in energy homeostasis by promoting glycolysis, lipogenesis and adipogenesis[15-19]. Functionally, SREBP-2 gene activation leads to enhanced Chol uptake and biosynthesis, while SREBP-1 is primarily involved in fatty acid and glucose metabolism[20-22]. Mechanistically, it is thought that when cells are deprived of Chol, SREBPs are cleaved by two proteolytic steps. First, the SREBP precursor is transported to the Golgi by the chaperone protein SCAP and cleaved via two proteases to release the mature, transcriptionally active 68 kDa amino terminal domain[11,12]. This domain is then released from the endoplasmic reticulum membrane and transported into the nucleus, where it binds to specific nucleotide sequences in the promoters of the LDLR and other genes regulating Chol and TG homeostasis[10].

While disorders of Chol metabolism and related lipoproteins occupy a pivotal position in events leading to CAD, other important contributors include those that regulate the viability of blood vessels affecting vascular function leading to the formation of plaques. This is particularly true for coronary arteries, for example, in which an imbalance in a number of these processes triggers a proatherogenic state initiating the progression of atherosclerosis. Several disease pathways associated with regulation of blood pressure and glucose metabolism are involved in intricate ways. The metabolic syndrome poses a major public health problem by predisposing individuals to CAD and stroke, the leading causes of mortality in developed countries. Its impact on the risk of atherosclerotic cardiovascular disease is greater than that of any of its individual components. Frequently, many of these metabolic manifestations, precede the development of overt diabetes by many years[23]. This syndrome is manifest clinically by such cardiovascular risk factors as hypertension, dyslipidaemic, and coagulation abnormalities. This abnormal metabolic milieu contributes to the high prevalence of macrovascular complications including CAD as well as more generalized atherosclerosis. It is frequently seen in obese individuals, and characterized by glucose intolerance, hyperinsulinemia, a characteristic dyslipidaemic (high TGs; low HDL-C, and small, dense LDL-C), obesity, upper-body fat distribution, hypertension, increased prothrombotic and antifibrinolytic factors, and therefore an increased risk of CAD[23]. However, while the conventional risk factors, insulin resistance parameters, and metabolic syndrome are important in predicting CAD risk, in some population environmental factors may be determinant in the ultimate manifestation of the disease.

Apart from the PPARs, the Forkhead transcription factor (Foxo1) is also believed to play an essential role in controlling insulin-dependent regulation of microsomal TG transfer protein (MTP) and apolipoprotein C-III (Apo C-III), two key components that catalyze the rate-limiting steps in the production and clearance of triglyceride-rich lipoproteins[24,25]. Under physiological conditions, Foxo1 activity is inhibited by insulin, while under insulin resistant conditions Foxo1 becomes uncontrolled, contributing to its hyperactivity in the liver[24]. This effect contributes to hepatic overproduction of VLDL and impaired catabolism of triglyceride-rich particles, accounting for the pathogenesis of hypertriglyceridemia. Thus, augmented Foxo1 activity in insulin resistant livers promotes hepatic VLDL overproduction and predisposes to the development of hypertriglyceridemia[25], offering a possible route for this manifestation.

As such the contributions of the individual disease pathways such as diabetes or hypertension may manifest themselves independently or in combination with other disorders, leading to other complications with added risk as is the case with the metabolic syndrome. Among these, type 2 diabetes mellitus (T2DM) constitutes probably the most important risk disease for CAD. In contrast to type 1 diabetes mellitus, the type 2 endocrinopathy is clustered in minority populations and has both strong genetic and environmental components that influence its manifestation. This disease is a heterogeneous disorder and patients are often characterized by features of the insulin resistance syndrome, also referred to as the metabolic syndrome. This syndrome is defined as a cluster of interrelated common clinical disorders, including obesity, insulin resistance, glucose intolerance, hypertension, and dyslipidaemic (hypertriglyceridaemia and low HDL-C levels), exhibiting rising incidence to epidemic levels in the developed world. Among others, insulin has important vascular actions to stimulate production of nitric oxide from endothelium. This leads to capillary recruitment, vasodilatation, increased blood flow, and subsequent augmentation of glucose disposal in classical insulin target tissues, such as the skeletal muscle. Individuals displaying three of the features of insulin resistance (elevated plasma insulin and apolipoprotein B concentrations and small, dense LDL particles) show a remarkable increase in CAD risk and the increased risk associated with having small, dense LDL particles may be modulated to a significant extent by the presence/absence of insulin resistance, abdominal obesity and increased LDL particle concentration[26]. They influence risk for CAD through promoting endothelial dysfunction and enhanced production of procoagulants by endothelial cells[27].

Systems regulating the coagulation mechanisms also have their fair share of disease pathways leading to CAD. To begin with, blood platelets play a crucial role in physiological haemostasis and in the pathology of prothrombotic states, including atherosclerosis. Platelets are anucleate cells with no DNA. The differentiation of their precursor, the megakaryocyte, is characterized by nuclear polyploidization through a process called endomitosis. Changes in the megakaryocyte-platelet-haemostasis axis may precede acute thrombotic events. Thereby, the changes in megakaryocyte ploidy distribution may be associated with the production of large platelets. Large platelets are denser and more active haemostatically. Mean platelet volume, an important biological variable determinant of platelet reactivity, is increased in patients after MI and is a predictor of a further ischaemic event and death following MI[28]. Apart from platelets, changes also in the parental megakaryocyte are associated with chronic and acute vascular events[29]. The regulation of megakaryocytopoiesis depends on several haematopoietic factors such as thrombopoietin. In T2DM, platelet abnormalities, including altered adhesion and aggregation, render the cells hypersensitive to agonists. Besides, disturbed carbohydrate and lipid metabolism may lead to physicochemical changes in cell membrane dynamics, and consequently altered exposure of surface membrane receptors. These manifestations, together with increased fibrinogen binding, prostanoid metabolism, phosphoinositide turnover and calcium mobilization often present in diabetic patients, contribute to enhanced risk of small vessel occlusions and accelerated development of atherothrombotic disease of coronary, cerebral and other vessels in diabetes. The disease has emerged as an important condition of older patients in which both microvascular and macrovascular complications are a common cause of morbidity and mortality. Microvascular complications have only been recently recognized as an important and frequent complication of T2DM[30].

Additionally, environmental factors, such as food consumption, constitute important components regulating pathways to complex diseases such as CAD and cancer. Dietary Chol absorption, endogenous Chol synthesis and biliary Chol excretion regulate whole body Chol balance as a result of biotransformation into bile acids or direct Chol excretion. Nuclear hormone receptors, such as the liver X, farnesoid X and retinoid X receptors, regulate the absorption of dietary sterols by modulating the transcription of several genes involved in Chol metabolism[31]. The ABC proteins transport dietary Chol from enterocytes back to the intestinal lumen, thus limiting the amount of absorbed Chol. By means of the same mechanism, ABC transporters also provide an efficient barrier against the absorption of plant sterols[31], which may vary among different ethnic populations. For example, it appears that some ethnic groups are at higher risk than others for the development of obesity and obesity-related non-communicable diseases, including insulin resistance, the metabolic syndrome, T2DM and CAD. Put together therefore, because of the various interactive factors regulating the functionality of coronary vascular beds, many risk factors may contribute to an individual acquiring the disease.

2.1 Coronary artery disease manifestation in the adult

These risk factors for CAD can be classified into those that regulate the levels of circulating lipoproteins, and those that regulate the susceptibility of arterial walls. Factors regulating lipoprotein levels include high circulating Chol and saturated fats in diet, obesity and emotional and neurogenic factors and those that regulate arterial susceptibility are insulin resistance, diabetes, hypertension, smoking and age (Figure 2). All these factors contribute to the pathways leading to atherosclerosis, oft in combination with environmental factors. Apart from the fact that most of the predisposing diseases are themselves complex ailments, combinations of some of these disorders can cluster to induce other forms of maladies, such as the metabolic syndrome, which in themselves constitute an added risk for coronary disease.

For almost all of these disease pathways, their impact on CAD manifestation can be classified as major or minor, depending on their assessed contribution (Figure 2). For example, in the regulation of blood pressure homeostasis insulin-resistant diabetes mellitus and essential hypertension are among the primary culprits, while angiotensin converting enzyme (ACE) and angiotensin 1 make up secondary causative factors. Furthermore, a great majority of these risk factors (e.g. hypertension, diabetes, hyperlipidaemia) are themselves complex disorders underlying a variety of etiologies. In essence therefore, CAD is shaped by a whole spectrum of phenotypic expression evolving through various events that lead to the formation and progression of atherosclerotic plaque in the inner lining of an artery causing it to narrow or become blocked and finally exude circulatory complications. The ultimate disease manifestation is an expression of the shift in the balance of interactions among factors influencing various aspects of coronary artery function and structure with prevalent genetic factors.

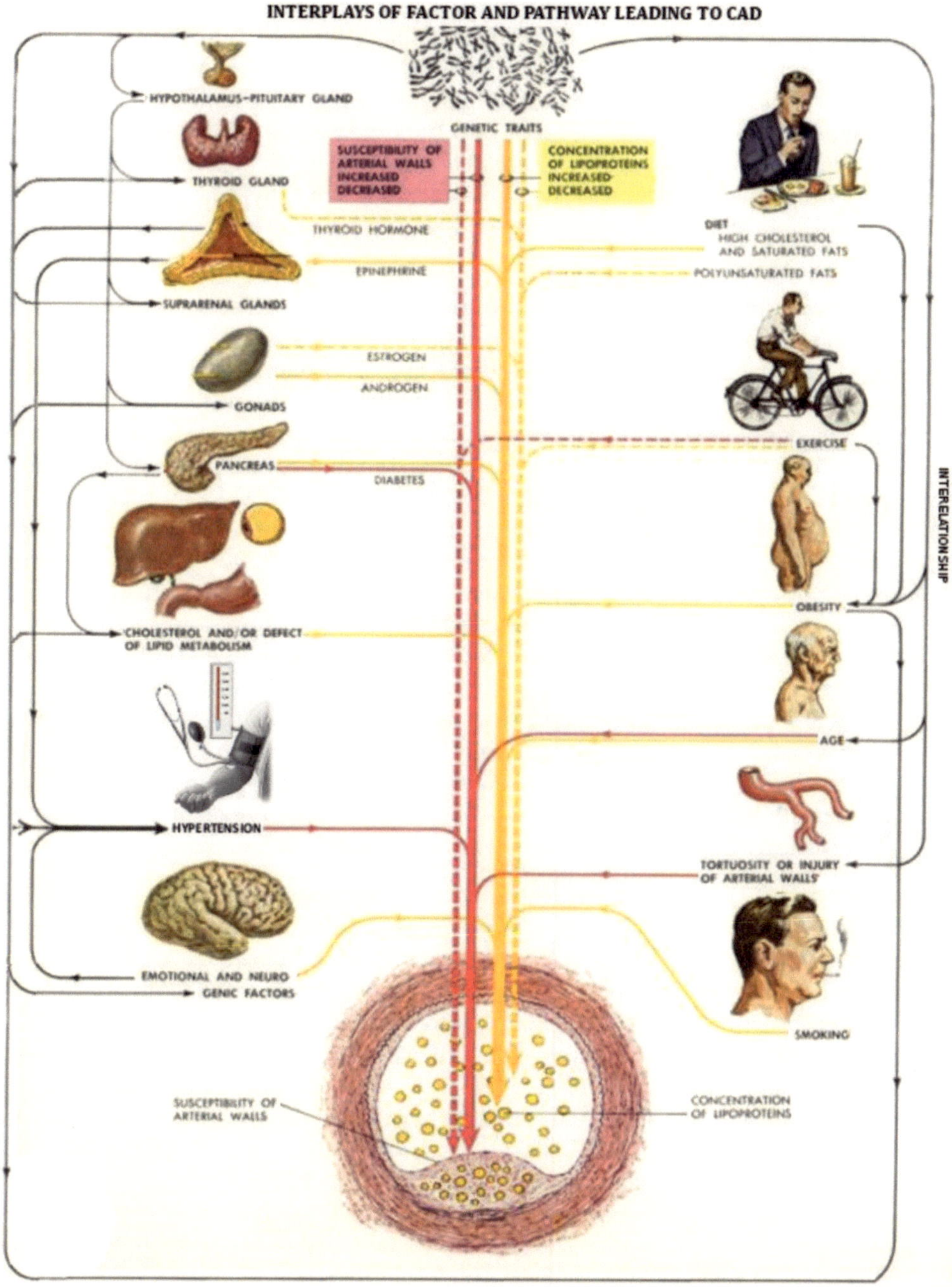

Fig. 2. The risk factors contributing to coronary artery disease pathways. The pathways may lead to either an increase in in circulating lipoproteins, influence susceptibility of the vessel walls or both components of atherosclerotic plaque formation.

2.1.1 Lipid metabolism and manifestation of coronary artery disease

As stated above, defects in lipid metabolic pathways, leading to increased circulating Chol levels constitutes the major underlying cause of CAD. Hyperlipidaemia, also sometimes referred to as hyperlipoproteinemia or dyslipidaemia, is the condition in which the blood lipid levels are too high, often leading to various cardiovascular disorders, particularly CAD. These disorders exist as hypercholesterolaemia, which is characterized by increased LDL levels, hypertriglyceridaemia characterized by increased chylomicrons or VLDL levels or combined disease manifest as increased LDL and VLDL, or VLDL and chylomicrons. Affected individuals may also have hypercholesterolaemia or chylomicron abnormalities of VLDL origin, with normal LDL-C levels, which is also defined as hyperlipoproteinemia.

Six subtypes of hyperlipoproteinemia types (I, II, III, IV, V and unclassified forms) have been characterized to date. Type I (also known as Buerger-Gruetz syndrome, primary hyperlipoproteinemia, or familial hyperchylomicronemia) is a very rare form due to a deficiency of lipoprotein lipase (LPL) or altered apolipoprotein C2. It results in elevated chylomicrons, the particles that transfer fatty acids from the digestive tract to the liver, exhibiting a prevalence of 0.1% of the population. Hyperlipoproteinemia type II, by far the most common form, is further classified into type IIa and type IIb, depending mainly on whether there is elevation in the TG level in addition to LDL-C. Thereby type IIa is known as familial hypercholesterolaemia. This form may be sporadic (due to dietary factors), polygenic, or truly familial as a result of a mutation either in the LDLR gene on chromosome 19 (0.2% of the population) or the Apo B gene (0.2%). In type IIb, the high VLDL levels are due to overproduction of substrates, including TGs, acetyl CoA, and an increase in Apo B synthesis. They may also be caused by the decreased clearance of LDL, with a prevalence of 10% in the population. These include (a) familial combined hyperlipoproteinemia (FCH) and (b) secondary combined hyperlipoproteinemia (usually in the context of metabolic syndrome, for which it is a diagnostic criterion). Hyperlipoproteinemia type III, also known as broad beta disease or dysbetalipoproteinemia, is due to high chylomicrons and intermediate density lipoprotein (IDL). It is due to the presence of elevated Chol-rich VLDL (β-VLDL) levels showing a prevalence of 0.02% in the general population.

The type IV form, also known as hypertriglyceridaemia (or pure hypertriglyceridaemia) is due to high TGs, with prevalence of 1%, while type V is very similar to type I, but with high VLDL in addition to chylomicrons. The rate of synthesis of TG-rich lipoproteins, LPL-mediated TG hydrolysis, and the hepatic capture of chylomicron remnants via the interaction of the lipoprotein receptor with Apo E and LPL, is key to the metabolism and modification of these lipoproteins. The modulation of such phenomena is influenced by both genetic and environmental factors, thus explaining their extraordinary individual variance[32]. Non-classified forms are extremely rare. They include hypo-alpha lipoproteinemia and hypo-beta lipoproteinemia with a prevalence of 0.01 - 0.1%. In subjects with and T2DM, the ability of insulin to regulate VLDL production becomes impaired due to insulin resistance in the liver, resulting in excessive VLDL secretion and accumulation of TG-rich particles in the blood. Such abnormality in lipid metabolism characterizes the pathogenesis of hypertriglyceridaemia and accounts for increased risk of CAD in obesity and T2DM. Accumulating evidence also points to hypertriglyceridaemia as a marker for increased risk for CAD, and in fact, several atherogenic factors, such as increased concentrations of TG-rich lipoproteins, the atherogenic lipoprotein phenotype, (or lipid triad) and the metabolic syndrome[33,34]. The lipid triad consists of elevated serum TGs, small LDL particles, and HDL-C. The metabolic syndrome includes the coexistence of the lipid triad, elevated blood pressure, insulin resistance (plus glucose intolerance), and a prothrombotic state. However, the molecular basis that links insulin resistance to VLDL overproduction remains poorly understood.

Pathway	Primary risk determinants	Secondary risk determinants
Lipid metabolism	Familial dyslipidaemic disorders, including familial hypercholesterolaemia, familial defective apopliporptein B-100; Apopliporptein B-100; Sitosterolemia; Type III Hyperlipoproteinemia, Homocystinuria, Familial HDL deficiencies (apolipoprotein A1), Familial Combined Hyperlipidemia Apopliporptein B-100;.	Lipoprotein lipase; Hepatic lipase;, Lysosomal acid lipase; Sphingomyelinase; Lecithin-cholesterol acyltransferase; Apolipoproteins AII, AIV, CII, and CIII; proprotein convertase subtilisin/kexin type 9; ATP binding cassette protein subtype G5/8; Niemann-Pick type C1
Homeostasis of blood pressure	Insulin-resistant diabetes mellitus with acanthosis nigricans and hypertension Peroxisome proliferator-activated receptor-α; Angiotensinogen; ; Angiotensin converting enzyme; Primary hypertension;	Angiotensin II; Angiotensin II receptor, 11ß-ketoreductase; Cytochrome P450, family 1, subfamily B, polypeptide 1; Aldosterone synthase; Adducin; Nitric oxide synthase; Metafolin folate receptor; Thrombospondin
Glucose metabolism	Monogenic disorders leading to type 2 diabetes mellitus (e.g. insulin receptor, glucokinase); Peroxisome proliferator-activated receptor-α, -γ, -β;	Glucose transportersHuman leukocyte antigen locus DQ; Adiponectin; leptin receptor, melanocortin receptor 4; transcription factor 7-like 2; E-selectin
Hemostasis	Prothrombin; Factor V Leiden; Blood clotting disorders in conjunction with open foramen ovale; platelet-derived growth factor	Clotting factors II, V, VII; Fibrinogen; Plasminogen activator inhibitor-1; Thrombomodulin; transforming growth factor-β1
Inflammatory response genes	IInterleukin-6 and nuclear factor kappa-light-chain-enhancer of activated B cell; connexin 37;	Pyrin; Epithelial cell adhesion moleculeapolipoprotein *A*-I; Adenosine triphosphate-binding cassette transporter A1, and lecithin-cholesterol acyltransferase
Oxidative mediators	Homocystinuria; Paraoxone;, Methylenetetrahydrofolate reductase;	Cystathionine-beta-synthase; Nitric oxide synthase;
Adhesion mediators	Collagen IIIa; Glycoprotein IIIa, E-selectin; vascular cell adhesion molecule-1;	Epithelial cell adhesion molecule; Inter-cellular adhesion molecule 1
Gene regulators/ Transcritpion factors	Peroxisome proliferator-activated receptor-α,γ; Myocyte-specific enhancer factor 2A; Paraoxonase 1; GATA transcription factor-2	Sterol regulatory element binding protein; Hepatocyte nuclear factor 1-5; transcription factor 7-like 2

Table 1. Summary of the important risk genes and disease pathways leading to the manifestation of coronary artery disease.

Familial hypercholesterolemia (FH) is a clinical expression for the presence of elevated concentrations of LDL, deposition of LDL-derived Chol in tendons, skin xanthomas, and premature CAD, and an autosomal dominant trait of either increased serum Chol or premature CAD. It is also characterized by increased levels of total Chol and LDL-C, which result in excess deposition of Chol in tissues, leading to accelerated atherosclerosis and increased risk of premature CAD. Autosomal dominant FH is caused by LDLR deficiency and defective Apo B, respectively. Deficient LDLR activity results in elevated circulating LDL-C leading to its accumulation within blood vessel walls, which may result in arterial plaque formation, and therefore eventually occlude the arterial lumen. As such, HDL-C is often reduced in homozygous FH, while Lp(a) levels are high when corrected for Apo A isoforms[35]. While this phenomenon is likely to underlie genetic factors, the greater majority of these genes remain to be identified.

Autosomal recessive hypercholesterolemia (ARH) is a rare Mendelian dyslipidaemia characterized by markedly elevated plasma LDL levels, xanthomatosis, and premature CAD. LDLR function is normal, or only moderately impaired in fibroblasts from ARH patients, but their cultured lymphocytes show increased cell-surface LDL binding, and impaired LDL degradation, consistent with a defect in LDLR internalization[36]. Although the clinical phenotypes of ARH and homozygous FH are similar, autosomal recessive hypercholesterolaemia seems to be less severe, more variable within a single family, and more responsive to lipid-lowering drug therapy. In some individuals, the cardiovascular complications of premature atherosclerosis are delayed and involvement of the aortic root and valve is less common than in homozygous FH.

Another form of FH, heterozygous familial hypercholesterolemia (HFH) is an autosomal dominant disorder known to be associated with elevated Chol levels and increased risk of premature CAD. The estimated prevalence of HFH is 0.2% in most populations of the world. Apparently, the prevalence of peripheral arterial disease is increased dramatically in FH subjects compared with non-FH controls. In addition, the intima-media thickness of the carotid and/or femoral artery is increased in FH subjects.

Familial combined hyperlipidaemia (FCH) is a common heterozygous complex metabolic disorder characterized by (a) increase in cholesterolaemia and/or triglyceridaemia in at least two members of the same family, (b) intra-individual and intrafamilial variability of the lipid phenotype, and (c) increased risk of premature CAD. It is thought that in FCH elevated circulating levels of chylomicrons are broken down to produce atherogenic remnants through lipolysis of adipose cells, thereby contributing to the formation of atherosclerotic plaques. Thus, FCH is a common complex dominant disease condition associated with mixed hyperlipidaemia that accounts for up to 20% of premature CAD. The disease is sensitive to environmental effects. One of the roles of lipoprotein lipase is in the LDLR-like protein-mediated uptake of lipoprotein remnants in the liver and up to 20% of FCH patients show a genetic abnormality of this enzyme. FCH is very frequent (estimated prevalence: 0.5%-2.0%) and is one of the most common genetic hyperlipidaemias in the general population, being the most frequent in patients affected by CAD (10%) and among acute MI (AMI) survivors aged less than 60 (11.3%). The disease is subject to wide-scale environmental confounding traits such as obesity and the metabolic syndrome which remain to be elucidated.

Hypertriglyceridaemia represents one of the attributes of metabolic syndrome and is present in the most common genetic dyslipidaemia, the FCH. The disease also appears to underlie the phenomenon of small dense LDL in most instances. These particles are found in families with various disorders including premature CAD and hyperapobetalipoproteinemia, FCP, LDL subclass pattern B, familial dyslipidaemic hypertension, and syndrome X, as components of the metabolic syndrome[37]. Their presence is often accompanied by increased TGs and low HDL. While overproduction of VLDLs by the liver and increased secretion of large, Apo B-containing VLDL is the primary metabolic characteristic of most of these patients, this atherogenic syndrome seems to encompass also subclinical inflammation and elevated procoagulants. Their production occurs as a result of TG hydrolysis by LPL in VLDL, leading to the generation of IDL and in turn LDL. In LDL, the Chol esters are then exchanged for TG in VLDL by the Chol ester transfer proteins (CETPs), followed by hydrolysis of TG by HL to produce the particles. Apparently, CETP mediates a similar lipid exchange between VLDL and HDL, producing a Chol ester-poor HDL. In adipocytes, a primary defect in the incorporation of free fatty acids into TGs may trigger reduced fatty acid trapping and retention by adipose tissue, leading to increased levels of free fatty acids in plasma, increased flux of free fatty acids back to the liver, enhanced production of TGs, decreased proteolysis of Apo B, and increased VLDL production. Alternatively, insulin resistance may promote reduced retention of free fatty acids by adipocytes also leading to the same process. These metabolic disorders are often accompanied by decreased removal of postprandial TGs. Genes regulating the expression of the major players in this metabolic cascade, such as LPL, CETP, and HL, may also modulate the expression of the small, dense LDL[37]. Irrespective of the source, small, dense LDL particles have a prolonged retention time in plasma, are more susceptible to oxidation because of decreased interaction with the LDLR, and enter the arterial wall more easily, where they are retained more readily.

2.1.2 Glucose metabolism and coronary artery disease manifestation

Glucose is the primary source of energy required for normal organ function. Its metabolism involves the processing of simple sugars in foods to be utilized to produce energy in the form of adenosine triphosphate (ATP). Once consumed, glucose is absorbed by the intestines and into the blood. Extra glucose is stored in the muscle and liver as glycogen, which is hydrolyzed to glucose through gluconeogenesis and released into the bloodstream when needed. While tissues such as the brain and red blood cells can only utilize glucose, others can also use fats. Glucose can also be produced from non-carbohydrate precursors, such as pyruvate, amino acids and glycerol. Insulin and glucagon work synergistically to keep blood glucose concentrations normal. Insulin is produced in the pancreas, where its secretion is increased by elevated glucose concentrations, gastrointestinal hormones and beta(β)-adrenergic stimulation and can be inhibited by catecholamines and somatostatin. Accordingly, an elevated blood glucose concentration results in the secretion of insulin and glucose is transported into body cells, while glucagon has an opposite effect. Insulin exerts several functions that may influence the regulation of coronary vessel activity. Poor glucose metabolism as observed in insulin resistance is a primary cause for T2DM. Insulin resistance presents the impaired ability of either endogenous or exogenous insulin to lower blood glucose. It is typically characterized by decreased sensitivity and/or responsiveness to metabolic actions of insulin constituting a central feature of T2DM, obesity and dyslipidaemia, as well as a prominent component of hypertension and atherosclerosis that are all characterized by endothelial dysfunction. In some insulin-resistant individuals, insulin secretion will begin to deteriorate under chronic stress (glucose toxicity) and overt diabetes will result. If not, individuals will remain hyperinsulinemic, with perhaps some degree of glucose intolerance, together with other hallmarks of the insulin resistance syndrome (IRS). Increased free fatty acids and lipid accumulation in certain organs are mediators of insulin resistance[38].

The insulin resistance syndrome (syndrome X, metabolic syndrome) is a multifactorial disorder with obesity, dyslipidaemia, atherosclerosis, hypertension, and T2DM acting together to shorten life spans[23]. While a growing number of single genetic diseases affecting energy metabolism have been found to produce the clinical phenotype, strong familial occurrences, especially in racially prone groups together with modern genetic approaches are beginning to unravel the polygenetic nature of the syndrome. However, the strong lifestyle factors of excessive carbohydrate and fat consumption and lack of exercise are important keys to its phenotypic expression. The natural history includes small foetal gestational age birth weight, excessive weight gains during childhood, premature puberty, an allergic diathesis, acanthosis nigricans, striate compounded by gynecomastia, hypertriglyceridaemia, hepatic steatosis, premature atherosclerosis, hypertension, polycystic ovarian syndrome, and focal glomerulonephritis appearing increasingly through adolescence into adulthood. T2DM, which develops because of an inherent and/or an acquired failure of an insulin compensatory response, is increasingly seen from early puberty onward, as is atheromatous disease leading to CAD and stroke[23]. A number of physiological alterations of glucose metabolism including hepatic overproduction of glucose, and reduced glucose utilization by peripheral tissues as a result of insulin resistance contribute to the development of the metabolic manifestations of this disease. Ultimately, pancreatic failure and reduced insulin secretion lead to hyperglycemia and the diabetic state.

Inherited metabolic disorders contribute importantly to adverse cardiovascular outcomes and affect all tissue types[39]. Primary defects in energy balance that produce obesity (and visceral adiposity in particular) are sufficient to drive all aspects of the metabolic syndrome. Common obesity is polygenic, involving complex gene-gene and gene-environment interactions, which explain the multi-factorial obese phenotypes. Obesity also leads to a proinflammatory and prothrombotic state that potentiates atherosclerosis. Fat-derived adipokines, including tumor necrosis factor-alpha (TNF-α) and adiponectin have also been recently implicated as pathogenic contributors or protective factors. Distinct MAPK-dependent insulin-signaling pathways (largely unrelated to metabolic actions of insulin) regulate secretion of the vasoconstrictor endothelin-1 from endothelium. Endothelial dysfunction is often characterized by pathway-specific impairment in phosphatidylinositol 3-kinase (PI3K)-dependent signaling that contributes to a reciprocal relationship between insulin resistance and endothelial dysfunction. Thus, for example, PI3K-dependent insulin-signaling pathways regulating endothelial production of nitric oxide share parallels with metabolic insulin-signaling pathways. These and other cardiovascular actions of insulin contribute to coupling metabolic and hemodynamic homeostasis under healthy conditions.

2.1.3 Blood pressure homeostasis and coronary heart disease manifestation

Blood pressure is the pressure exerted by circulating blood on vessel walls and presents one of the principal vital signs of life. In general, blood pressure refers to arterial pressure of the systemic circulation. It can be influenced by various factors including the heart pumping rate, blood volume, vascular resistance and blood viscosity[40]. Although the endogenous regulation of arterial blood pressure is not yet completely understood, a number of mechanisms have been defined. These include the baroreceptor reflex, the renin-angiotensin (RAS) system and aldosterone release. Hence, the renin-angiotensin-aldosterone system (RAAS) constitutes a hormonal system primarily responsible for regulating blood pressure and fluid balance. Low blood volume induces secretion of renin in the juxtaglomerular cells in the kidneys. Renin in turn stimulates the production of angiotensin I from angiotensinogen, which is converted to angiotensin II (Ang II) by the ACE. Ang II induces vasoconstriction of the vessels resulting in increased blood pressure. It also stimulates the secretion of aldosterone from the adrenal cortex, which mediates an increase in the reabsorption of sodium and water from the kidney tubules into the blood. This in turn increases the fluid volume in the body and therefore the blood pressure. Increased RAAS activity leads to high blood pressure, and therefore to hypertension.

Hypertension is a vascular disease that may influence the viability of blood vessels. The disease is inheritable (primary) or may underlie environmental causes such as high salt consumption level. Evidence also suggests that Ang II plays an important role in the regulation of structure and function of both the heart and vessel wall. Under pathologic conditions, the ability of the heart and vessel wall to generate Ang II is increased, because of increased ACE expression. Hypertension is thought to correlate with impaired glucose tolerance. However, although the mechanism is not yet fully understood, this has been partly attributed to rapid nutrition and lifestyle transitions contributing to acceleration of obesity-related non-communicable diseases in some ethnic populations[41]. These include body phenotypes, such as high body fat, high truncal, subcutaneous and intra-abdominal fat, and low muscle mass, biochemical parameters such as hyperinsulinemia, hyperglycemia, dyslipidaemia, hyperleptinemia, low levels of adiponectin and high levels of C-reactive protein as well as procoagulant state and endothelial dysfunction[41]. Major atherogenic risk factors are likely mediators in the oxidative modification of DNA, and an increase in oxidative stress may derive from oxidatively damaged mitochondria[42].

2.1.4 Regulation of inflammatory processes and coronary artery disease

Inflammation is part of the complex biological response of vascular tissue to harmful stimuli, such as pathogens, damaged cells and irritants[44]. It is a protective mechanism the organism employs to remove injurious stimuli and to initiate the healing process. Inflammation can be classified as acute or chronic, whereby it presents the initial response of the body to harmful stimuli. This is achieved by the increased movement of plasma and leukocytes (especially granulocytes) from the blood into the injured tissues. A cascade of biochemical events propagates and matures the inflammatory response, involving the local vascular system, the immune system and various cells within the injured tissues. Prolonged inflammation, known as chronic inflammation, leads to a progressive shift in the type of cells present at the site of inflammation and is characterized by simultaneous destruction and healing of the tissue from the inflammatory process. Vascular endothelial dysfunction underlies the genesis and progression of numerous diseases. Among others, it has recently emerged as an early step in the development of atherosclerosis and is mainly characterized by a reduction in the bioavailability of nitric oxide. All of the traditional cardiovascular risk factors, including dyslipidaemia, arterial hypertension, hyperglycemia and diabetes, are associated with endothelial dysfunction, and oxidized LDLs, the renin-angiotensin axis and insulin resistance play important roles in the pathogenesis of impaired endothelial function. The increased expression of adhesion molecules and pro-inflammatory cytokines leads to abnormal endothelium-dependent vasodilatation. Apart from perturbation in systems regulating vasoconstriction and vasodilatation, ailments such as diabetes mellitus contribute equally to the formation of the plaque in blood vessels. Also, the immune system has recently been implicated in the pathogenesis of endothelial dysfunction and atherosclerosis with a particular regard towards autoimmunity due to the high prevalence of the atherosclerotic process in systemic autoimmune diseases. Dysfunction of HDL and its APOs A-I, A-II, and C-III has been observed in general populations, whereby high concentrations of HDL or Apo A-I in individuals with diabetes or CAD were found to reveal dysfunction in some population-based studies. It has been suggested that dysfunctional HDL particles even become proinflammatory or lose atheroprotective properties. While HDL dysfunctionality has been closely linked to obesity and low-grade inflammation, it appears nonetheless to act partly independently of them[45].

Chemokines are important mediators of angiogenesis, hematopoiesis and leucocyte trafficking. Chemokine Ligand-18 (CCL18)/pulmonary and activation-regulated chemokine (PARC) is a circulating chemokine that plays a role in injury healing, physiological homing of mononuclear blood cells and inflammatory responses. CCL18/PARC is also expressed in atherosclerotic plaques, and its levels have been associated with decreased cardiac function, decreased exercise capacity and increased inflammatory parameters including interleukin-6 (IL-6) and high sensitive C-reactive protein[46]. More importantly high CCL18/PARC levels appear to present an independent predictor of future cardiovascular events[46]

2.1.5 Environment and coronary artery disease management

Like all other risk factors of CAD, the type of food one consumes and style of life an individual leads, are equally important components for pathways leading to the disease, as they affect directly some of the risk factors, such as increased circulating Chol and predisposition to obesity. This is a chronic disease with a multifactorial etiology including genetics, environment, metabolism, lifestyle, and behavioral components which have been shown to contribute to the development of obesity[45]. Elevated body mass index, particularly caused by abdominal or upper-body obesity, has been associated with a number of diseases and metabolic abnormalities, many of which have high morbidity and mortality. These include hyperinsulinemia, insulin resistance, T2DM, hypertension, dyslipidaemia, CAD, and certain other malignancies. Besides, it appears that sedentary subjects with upper-body and visceral obesity who have the metabolic syndrome tend to be at higher risk for hypertriglyceridaemia in response to high-sucrose and high-carbohydrate diets[47]. Thereby, moderate weight loss mitigates the effect. Hyperinsulinemia or insulin resistance may play a role in promoting higher rates of VLDL synthesis and hypertriglyceridaemia in obesity, but the mechanisms remain unclear[47]. Some of these effects may be gender-related. For example, high dietary glycemic load is associated with higher serum triacylglycerol concentrations and greater risk of CAD in women[47], and cigarette smoking in overweight women with low-grade inflammation appears to offer limited protection against cardiometabolic risk[45].

Postprandial lipemia is traditionally defined by the extent and duration of the increase in plasma TGs in response to a fat-enriched meal. Alimentary lipemia has been associated with CAD, in a fashion that is influenced by both genetic and environmental factors. Disease processes, such as dyslipidaemia, hypertension, glucose and insulin metabolism, lifestyle habits, such as eating and exercise patterns, as well as socioeconomic status aggregate in families with CAD. The degree of risk associated with a family history varies with the degree of relationship and the age at onset of disease. Postprandial lipoprotein metabolism is modulated by background dietary pattern as well as meal composition including fat amount and type, carbohydrate, protein, fibre, alcohol, and several lifestyle conditions such as physical activity, tobacco use, physiological factors including age, gender, menopausal status and pathological conditions such as obesity, insulin resistance, diabetes mellitus. Overall, the variability in postprandial response is important and complex, and the interactions between nutrients, dietary or meal compositions and gene variants need further investigation. Furthermore, extremely low fat dietary habits or major gene interactions may influence the lipid profile and the excess cardiovascular mortality observed in heterozygous FH, whereas minor gene determinants do not seem to play any significant role. All other factors put into consideration, the prevalence of the disease may vary among populations, due to differences in the awareness of the disease in a given population.

2.2 Early onset coronary artery disease

Acute coronary syndrome (ACS) is a manifestation of myocardial infarction (MI) at young age, usually described as being under 45 years of age. It is usually associated with coronary thrombosis, and chest pain can also be precipitated by anemia, bradycardias or tachycardias. AMI represents the main thrombotic complication of CAD, with a presence of approximately 9% of the new events of MI occurring in patients. The condition is produced by development of a thrombus at the site of an atherosclerotic plaque that initiates abrupt arterial occlusion, with ischemia and cell death. Evidence of significant disease at coronary angiography suggests the presence of a premature atherosclerotic process. Based on the appearance of the electrocardiogram (ECG), they are also defined as non-ST elevation myocardial infarction (NSTEMI) and ST segment elevation myocardial infarction (STEMI) or unstable angina[48], whereby STEMI constitutes about 30%, NSTEMI 25% and unstable angina 38% of the affected individuals. Unstable angina occurs suddenly often at rest with minimal exertion, or at lesser degrees of exertion than a previous angina. MI at a young age is commonly characterized by evidence of multiple cardiovascular risk factors and by a favorable prognosis in short- and medium-term follow-up. Thus, AMI reflects a degree of damage to the coronaries by atherosclerosis. Apparently, the type of ischemic event shows gender-specific differences. Thus, in women it appears to present more frequently with unstable angina and NSTEMI, whereas men will have ACS with STEMI[48-50]. However, it is still questionable whether this gender association has any genetic background to it.

Several modifiable factors such as hypertension, diabetes, smoking, obesity, and hypercholesterolemia are involved in AMI manifestation. However, in a large number of patients with AMI, modifiable risk factors are not present. Furthermore, apart from early onset of CAD, recurrent coronary events in the young also present an important problem. Recently, the role of Lp(a), homocysteine, inflammation and infection as prime culprits in the pathogenesis of CAD has become a subject of intense research and debate. Specifically, hyperhomocysteinemia is a risk factor of recurrent coronary event in the young and an element of gene-environment interaction may also contribute significantly to its manifestation. Monogenic disorders are seen in approximately 5% of premature CAD cases, and this prevalence is higher in populations with the founder effect. Family history of MI is positively associated with the risk of early MI in women. While the association with parental history of MI is mediated through the clustering of other common risk factors, the association of sibling history of MI with early-onset MI in young women is only partially explained by the clustering of established and newly-identified risk factors[51].

Heredity has a significantly great share in AMI. Particularly, familial lipidaemic disorders play a pivotal role in early onset of CAD. Familial lipoprotein disorders are seen frequently in subjects with premature CAD. In FH, early CAD is a complex trait that results from a large monogenic component of susceptibility due to elevated LDL-C even in the absence of any other risk factors. Increased LDL and decreased HDL-C predict premature CAD, as do elevated levels of Apo B or reduced levels of Apo A. The metabolic abnormality in many FH-affected individuals is overproduction of Apo B-containing lipoproteins causing elevated levels of plasma Chol, TGs, or both. Low levels of HDL-C and an abundance of dense LDL particles are other features contributing to the high association of this disorder with premature CAD. Although for most children the process of atherosclerosis is subclinical, dramatically accelerated atherosclerosis occurs in some pediatric disease states, with clinical coronary events occurring in childhood and very early adult life. A striking example is found in children who have the homozygous form of FH with extremely high levels of LDL-C, whereby severe atherosclerosis and CAD often develop during the first decades of life.

Among patients with CAD onset before the age of 55, about 5% of cases are attributable to HFH, a monogenic disorder that affects about 1 in 500 people, with a higher prevalence in certain subpopulations. The disease manifests with severe hypercholesterolemia since birth (Chol levels >5-6 the upper normal limit), which, if untreated, leads to early onset accelerated atherosclerosis and premature coronary death, usually before the second or third decades of life. It occurs primarily as an autosomal dominant disorder with a gene-dosage effect. The clinical phenotype of HFH is characterized by increased plasma levels of total Chol and LDL-C, tendinous xanthomata, and premature symptoms of CAD. The disease is characterized by Chol deposits affecting the corneas, eyelids and extensive tendons, elevated plasma concentrations of LDL-C and accelerated vascular disease, especially CAD. It is inherited as an autosomal dominant disorder with homozygotes having a more severe phenotype than do heterozygotes. Dyslipidaemic states associated with premature atherosclerotic disease and high cardiovascular risk are characterized by a disequilibrium related to an excess of circulating concentrations of atherogenic lipoproteins relative to those of atheroprotective HDL, thereby favouring arterial Chol deposition and enhanced atherogenesis. In such states, CETP activity is elevated and contributes significantly to the Chol burden in atherogenic Apo B-containing lipoproteins[6,7].

3. The genetic basis of coronary artery disease

Variation in human genes is a result of structural alteration(s) in the sequence of the gene due to a modification in any one of the DNA bases, producing different forms of the gene known as polymorphisms. These polymorphic changes may or may not lead to changes in amino acids, consequently constituting an alteration in the functional expression of the resultant protein. The types of gene variants are defined as missence, silent, nonsense or Frameshift mutations, depending on the resultant effect of the changes on the protein product. These sequence variations are classified as large-scale or small-scale mutations, and may influence any type of protein, including structural, signaling, or enzymes engaged in various functions. Large-scale mutations usually lead to a gain or loss of chromosomal regions or translocation of parts of a chromosome, whereas small-scale mutations are nucleotide-based substitutions, deletions or insertions leading to new gene products, as well as gene, protein and phenotypic expression. One of the most important findings in recent times is the recognition of the fact that sequence variations in the human genes are confined to single nucleotide polymorphism (SNPs). The number of SNPs varies within one gene from one population to another. It is also thought that more than 50% of all coding SNPs produce a predictable change in the protein sequence. This fact points to a high level of human protein diversity, with potentially great impact on disease manifestation and modes by which patients respond to drug therapy.

Sequence variations implicated in complex diseases such as CAD are often found in genes regulating diverse mechanisms (e.g. lipid metabolism, glucose handling, blood pressure regulation, or vascular contractility). Indeed, virtually all risk factors for the disease themselves underlie genetic background. Besides, many of these risk factors seem to share some genomic regions and/or gene variants among themselves as well as with CAD, pointing to common loci and possible gene-gene interactions as a mechanism for such complex diseases. An added intricacy to the situation with complex diseases, such as CAD, is the fact that changes in various genes may be related to clusters of dysfunctions that also contribute to the disease, rendering it oft difficult to decipher exactly which factors may be the primary or secondary culprits. Hence, ultimately manifestation of CAD is a product of interaction of environmental factors with alteration in genes that regulate numerous pathways. This section summarizes some of the important genes engaged in the different pathways leading to its manifestation. The catalogue of gene discussed is far from being exhaustive, but simply intended to reflect on some of the established pathways, as well as findings that have recently stimulated further search into their relevance for CAD.

3.1 Pathways regulating lipid metabolism

Understandably, alterations in genes regulating circulation Chol levels and its metabolites should occupy a key position among the disease pathways leading to CAD manifestation. As such, lipidaemic disorders leading to an increase in circulating Chol could theoretically result from mutations in genes involved in any of the various pathways regulating its homeostasis. Hence, perhaps by far the most well-studied risk pathways for CAD are those leading to FH, an autosomal defect related to mutations in the LDLR, the Apo B and the PCSK9 genes. However, mutations in several other genes, such as LDLR adapter protein 1 (LDLRAP1) Apo A-I, Apo A-IV, Apo A-V, Apo C-III, can also lead to a phenotype similar to the disease. In humans, *LDLR* mutations induce hypercholesterolemia and, subsequently, Chol deposition to a variable degree, not only confirming the pathogenetic role of *LDLR* but also highlighting the existence of additional factors in determining the phenotype. Apparently, receptor-negative mutations result in a more severe phenotype than do receptor-defective mutations[52]. At least five specific monogenic disorders, are known to be related to this phenomenon. These are familial hypercholesterolemia, familial ligand-defective Apo B, autosomal recessive hypercholesterolemia, sitosterolemia and cholesterol 7-alpha-hydroxylase deficiency. The diseases may occur in the form of a Mendelian (caused by a defect in a single gene) or as a complex trait (resulting from an interaction of genetic predisposition and environmental factors). Several loci including LDLR-associated protein, PCSK9 and ATP-binding cassette transporters ABCG5 and ABCG8 have been identified for monogenic hypercholesterolemia. Functionally, ABCG5 and 8 pump sterols out of the hepatic and intestinal cells into bile and intestinal lumen, respectively. A number of PCSK9 variants have been identified, some of which are gain-of-function mutations causing hypercholesterolemia by a reduction of LDLR levels, while loss-of-function variants have been associated with a reduction of LDL-C levels and a decreased risk of CAD[53]. Furthermore, at least nine of the apolipoproteins known to play a major role in lipid metabolism have been implicated in influencing plasma levels of HDL, VLDL, LDL chylomicrons or TGs[54]. Mutations in the Apo B gene can result in a phenotype that is clinically indistinguishable from FH, and have also been shown to be associated with CAD. Although many studies indicate that the FH phenotype is influenced by other genetic and environmental factors, it remains unclear whether or not these are synergistic interactions or simply additive effects[52]. Furthermore, although HFH is genetically heterogeneous, it is most often caused by heterozygous mutations in the gene encoding the LDLR.

Another form of FH, the ARH has been associated with the insertion mutation in a phosphotyrosine binding domain of the so-called ARH protein[55], encoding a cellular adaptor protein required for LDL transport, and consequently for internalization of LDLs in the liver. This protein is thought to function as an adaptor protein that couples LDLR to the endocytotic machinery[36]. The phenotypic expression of this homozygous FH appears to be dominated by the consequences of the *LDLR* gene mutations. An autosomal recessive form of FH caused by loss-of-function mutations in *LDLRAP1a* has also been reported. In heterozygous FH, however, the underlying mutational *LDLR* type determines only to a much lesser extent, if any, the variable phenotypic expression. Conversely, some *PCSK9* loss-of-function mutations resulting in low levels of LDL-C appear to protect against CAD[56 57]. However, despite compelling evidence indicating that PCSK9 impairs the LDLR pathway, its role in Chol metabolism remains incompletely defined. Additional atherogenic risk factors of environmental, metabolic, and genetic origin are presumed to influence the clinical phenotype in FH. Other risk factors include the *LPL* gene which is thought to present a risk factor for dyslipidaemia, characterized by hypertriglyceridaemia and low HDL-C levels which increases with age and weight gain, and is associated with CAD and T2DM.

The HDL-C levels are under considerable genetic control with heritability estimates of up to 80%, and low HDL-C syndromes have generally been correlated with an increased risk of CAD. The cardioprotective effects of HDL-C have been attributed to its role in reverse Chol transport, its effects on endothelial cells, and its antioxidant activity[58]. On the other hand, relative HDL-C deficiency states have been associated with the ATP binding cassette protein (ABCA1), Apo A1 and lecithin cholesteryl acyl transferase defects. However, although numerous candidate genes contribute to the low HDL-C phenotype, their impact on CAD is heterogeneous, single gene abnormalities responsible for HDL-C deficiency states may have variable effects on atherothrombotic risk, reflective of diverse gene-gene interactions and gene-environmental relationships. Other potentially important candidates involved in low HDL-C syndromes in humans include *Apo C3*, *LPL*, sphingomyelin phosphodiesterase 1, and glucocerebrosidase. Molecular variation in ABCAI and Apo AI and partly lecithin cholesteryl acyl transferase deficiency have been associated with increased CAD, while some of the *Apo A1* variants, such as Apo A1 Milano and Apo A1 Paris have been associated with reduced risk. Endothelial lipase gene polymorphisms have also been associated with HDL-C concentrations[59]. This lipase participates in HDL metabolism by promoting the turnover of HDL components and increasing the catabolism of Apo A-I[59], which distinguishes itself from other TG lipases in showing the highest activity on HDL[59]. Similarly, mutations in the *CETP* gene associated with CETP deficiency are characterized by high HDL-C levels and reduced cardiovascular risk.

In contrast to FH, which is caused by mutations in a number of affected genes, the genetics of FCH have remained obscure and very few definite candidate genes have been identified thus far. Of these, the strongest evidence links the lipid components of FCH to intronic variants in the upstream transcription factor 1 (*USF1)* gene on chromosome 1q21-23. Modifying genes, particularly those that influence the high TG trait, include apo C3 and apolipoprotein A5 (*apo A5*). *Apo A5* is a member of the apolipoprotein *Apo A1/C3/A4* gene cluster, and is important in regulating plasma TG levels. It also represents a downstream target of USF1, implicating a USF1-dependent pathway in the molecular pathogenesis of dyslipidemias[60]. However, the relationship of *USF1* polymorphisms with diabetes and the metabolic syndrome, which co-localize to this region and are also associated with mixed hyperlipidaemia, has yet to be defined. Additionally, Apo AV is an activator of LPL, linked to familial hypertriglyceridaemia and FCH to upstream stimulatory factor 1[61]. A case study of a patient with αβ-lipoproteinaemia suggested that the hypertriglyceridaemia seen in patients with FCH may result from an abnormality in microsomal TG transport protein function. A direct relationship between the post-prandial TG levels and LDL-C levels in the fasting state of patients with FCH and sporadic hypercholesterolaemia has also been postulated, which increases considerably when all the MI survivors are considered independent of age. The *USF1* has been linked with familial combined hyperlipidaemia in some ethnic groups. Currently, genetic and functional evidence is supportive of a role for the *USF1* in the etiology of FCP and its component traits, although the mechanism still remains largely unknown[62]. While the genetic defect remains unknown, linkage to the region of the Apo *AI- CIII- AIV* gene cluster on chromosome 11 has been implicated.

Other mutations, especially the truncation-causing mutations in Apo *B* and MTP can cause familial hypobetalipoproteinemia, characterized by hypercholesterolemia and resistance to atherosclerosis[63]. Therefore, in genetic dyslipidaemia elevated Apo B levels and reduced Apo A levels (or increased Apo B/AI ratio) differ and predict premature CAD[64]. One of the most extensively studied lipoprotein genes in this respect is the *apo E*, which has been linked with various forms of lipidaemic disorders. An example of an *apo E*-mediated, autosomal recessive, lipid disorder is familial dysbetalipoproteinemia (FD). The gene exists in three allelic forms (epsilon2 (ε2), ε3 and ε4 coding for isoforms E2, E3, and E4 and having different binding affinities for the apo E receptors. This genetic variation is associated with different plasma lipoprotein levels, different response to diet and lipid-lowering therapy, and a variable risk for cardiovascular disease and Alzheimer's disease. While the ε2 allele is associated with elevated TG levels, the ε4 allele is associated with increased Chol levels. The ε2/ε2 genotype is thought to present the most common cause for hyperlipoproteinemia type III. However, although several studies support the role of *apo E* polymorphism in CAD either directly or indirectly via its influence on lipid and lipoprotein levels, there are some studies which show lack of such relationships.

3.2 Pathways regulating blood pressure

Given that hypertension, diabetes, dyslipidaemia, and obesity exhibit a substantial heritable component, it is to be expected that important genes encoding proteins related to these pathways may predispose individuals to this cluster of cardiovascular risk factors. Specifically, as the core regulator of systemic blood pressure, and being involved in the cardiovascular homeostasis, several polymorphisms in genes of the RAAS system have been found to have pleiotropic effects on cardiovascular disorders. A constituent of this system is angiotensinogen (*AGT*), a serum renin substrate glycoprotein synthesized in the liver, which is released as the precursor of angiotensin, the hormone that forms part of the systemic blood pressure regulatory system. Risk variants in this gene have been identified that lead not only to hypertension[65,66], but also to CAD[67-70]. Apart from the *AGT*, several other genes engaged in regulating components of the RAAS pathway have also been identified as constituting risk for primary hypertension. These include among others, the alpha(α-) adducin *(ADD1)*[71], *ACE*[72-75], nitric oxide synthase[76], metafolin folate (methyl tetrahydrofolate; MTHF) receptor *(MTFHR)*[77] and thrombospondin *(THBS)* genes[78,79]. The *THBS*s are a 5-member gene family that mediates cell-cell and cell-matrix interactions. These proteins are either trimers or pentamers, and their functions depend on their abilities to interact with numerous extracellular ligands and cell surface receptors through the multiple domains that compose each subunit. Thus, polymorphisms in 3 *THBS* genes encoding *THBS1*, *THBS2*, and *THBS4* were proposed to modulate the risk of premature CAD[78,79] and MI[80-82]. Interestingly, literally all of these genes have also been implicated in CAD manifestation. However, the important question remains as to whether their role in CAD is by virtue of their influence on the blood pressure control or some other signaling links may exist among the pathways involved in the disease process.

3.3 Pathways regulation glucose metabolism

The impact of T2DM as a primary cause for CAD has now become common knowledge. In fact, diabetic patients are thought to have a 3-fold higher risk of developing atherosclerosis and its clinical complications as compared to non-diabetic individuals. Part of the cardiovascular risk associated with this disease is probably due to genetic determinants influencing both glucose homeostasis and the development of atherosclerosis. Besides, T2DM frequently coexists with other cardiovascular risk factors like arterial hypertension, central obesity and dyslipidaemia in the manifestation of CAD. Several genes including *ADIPOQ* and peroxisome proliferator-activated receptor (*PPAR*) genes have been implicated in manifestation of metabolic syndrome (MS)[83,84]. Adiponectin (*ADIPOQ*) is an adipocyte-derived hormone and an essential modulator of insulin sensitivity. It is abundantly secreted by adipocytes, plays important roles in lipid and glucose metabolisms, and has direct anti-inflammatory and anti-atherogenic effects. Since it modulates several metabolic processes, it is thought to play an important role in the suppression of the metabolic derangements that may lead to MS. It may serve as an important biomarker for metabolic syndrome, and some of its common polymorphisms have been associated with the phenotypes related to body weight, glucose metabolism, insulin sensitivity, and risk of T2DM and CAD[85]. While circulating ADIPOQ is involved in the atherosclerotic process and has been associated with cardiovascular disease as well as obesity, insulin resistance, metabolic syndrome, and T2DM[83,84,86,87], its relationship with the early onset of atherosclerosis in hyperlipidaemia is still not completely understood.

The PPAR-α, -γ, -β are members of the nuclear receptor superfamily of ligand-activated transcription factors that have central roles in the storage and catabolism of fatty acids. All three PPARs are activated by naturally occurring fatty acids and fatty acid metabolites, indicating that they function as the fatty acid sensors of the body. Hence, they constitute major regulators of energy homeostasis. They not only control lipid metabolism, but also regulate vascular diseases, such as atherosclerosis and hypertension, as well as the expression of genes involved in fatty acid β-oxidation. Specifically, PPAR-γ plays a critical role in adipocyte differentiation and serves as the receptor for the glitazone class of insulin-sensitizing drugs used in the treatment of T2DM. *PPARβ* polymorphisms are associated with plasma lipid levels, body mass index and the risk for diabetes and CAD[88]. *PPARγ2* variants have also been shown to influence insulin sensitivity in interaction with *ADIPOQ* or to influence plasma ADIPOQ levels. It has recently been suggested that PPARs may present a functional link between obesity, hypertension and diabetes. However, in contrast to PPARα and PPARγ, relatively little is known about the biology of PPARβ, although recent findings suggest that this subtype has a role in lipid homeostasis also.

Candidate gene variants for polygenic obesity appear to disrupt pathways involved in the regulation of energy intake and expenditure and include adrenergic receptors, uncoupling proteins, PPARG, POMC, MC4R and a set of variants in the FTO locus. Notably, the FTO gene is the most robust gene for common obesity characterized to date, and recent data shows that the FTO locus seems to confer risk for obesity through increasing energy intake and reduced satiety. Gene variants involved in pathways regulating addiction and reward behaviours may also play a role in predispositioning to obesity[89]. Other obesity-related genes including *ADIPOQ*, leptin receptor, and fat mass obesity-related genes have also been described with respect to manifestation of metabolic syndrome and CAD/MI[90]. While genes, such as the *PPARs*[91] have been discussed as independent risk for CAD[88], several of them may share common variants for metabolic syndrome with CAD/MI, among themselves and/or with others, including *Ang II*[92], AMP deaminase-1[93] and *ACE*[91] genes. For example, the risk of acquiring CAD in patients with T2DM appears to increase significantly in the presence of the several gene variants such as those of the transcription factor 7-like 2 (*TCF7L2*)[94] and E-selectin genes[95]. Other genes associated with CAD include the *C5L2*, a stimulator of TG synthesis or glucose transport and constitutes a functional receptor of acylation-stimulating protein[96]. Together, these data only reveal the complexity of mechanism involved in disease pathways regulating CAD and its risk factors.

A rare genetic form of insulin resistance is Dunnigan-type familial partial lipodystrophy (FPLD), which is characterized by loss of subcutaneous fat from extremities, trunk, and gluteal region. It is always accompanied by insulin resistance and hyperinsulinemia, often with hypertension, dyslipidaemia, T2DM and early endpoints of atherosclerosis. FPLD is thought to result from mutated *LMNA*, which encodes nuclear lamins A and C. Familial studies indicate that dyslipidaemia precedes the plasma glucose abnormalities in FPLD subjects with mutant *LMNA*, and that the hyperinsulinemia is present early in the course of the disease. Plasma leptin is also markedly reduced in subjects with FPLD due to mutant *LMNA*. Thus, a defect in the structure and function of the nuclear envelope can result in a phenotype that shares many aspects with the common syndrome of insulin resistance.

3.4 Pathways regulation smooth muscle cellular viability and function

Since inflammatory mechanisms play a central role in mediating all phases of atherosclerosis, genes encoding for inflammatory or anti-inflammatory molecules are candidates for the risk of developing atherosclerosis. Genetic variability affecting many functional areas such as lipid and energy metabolisms, hypertension and haemodynamic mechanisms, blood clotting homeostasis, inflammation, and matrix turnover in the vascular wall will have an impact on the development of macrovascular complications in diabetic patients. During atherogenesis intercellular communication via gap junctions as well as cell membrane channels linking the cytoplasmic compartments of adjacent cells play a critical role. The component protein subunits of these channels, called connexin (Cx), belong to a multigene family. Cx37 is involved in growth, regeneration after injury and ageing of the endothelial cells, pointing to a potential role in atherosclerosis. A variant of the Cx37 gene has been associated with thickening of the carotid intima and therefore CAD[97]. Recently a higher prevalence of pro-inflammatory polymorphisms of several genes including pyrin, epithelial cell adhesion molecule (*EPCAM)*, *Cx37* and *PCR* genes and a lower prevalence of anti-inflammatory polymorphisms, such as the *TLR4, IL10* and *CCR5Δ32*) has been documented[98,99], suggesting early MI could be associated with a genetic predisposition to an intense inflammatory response, linked also to an hyperviscosity syndrome[98,99]. Intima media thickness studies have provided evidence that hypoalphalipoproteinemia due to mutations in apo *A-I, ABCA1,* and *LCAT* is associated with increased progression of atherosclerosis[100]. In contrast, hyperalphalipoproteinemia as a result of loss of CETP function is associated with unaltered atherosclerosis progression.

The generation of oxidative stress is believed to be an important cause of DNA damage in atherosclerosis. Under oxidative stress, both blood monocytes and plasma lipoproteins invade the arterial wall, leading to their exposure to atherogenic modifications[101,102]. Hence, increased oxidative stress has been implicated in the pathogenesis of the atherothrombotic process. A recent addition to the list of genes thought to be involved in oxidative stress are the paraoxonases (*PONs*), a family of closely related antioxidants encoded by at least three clustered genes (*PON1,* PON2 and PON3) on chromosome 7q. The human PON1 is an HDL-associated arylesterase that hydrolyzes paraoxon[103]. It is thought to exert an antiatherogenic effect by protecting LDLs against oxidation[104,105] partly by slowing down the accumulation of lipid peroxides in LDLs under oxidizing conditions. Understandably therefore, alterations in the *PON1* gene are implicated in dyslipidaemic disorders. Furthermore, free radical production in the immediate postrecanalization phase after thrombotic occlusion of a major coronary artery in humans is associated with MI[106]. The NADPH oxidase system as a main source of reactive oxygen species in vascular cells has been implicated in development and progression of CAD. In contrast, some gene variants, such as c.-930A>G in the promoter region of p22-PHOX gene have been shown to have protective effects[107].

Apart from inflammatory processes, alterations in genes regulating blood cell formation (hematopoiesis) and blood coagulation mechanisms constitute important cell function-related risk for CAD. The fraction of immature platelets is increased in ACS, especially in the acute phase of STEMI[108]. Immature platelets with an increased hemostatic potential may contribute to coronary thrombus formation. Recently a quantitative trait locus 12q24 associated with mean platelet volume and platelet count has been implicated as a risk locus for CAD[109]. Polymorphisms in genes regulating various aspects of hematopoiesis and blood coagulation processes including leptin[110], the GATA transcription factor *GATA-2* have also been implicated in CAD. GATA-2 is an important regulator of hematopoiesis. Among others, glycoprotein growth factors regulate the proliferation and maturation of the cells that enter the blood from the marrow, as well as causing cells in one or more committed cell lines to proliferate and mature. Other recently added culprits for CAD include the lipase A, lysosomal acid, cholesterol esterase (*LIP*A), platelet-derived growth factor (*PDGF*), *ADAMTS7-MORF4L1*, and KIAA1462[111] genes.

3.5 Gene and mRNA regulatory pathways

One of the most exciting findings in recent times is the discovery of several loci in DNA regions that regulate transcription rather than the coding regions for protein as risk sequences for disease. As such, several transcription factors (TFs) have been associated with CAD/MI, some of which have been discussed above. These include the *GATA2*[112], myocyte-specific enhancer factor 2A (*MEF2A)*[113-115], proteasome subunit alpha 6 (*PSMA6)*[116,117], transcription factor 7-like 2 (*TCF7L2*) genes, among others. GATA-2 constitutes a target gene ensemble consisting of genes encoding key determinants of endothelial cell identity and inflammation. These sites characteristically contained motifs that bind activator protein-1 (AP-1), a pivotal regulator of inflammatory genes[118]. It plays an essential role in the establishment and maintenance of adult hematopoiesis, and is present in hematopoietic stem cells, as well as cells that make up the aortic vasculature, such as the aortic endothelial and smooth muscle cells. Several of the *GATA2* gene variants have been associated with familial early onset of CAD[112]. The *MEF2* is a member of the MADS gene family (name for the yeast mating type-specific transcription factor MCM1, the plant homeotic genes 'agamous' and 'deficiens' and the human serum response factor SRF, a family that also includes several homeotic genes and other transcription factors, all of which share a conserved DNA-binding domain). This proteasome is a multicatalytic proteinase complex distributed throughout eukaryotic cells at a high concentration, and cleaves peptides in an ATP/ubiquitin-dependent process in a non-lysosomal pathway. An essential function of a modified proteasome, the immunoproteasome, is the processing of class I MHC peptides. Interestingly, a great majority of entities associated with disease reside in the untranslated regions (UTRs), particularly the 3 prime (3′-UTR) of these genes. Thus, for example, the *MEF2A* gene is highly polymorphic and harbours several deletions in the 3′-UTR that are implicated in CAD/MI[113]. The 3′-UTR regions contain sequences involved in gene regulatory and mRNA maturation processes. It also harbours binding sites for micro RNAs, which are involved in transcriptional and protein processing mechanisms. While the exact mechanisms are still to be elucidated, it appears nonetheless that changes in transcription factors, gene regulatory and mRNA maturation mechanisms exert important influence impacting disease pathways of complex diseases, such as CAD. Hence, the speculation that the disease-causing loci are more likely to be in DNA regions that regulate transcription rather than being in coding regions for protein[119]. Besides, novel genes also continue to be uncovered through genome-wide studies which do not belong to the canonical pathways of CAD, lipid metabolism or any of its other risk factors.

3.6 Gene-gene and gene-environmental interaction in manifestation of coronary artery disease

The fact that several pathways commonly lead to CAD points to the possibility of interactions of these risk factors at various levels in the path to disease manifestation. Besides, the exceedingly high prevalence of risk factors such as T2DM, dyslipidaemia and hypertension in CAD individuals raises the question as to which pathway(s) or mechanism may be the primary cause of disease in cases harbouring combinations of such factors. This is compounded by the fact that, for example, the set of metabolic and physiologic risk factors associated with elevated cardiovascular disease risk including hypertriglyceridaemia, low HDL-C levels, hypertension, abdominal obesity, and insulin resistance all contribute to similar ailments, each of which may underlie genetic factors. The expression of each one of the major factors is now known to be the result of complex interactions between genetic and environmental factors. For example, as discussed above, obesity may play a major role in triggering the metabolic syndrome by interacting with variants in candidate genes for dyslipidaemia, hypertension and insulin resistance.

Not surprisingly, in the last decade, a sizeable portion of research interest has focussed on trying to understand possible interactions among individual disease-causing variants or genes on complex disease manifestation. One of the most well studied systems is the RAAS pathway, which has been evaluated with respect to interactions among its risk variants/genes as well as with other genes in triggering CAD. Significant two-way and three-way gene-gene interactions between ACE I/D, AT1R A1166C polymorphisms and AGT gene haplotypes have been associated with CAD in a number of studies[120]. One study has described several synergistic effects between the studied polymorphisms and classical risk factors such as hypertension, obesity, diabetes and dyslipidaemia[121]. Thus, the presence of the DD genotype of ACE I/D (and also ACE11860 GG) increased the odds of developing CAD when related to each one of these classical risk factors, particularly in the male and early onset CAD subgroup analysis. Interactions have also been observed between ACE DD or ACE 8 GG with PON1 192RR in increasing the risk of CAD[122,123]. Concomitant presence of ACE DD and AT1R 1166 CC genotypes has also been reported to synergistically increase the predisposition to diastolic heart failure[126]. Significant interaction between APOE and LPL variants and HDL-C levels was also reported[130], furnishing support to the idea that several polymorphisms in apolipoprotein genes may by themselves and/or in interaction with other polymorphisms contribute to risk for CAD in men[130]. Interaction of the GNB3 825T allele with the ACE D allele was also reported in MI[131].

Apart from the RAAS system, interactions have also been evaluated involving multiple gene variants with respect to CAD manifestation. One such a study linked increased risk of the disease in association with changes in genes belonging to different enzymes compared to the isolated polymorphisms[122]. Another study suggested that several polymorphisms in apolipoprotein genes may by themselves and/or in interaction with for example the *PPARγ* C161-->T variant and apo ε4 genotype influence serum Chol level, in which the impact of the later on CAD was attenuated through the former genotype[125]. Epistatic, high-order, gene-gene interactions between RAS gene polymorphisms and CAD has also been discussed[127]. Similar interaction between variations in the ACE and ATR2 genes has been hypothesized in relation to the extent of coronary atherosclerosis[129].

Other studies have addressed the possible interactions of various gene variants with risk diseases, such as hypertension or T2DM in acquiring CAD. For example, the AGT235 TT increased the CAD risk in the presence of hypertension and dyslipidaemia, while AT1R1166 interacted positively with hypertension, smoking and obesity[121]. An interaction between RAAS predisposing genes and some biochemical/environmental risk factors was also reported in CAD onset, pointing to a significant enhancement of the effects of classical markers especially by ACE I/D and ACE11860[121].

One form of interaction currently attracting great attention is that of the haplotypes versus individual risk variants. Such an interaction would involve nucleotide changes occurring in the same genomic region, either within a single gene or in several genes at the same locus. Generally, it can be acknowledged that in many cases, haplotyping has been found to be more meaningful than individual variants. One study involving methylenetetrahydrofolate reductase C677T, plasminogen activator inhibitor 4G/5G, and endothelial nitric oxide synthase 3-27 base pair repeat polymorphism in patients with early-onset CAD suggested the coexistence of high-risk alleles as augmenting the severity of the disease[128]. These results are a manifestation of the relevance of the concept of multilocus and multi-gene effects in complex diseases, such as CAD.

Besides, a number of genes are linked with changes in environmental factors affecting disease outcome. Thus, variables such as the postprandial lipid response have been shown to be modified by polymorphisms within multiple genes for the apolipoproteins, *LPL*, *HL*, fatty acid binding and transport proteins, *MTP* and scavenger receptor class B type I[132], while several other genes including the a*po A1/C3/A4/A5* cluster, *ABCA1*, *CETP*, human glucokinase regulatory protein (*GCKR*), *HL*, IL-6, *LPL*, lipid-droplet associated protein, perilipin, and *TCF7L2* have all been implicated in the modulation of the postprandial lipid metabolism[133]. All these genetic changes in combination with other disease-causing elements are likely to exacerbate CAD. Furthermore, it has been suggested that the interplay of genetic and environmental factors places first-degree relatives of individuals with premature CAD at greater risk of developing the disease than the general population. However, the data on this subject is still very limited. Besides, reliability of available data on these interactions is not established, since replication studies are still lacking in the literature.

4. Genetics of acute coronary syndrome in the young

Acute myocardial infarction AMI in young individuals presents a typical pattern of risk factors, clinical, angiographic and prognostic characteristics that differ from those related to adult disease manifestation. An important feature of early onset is a positive family history, which has become a recognized cardiovascular risk factor. Cutaneous and tendinous xanthomata develop in childhood and are the most common reason for initial presentation. However, the pathogenic mechanisms are multifarious and complex. The frequency of FH is estimated to be 1 in 500. About 50% of individuals with FH die before the age of 60 due to MI.

Since CAD manifests itself both as an early and late onset event, different risk factors may determine the stages at which the disease becomes apparent. A most useful approach for identifying genes associated with the condition involves linkage studies, which provide leads through potential genomic loci that can be mined for candidate genes. A wealth of data pointing to several genomic links for ACS at a young age has already been produced in different laboratories. Examples include linkage to the 2q36-q37.3, 3q26-q27 and 20q11-q13[134], for which a number of gene are currently being targetted for further investigation. Among the suspect genes described thus far is the insulin receptor substrate-1 gene, thought to present a locus for combined disease processes of atherosclerosis, plaque instability, and coronary thrombosis[134].

The natural link between familial dyslipidaemic disorders and early onset of CAD has placed genes involved in lipid metabolism at the focus of research interest. These studies have led to the discovery of several polymorphisms in the *Apo B*, *LDLR* and *PCSK9* genes among others. Missense mutations in the LDLR-binding domain of Apo B are believed to cause familial ligand-defective Apo B, characterized by hypercholesterolemia and premature CAD. Heterozygosity of the LDLR is relatively common, and gain-of-function mutations in PCSK9 also cause autosomal dominant hypercholesterolemia, through elevation of plasma Chol concentrations associated with low-density lipoproteins (LDLs). Other gene polymorphisms involved in the increase in LDL include those in the *Apo B*, *Apo E* and *LPL* genes. The *Apo* ε4 has also been linked to an increased risk of AMI as well as independent predictor of adverse events at young age[135]. Familial LPL deficiency is a rare inborn error of metabolism caused by mutational changes within the *LPL* gene, leading to massive hypertriglyceridemia and reduced HDL-C, both of which are risk factors for the development of CAD. Besides, human HL deficiency as a second causative factor for hyperlipidaemia is also strongly associated with premature CAD[43].

Apart from the regulation of lipid metabolism, several other genetic variants have surfaced as risk for AMI in the last decade. Cross-sectional studies endeavouring to identify variants in candidate genes for early development of CAD and AMI have focused primarily on polymorphisms influencing certain biological functions, such as coagulation and fibrinolysis, platelets, vascular function, lipid metabolism and inflammation. Indeed various genes have been identified encoding coagulation proteins, fibrinolytic proteins, platelet receptors, homocysteine metabolizer, and those related to endothelial dysfunction, abnormal blood flow and oxidative stress[136]. Examples include genes encoding the prothrombin, apo E, Factor V Leiden, Factor VII, and transforming growth factor-β1 (*TGF-β1*) genes[137]. Limited and controversial data also exists on the impact of the plasminogen activator inhibitor-1 (*PAI-1*) gene polymorphism in the pathogenesis of AMI. Thereby, some studies suggest that young patients <35 years possessing the 4G allele exhibit higher PAI-1 plasma levels but lower Lp(a) levels compared to 5G/5G homozygotes, indicating that the 4G allele of the *PAI*-1 4G/5G polymorphism is less frequent among survivors of MI at very young age compared with matched controls[138]. It has further been argued that AMI at young age could be also caused by a reduction of the fibrinolytic activity, in the presence of the *PAI* 4G allele.

Because ischemic stroke with arterial occlusion or undetermined etiology is more likely to be related to a genetic prothrombotic state, polymorphic changes in genes regulating clotting processes have attracted attention as potential culprits of ACS. Thus, the platelet membrane receptor glycoproteins (GPs) are essential for the platelet activation process, and the genetic polymorphisms in the encoding genes may influence the risk of ACS and atherosclerosis. Recently, a metaanalysis implicated platelet glycoprotein IIb/IIa (GPIIb-

IIIa), a membrane receptor for fibrinogen and von Willebrand factor and thrombopoetin variants in AMI[98]. The GP IIIa PI A2 allele has also been strongly associated with a previous history of MI, as well as the severity of disease, while in young smokers, the PAI-1 4G allele appears to present a mild risk factor for the development of MI[139]. Other gene variants including the GPIIb W86R mutation which produces a nonfunctional enzyme associated with elevated TG levels in the affected individual[140], and the prothrombin G20210A variant which displayed a modest but significant risk factor for AMI at young ages[141] have also been associated with the syndrome. An important aspect of the impact of these risk genes on ACS is the influence of the environmental components such as smoking, gender and socioeconomical factors. An example is the suggestion that the impact of the dominant mode for the thrombomodulin -33G/A polymorphism (GA+AA genotype) on a combination of CAD risk factors such as MI, hypertension and T2DM may be related to smoking in young individuals[142 143]. Thrombomodulin is an endothelial cell surface receptor for thrombin, which plays an important role in the regulation of blood coagulation by decreasing thrombin activity and activating protein C. A case study also reported an association of the Apo E (p.Arg136Cys) mutation and obese gene carriers, but with no severe dyslipidaemia in young smokers[144]. Also, synergistic effect of the *MMP-3* 5A/6A variant in the promoter region with smoking on the onset of AMI has been described in young patients with MI[145]. Furthermore, the contribution of the activated protein C resistance (APCR) as an increased risk for AMI has been described specifically in women smokers.

Other studies also point to the metafolin folate (methyl tetrahydrofolate; *MTHF*), *CD14*, E-selectin, *eNOS* and the *PECAM1* genes as potential candidates for ACS[98]. Apart from being implicated in the onset of CAD, the MTHF C677T variant has been associated with the risk for recurrent coronary events. Elevated plasma homocysteine level at admission is considered to be an independent risk factor for these events after the first episode of ACS in young patients, irrespective of the status of this variant[146]. Interestingly, while an increased risk of developing coronary artery lesions was described in the presence of a mannose-binding lectin (MBL2) variant in pediatric patients, in patients older than one year, an increased risk of the lesions was observed in wild-type genotype carriers, leading to the suggestion that MBL has an ambiguous role in Kawasaki disease and contributes differently to the pathophysiologic development CAD[147]. Another gene variant, the annexin V -1C/T seems to have a minor effect in bleeding disorders, but to play a protective role against AMI, reducing the risk of developing the disease[148].

Apart from genes regulating lipid metabolism and coagulation pathways, other gene families of importance in ACS include those encoding growth factors, proteins for proinflammatory processes, dyslipidaemia and obesity-related genes. These include two *TGF-β1* variants that have been linked AMI in young patients[149]. Associations between obesity-related variants, metabolic syndrome and AMI include those of *ADIPO Q*, *LEPR* *MC4R* and *FTO* polymorphisms. Furthermore, in a couple of case-control studies, Cx37 was implicated in AMI[97]. Also, a case-control study involving young patients with a first event of acute CAD or ischemic stroke, suggested that common variants in the VWF gene were associated with VWF levels and the risk for cardiovascular disease[150]. However, information on the contribution of common VWF gene variants to VWF levels and cardiovascular disease risk is still limited.

Plaque rupture is a well established critical factor in the pathogenesis of AMI. Recently, interest has also focussed on the relationship between inflammation and manifestation of atherosclerosis, leading to the identification of stromelysin-1 (i.e. matrix metalloproteinase-3; MMP-3) as a risk gene. MMP-3 can degrade extracellular matrix and has been identified extensively in human coronary atherosclerotic plaques. It may contribute to the weakening of the cap and subsequent plaque rupture. Also, the aldosterone synthase (*CYP11B2*) -344 C/T gene variant, which may influence plasma aldosterone levels, has been reported to strongly influence left ventricular diameters and mass in young adults and arterial stiffness in essential hypertensives.

However, since CAD is a multifactorial disease, single mutations are likely to provide a small or modest contribution to risk, which may depend on interaction with other genes and/or a particular environment. Besides, there is still some controversy or uncertainties with regards to the role of some individual pathways or gene variants in ACS, such as those encoding some of the obese-related or RAAS genes[90]. For example, a borderline association for AMI with the ACE D/I polymorphism was described as a risk only in the occurrence and the long-term prognosis of AMI at young age in one study[151], leading to the conclusion that polymorphisms in RAAS genes may be important in the onset of a first AMI in young patients, but not in the disease progression after a long follow-up period[151]. Besides, the role of some of the genes/ gene variants has been refuted by a number of studies. This includes the role of Factor V Leiden, where some studies reported protective effects of certain variants initially thought to be causative. A metaanalysis also refuted the association between the PlA1/A2 of the *GP IIIa* gene and young AMI, which had been implicated in a number of studies. The prothrombotic gene polymorphisms did not appear to have a significant influence on the prognosis in young ischemic stroke due to arterial occlusion of undetermined causes in a Taiwanese study[152]. However, these facts only stress the importance of replication of studies especially those that involve small numbers. More importantly, they reveal the importance of environmental factors especially for complex diseases such as CAD. Furthermore, this scenario points to the fact that not everything is known yet about the gene/gene variant responsible for CAD and its risk factors. Identifying such genes should greatly enhance our understanding of the intricacy of CAD manifestation, to identify individuals at risk and more importantly facilitate the development of more efficacious treatment strategies and introduction of early preventive measures. Thus, research efforts continue to address the identification of acquired and inherited risk factors of this complex disease.

5. Genetics and drug therapy of coronary artery disease

Treatment of coronary artery disease entails among others, lowering of circulating cholesterol, antiplatelet therapy representing the basis of treatment for the short- and long-term prevention of atherothrombotic disease processes, as well as measures to prevent or treat hypertension, heart failure and T2DM. Factors involved in inflammation (cytokines, TNF), proliferation of smooth muscle cells and vasoactivation are also important. In all these incidences however, it is well established that patients often respond differently to drug therapy. For example, in the treatment of lipidaemic disorders, not all patients respond equally well to therapy with statins. There are several reasons why patients respond in different fashions to drug therapy. One major explanation is the mode by which the drugs are metabolized by the various enzymes. It is now well recognized that genetic variations can contribute to these differences in drug disposition and, consequently, clinical efficacy at the population level. Thus, the metabolism may occur too rapidly, thereby leading to accelerated elimination from the body before it has had enough time to exert its effect. The opposite may equally be true that the drug is broken down too slowly resulting in its accumulation and therefore toxicity. Furthermore, the ability of the drug to bind to its receptor site may be hampered by changes in functional motifs of the target protein. Moreover, the level of the signalling message may be influenced by changes in the amount of target protein produced in different patients. All these factors could be due to sequence variations in human genes.

With respect to cardiovascular disease per se, statins are probably the most frequently prescribed class of drug, and understandably great effort has been invested in trying to understand the genetics of variations in patient response as well as toxicity of these drugs. To begin with, the fact that considerable interindividual variation exists in response to statin therapy, in terms of both lipid-lowering and adverse drug reactions has been demonstrated in several candidate gene studies as well as meta-analyses from several primary and secondary intervention studies. Notably, most statins are the substrates of several cytochrome P450s (CYPs), and polymorphisms in these enzymes appear to be responsible for variations in their hypolipidemic activity. Strong association of sequence variants of several genes including *HMGCR, CETP, SREBF1 and ABCG8* genes with the alteration in LDL-C reduction capability of different statins appears to be well-established[153]. Besides, drugs such as pravastatin and rotuvastatin are not susceptible to CYP inhibition, but are substrates of the a hepatic transporter and solute organic anion-transporting polypeptide (OATP) 1B1 (encoded by the *SLCO1B1* gene) which is responsible for liver transportation of the statins[154]. Variants of the apolipoprotein, particularly the apo E and apo A5 also have their share in these processes[155-158]. Similarly, genetically impaired ABCG2 transporter efflux activity results in a marked increase in systemic exposure to various statins[159]. Importantly, the effects of these genetic polymorphisms differ depending on the specific statin that is used. With respect to reduction of MI though the use of statin, defective interaction may occur with a number of variants in several genes including the scavenger receptor class B member 1 (*SCARB1*) *HMGCR, SREBF1, ABCG5/8, PCSK9,* hepatic triglyceride lipase *(LIPC*), *ABCA1, PPAR,* LDLR-related protein 1 (*LRP1*) and *SOAT1*[160 161 162]. Other important features of statin pharmacokinetics include calmin gene polymorphism, which may exhibit differences on the actions of simvastatin, pravastatin and artovastatin on total and LDL-C reduction[163] and ABCG2 which is associated with significantly greater LDL-C reduction with rosuvastatin compared to other statins [164].

Furthermore, despite the high efficacy and almost universal use of statins in cardiovascular disease prevention, their adverse actions appear to be their greatest disadvantage. In this regard, the use of high dose of statins in combination with other drugs is also not without problems, since their pharmacokinetics may be altered, leading to increasing blood levels with consequent risk of liver or muscle toxicity as demonstrated most commonly for agents metabolized by the CYP450 3A4 enzyme. Specifically, simvastatin has been associated with an increased risk of rhabdomyolysis when taken in combination with multiple inhibitors of CYP3A4[161]. Moreover, while the safety data for the statins suggest a very low incidence of severe adverse reactions, such as rhabdomyolysis and myopathy, myalgias without serum creatine kinase elevation remains a common side effect and the important reason for discontinuation of therapy. Myopathy has been reported in a considerable number of patients, but the mechanisms underlying muscle injury have yet to be fully characterized. These mechanisms may include statin-induced differences in Chol:phospholipid ratio, isoprenoid levels, small GTP binding proteins and apoptosis[165]. Furthermore, while depletion of Chol within the myocyte cell wall and/or the depletion of key intermediates within its synthesis pathway are hypothesized as possible mechanisms of statin-associated adverse drug actions (ADRs), pharmacogenetic variability may also contribute as a risk for ADRs[155]. These may include, for example, enzymes, transporters, cell membrane receptors, intracellular receptors or components of ion channels that contribute to the pharmacokinetics or pharmacodynamics of response to a particular drug. One of the genes identified thus far as likely to contribute to the development of simvastatin-induced myopathy and myalgia is the *SLCO1B1* gene[161,166]. Thereby, the *SLCO1B* variant increases the risk of statin-induced myopathy by reducing the hepatic uptake of the statins. Essentially all statins are, in fact, substrates of membrane transporters, whereby *SLCO1B1* polymorphisms can decrease the liver uptake, as well as the therapeutic potential of these agents, and may be linked to their muscular side-effects. Elevated levels of simvastatin metabolites (but not pravastatin) have been observed among carriers of *SLCO1B1*5* allele, pointing to a genetic susceptibility to both myopathy and statin-induced myalgias in the absence of elevated serum creatinine kinase[167]. The risk of myalgia among *SLCO1B1* carriers appears to be unique for artovastatin. Also, polymorphic changes in the CYPs, *CYP2D6, CYP3A4* and *CYP3A5* are linked with statin-induced myopathy and show variable effects on altering the pharmacokinetic profile of statin metabolism. Furthermore, although myalgia appears to be associated with the whole group of drugs, there is a significant amount of variability within the class[168 169].

The major site of statin action is within hepatocytes and recent interest has also focussed on seeking the explanation for the differences in the impact of genetic variations in hepatic influx and efflux transporters[170]. Among the most promising candidate genes for pharmacogenomic analysis of statin therapy is the *HMGCR* as a direct target gene and other genes modulating lipid and lipoprotein homeostasis such as *PPARs*. A synergist effect has also been reported in which attenuation in lipid-lowering response to simvastatin caused by some *LDLR* haplotypes was enhanced in the presence of *HMGCR* haplotypes[171], pointing to modulation of effects through gene-gene interactions.

Apart from statin therapy, antiplatelet therapy represents the basis of treatment for the short- and long-term prevention of atherothrombotic disease processes, in particular in high-risk settings such as in patients with ACS and those undergoing percutaneous coronary intervention. Currently, the most common treatment involves dual antiplatelet therapy with aspirin and clopidogrel. Specifically, clopidogrel is a prodrug that undergoes hepatic biotransformation by CYP2C19 into its active metabolite. However, a considerable number of patients continue to experience adverse outcomes, including both bleeding and recurrent ischemic events, possibly attributable, in part at least, to the broad variability in individual response profiles to this standard antiplatelet treatment regimen[172]. Gene polymorphisms affecting clopidogrel metabolic bioactivation and platelet function may be responsible. These include CYP2C19 *2, *3 and *17, CYP2C9 *2 and *3, MDR1*2, and functional variants in the genes encoding platelet membrane receptors and intracellular signaling proteins[173,174]. Moreover, gene polymorphisms may also have an important role in determining levels of platelet inhibition and provide a tool for identifying patients at risk of adverse events.

In ischemic heart disease, the most commonly suspected genes are those related to lipid metabolism, coagulation and fibrinolytic systems as well as the RAAS pathway. Drugs that modulate the RAAS play an important role in advanced cardiovascular disease prevention strategies. Inhibitors of the RAAS, in particular ACE inhibitors are beneficial in specific patient groups, including those with hypertension, heart failure, diabetes mellitus and stable CAD. Hence ACE inhibitors are among the most commonly used drugs in stable CAD since they have been proven to be effective for reducing the risk of cardiovascular morbidity and mortality. However, while clinical trials demonstrated some consistent beneficial effect of ACE inhibitors across groups of patients based on clinical characteristics, the variability in treatment response on the individual patient level is high. Just as in the treatment of lipidaemic disorders, a primary cause seems to be genetic variations. Furthermore, treatment of diabetes constitutes an integral part of regimens to control coronary vascular disorders, which is similarly subject to issues of differences in patient responses to therapy. Examples include the uncoupling protein variant which has been correlated with β-blocker response among ACS patients with diabetes[175], and the *SLCO1B1* gene variants also thought to be responsible for intolerance in diabetic patients[176]. Variability within the *SLCO1B1* and *ABCB1* genes are also linked with the modification of the effectiveness of statins in the prevention of the clinical outcome of MI[177].

However, while a great deal has been written about the potential of pharmacogenetic testing to informed therapy based on an individual's genetic makeup, and to decide the most effective choice of available drugs, or to avoid dangerous side effects, currently, there is little hard data for either in the field of cardiovascular disease. The usual approach has been the opportunistic use of drug trials in unrelated patients, and to look for differences in response or outcome by candidate gene genotype, for example, in those encoding drug metabolizing enzymes (activators and metabolizers), as well as enzymes and receptors involved in lipid metabolism, adrenergic response, among others. As with all association studies, initially promising results have often failed the test of replication in larger studies. An example is the attempt to employ relationship between the CETPTaq-I variant and response to statins, which has been ultimately withdrawn[178]. Nonetheless, ongoing exploration of genetic polymorphisms that influence response to drug therapy may one day allow the clinician to customize treatment strategies for patients in order to improve their success rate. In the treatment of CAD or ACS, greatest chance appears to have been accomplished in the area of regulating circulating lipids. The hope is that pharmacogenomic testing in future will allow risk stratification of patients to avoid serious side effects and enable clinicians to select lipid-lowering drugs with the highest efficacy resulting in the best response to therapy. The compounds include drugs indicated for dyslipidaemia, such as statins, fibrates, niacin and cholestyramine, as well as those used for other purposes, including calcium channel blockers, angiotensin receptor blockers and glitazones. Furthermore, currently available data from pharmacogenetic trials, a combined analysis of multiple genetic variants in several genes is more likely to give significant results than single gene studies in small cohorts. Thus, larger studies or combination analyses involving more than two different polymorphisms would enable us to find clinically or biologically more meaningful differences, and genes influencing Chol biosynthesis in the liver, such as ABCG5/G8,

CYP7A1, HMGCR, would be good candidates. In this regard, plasma TG concentration is also reemerging as an important cardiovascular disease risk factor. More complete understanding of the genes and variants that modulate plasma TG should enable development of markers for risk prediction, diagnosis, prognosis, and response to therapies and might help specify new directions for therapeutic interventions.

6. Summary

Atherosclerosis is a multifactorial, multistep disease that involves chronic inflammation at every step, from initiation to progression, and all the risk factors contribute to pathogenesis by aggravating the underlying inflammatory process. Despite well-invested efforts to minimize attributable risk from known contributors to the disease such as hypertension, dyslipidaemia, and smoking, CAD remains the number one cause of death in industrialized countries. Clinical trials have consistently demonstrated a family history of coronary disease to be predictive for future cardiovascular events beyond that which would be explained by traditional risk factors. These findings do not only support but also have prompted great interest to study the genomic basis of CAD and MI. Recent advances in genotyping technology have allowed for easier identification and confirmation of susceptibility genes for complex traits across different cohorts in the pathways leading to CAD. This has been facilitated through increased power of studies enhanced by faster accrual of cases and control subjects and more precise genetic mapping, and have allowed us define the genes contributing to a possibly great majority of population-attributable risk for T2DM, hypertension and ACS. Similar progress in replicating novel susceptibility genes for CAD and specifically MI is now advancing rapidly. Several genes have already been identified and more are in the pipeline. With improved resequencing technology and better phenotypic characterization of the CAD cases and control subjects, comprehensive identification and confirmation of genes associated with CAD risk appear to be around the corner, in order to allow us to better quantify CAD risk early enough in life and institute more effective therapy reducing the burden of an individual developing CAD. However, being a complex disease, the disease pathways to CAD are interwound in an intricate network, which together with environmental factors require complex tools to decipher. Such an in-depth knowledge of the various pathogenic mechanisms involved in the disease will significantly enhance our substantiation of the existing knowledge about the disease.

Furthermore, while substantial progress has been made in the identification of common DNA sequence variations in genes influencing the pharmacokinetics and pharmacodynamics of related drugs and in disease-modifying genes relevant for CAD, our present understanding of pathophysiological mechanisms does not offer a reliable approach to address the same at preclinical level. Pharmacogenomics can provide important insights into the therapy of CAD and related risk factors through elucidation of the genetic (or genomic) contribution to variable response to different drugs. The search for genetic polymorphisms may enable us to identify novel determinants of drug responsiveness by studying candidate gene belonging to the gene families that encode proteins involved in pharmacokinetics, the genes encoding proteins engaged pharmacodynamics and genes encoding proteins involved in the underlying disease condition or intermediate phenotype. A better understanding of the pathogenesis of CAD will enhance the advancement of pharmaceutical and lifestyle modifications for reducing mortality resulting from the disease.

7. References

[1] Park SW, Moon YA, Horton JD. Post-transcriptional regulation of low density lipoprotein receptor protein by proprotein convertase subtilisin/kexin type 9a in mouse liver. J Biol Chem 2004;279:50630-8.

[2] Maxwell KN, Breslow JL. Proprotein convertase subtilisin kexin 9: the third locus implicated in autosomal dominant hypercholesterolemia. Curr Opin Lipidol 2005;16:167-72.

[3] Cohen J, Pertsemlidis A, Kotowski IK, Graham R, Garcia CK, Hobbs HH. Low LDL cholesterol in individuals of African descent resulting from frequent nonsense mutations in PCSK9. Nat Genet 2005;37:161-5.

[4] Benjannet S, Rhainds D, Essalmani R, et al. NARC-1/PCSK9 and its natural mutants: zymogen cleavage and effects on the low density lipoprotein (LDL) receptor and LDL cholesterol. J Biol Chem 2004;279:48865-75.

[5] Li H, Li H, Ziegler N, Cui R, Liu J. Recent patents on PCSK9: a new target for treating hypercholesterolemia. Recent Pat DNA Gene Seq 2009;3:201-12.

[6] Le Goff W, Guerin M, Chapman MJ. Pharmacological modulation of cholesteryl ester transfer protein, a new therapeutic target in atherogenic dyslipidemia. Pharmacol Ther 2004;101:17-38.

[7] Le Goff W, Guerin M, Nicaud V, et al. A novel cholesteryl ester transfer protein promoter polymorphism (-971G/A) associated with plasma high-density lipoprotein cholesterol levels. Interaction with the TaqIB and -629C/A polymorphisms. Atherosclerosis 2002; 161:269-79.

[8] Sakai J, Rawson RB. The sterol regulatory element-binding protein pathway: control of lipid homeostasis through regulated intracellular transport. Curr Opin Lipidol 2001;12:261-6.

[9] Horton JD, Goldstein JL, Brown MS. SREBPs: transcriptional mediators of lipid homeostasis. Cold Spring Harb Symp Quant Biol 2002;67:491-8.

[10] Horton JD, Goldstein JL, Brown MS. SREBPs: activators of the complete program of cholesterol and fatty acid synthesis in the liver. J Clin Invest 2002;109:1125-31.

[11] DeBose-Boyd RA, Brown MS, Li WP, Nohturfft A, Goldstein JL, Espenshade PJ. Transport-dependent proteolysis of SREBP: relocation of site-1 protease from Golgi to ER obviates the need for SREBP transport to Golgi. Cell 1999;99:703-12.

[12] Nohturfft A, DeBose-Boyd RA, Scheek S, Goldstein JL, Brown MS. Sterols regulate cycling of SREBP cleavage-activating protein (SCAP) between endoplasmic reticulum and Golgi. Proc Natl Acad Sci U S A 1999;96:11235-40.

[13] Eberle D, Hegarty B, Bossard P, Ferre P, Foufelle F. SREBP transcription factors: master regulators of lipid homeostasis. Biochimie 2004;86:839-48.

[14] Edwards PA, Tabor D, Kast HR, Venkateswaran A. Regulation of gene expression by SREBP and SCAP. Biochim Biophys Acta 2000;1529:103-13.

[15] Eberle D, Clement K, Meyre D, et al. SREBF-1 gene polymorphisms are associated with obesity and type 2 diabetes in French obese and diabetic cohorts. Diabetes 2004;53:2153-7.

[16] Chirieac DV, Collins HL, Cianci J, Sparks JD, Sparks CE. Altered triglyceride-rich lipoprotein production in Zucker diabetic fatty rats. Am J Physiol Endocrinol Metab 2004;287:E42-9.
[17] Wang Z, Jiang T, Li J, et al. Regulation of renal lipid metabolism, lipid accumulation, and glomerulosclerosis in FVBdb/db mice with type 2 diabetes. Diabetes 2005;54:2328-35.
[18] Biddinger SB, Almind K, Miyazaki M, Kokkotou E, Ntambi JM, Kahn CR. Effects of diet and genetic background on sterol regulatory element-binding protein-1c, stearoyl-CoA desaturase 1, and the development of the metabolic syndrome. Diabetes 2005;54:1314-23.
[19] Lin J, Yang R, Tarr PT, et al. Hyperlipidemic effects of dietary saturated fats mediated through PGC-1beta coactivation of SREBP. Cell 2005;120:261-73.
[20] Amemiya-Kudo M, Shimano H, Hasty AH, et al. Transcriptional activities of nuclear SREBP-1a, -1c, and -2 to different target promoters of lipogenic and cholesterogenic genes. Journal of lipid research 2002;43:1220-35.
[21] Shimano H, Yahagi N, Amemiya-Kudo M, et al. Sterol regulatory element-binding protein-1 as a key transcription factor for nutritional induction of lipogenic enzyme genes. J Biol Chem 1999;274:35832-9.
[22] Yahagi N, Shimano H, Hasty AH, et al. A crucial role of sterol regulatory element-binding protein-1 in the regulation of lipogenic gene expression by polyunsaturated fatty acids. J Biol Chem 1999;274:35840-4.
[23] Ten S, Maclaren N. Insulin resistance syndrome in children. J Clin Endocrinol Metab 2004;89:2526-39.
[24] Kim DH, Zhang T, Ringquist S, Dong HH. Targeting FoxO1 for Hypertriglyceridemia. Current drug targets 2011;12:1245-55.
[25] Kamagate A, Dong HH. FoxO1 integrates insulin signaling to VLDL production. Cell Cycle 2008;7:3162-70.
[26] Lamarche B, Lemieux I, Despres JP. The small, dense LDL phenotype and the risk of coronary heart disease: epidemiology, patho-physiology and therapeutic aspects. Diabetes Metab 1999;25:199-211.
[27] Sitia S, Tomasoni L, Atzeni F, et al. From endothelial dysfunction to atherosclerosis. Autoimmun Rev;9:830-4.
[28] Kutti J, Weinfeld A. Platelet survival and platelet production in acute myocardial infarction. Acta Med Scand 1979;205:501-4.
[29] van der Loo B, Martin JF. Megakaryocytes and platelets in vascular disease. Baillieres Clin Haematol 1997;10:109-23.
[30] Khan MA, Collins AJ, Keane WF. Diabetes in the elderly population. Adv Ren Replace Ther 2000;7:32-51.
[31] Norata GD, Catapano AL. Lipid lowering activity of drugs affecting cholesterol absorption. Nutr Metab Cardiovasc Dis 2004;14:42-51.
[32] Perez-Martinez P, Lopez-Miranda J, Perez-Jimenez F, Ordovas JM. Influence of genetic factors in the modulation of postprandial lipemia. Atheroscler Suppl 2008;9:49-55.
[33] Grundy SM. Hypertriglyceridemia, atherogenic dyslipidemia, and the metabolic syndrome. The American journal of cardiology 1998;81:18B-25B.

[34] Grundy SM, Balady GJ, Criqui MH, et al. Primary prevention of coronary heart disease: guidance from Framingham: a statement for healthcare professionals from the AHA Task Force on Risk Reduction. American Heart Association. Circulation 1998;97:1876-87.

[35] Boes E, Coassin S, Kollerits B, Heid IM, Kronenberg F. Genetic-epidemiological evidence on genes associated with HDL cholesterol levels: a systematic in-depth review. Exp Gerontol 2009;44:136-60.

[36] Cohen JC, Kimmel M, Polanski A, Hobbs HH. Molecular mechanisms of autosomal recessive hypercholesterolemia. Curr Opin Lipidol 2003;14:121-7.

[37] Kwiterovich PO, Jr. Clinical relevance of the biochemical, metabolic, and genetic factors that influence low-density lipoprotein heterogeneity. The American journal of cardiology 2002;90:30i-47i.

[38] Moller DE, Kaufman KD. Metabolic syndrome: a clinical and molecular perspective. Annu Rev Med 2005;56:45-62.

[39] Wilcken DE. Overview of inherited metabolic disorders causing cardiovascular disease. J Inherit Metab Dis 2003;26:245-57.

[40] Richter WF, Whitby BR, Chou RC. Distribution of remikiren, a potent orally active inhibitor of human renin, in laboratory animals. Xenobiotica 1996;26:243-54.

[41] Misra A, Khurana L. Obesity-related non-communicable diseases: South Asians vs White Caucasians. Int J Obes (Lond);35:167-87.

[42] Andreassi MG. Coronary atherosclerosis and somatic mutations: an overview of the contributive factors for oxidative DNA damage. Mutat Res 2003;543:67-86.

[43] Connelly PW, Hegele RA. Hepatic lipase deficiency. Crit Rev Clin Lab Sci 1998;35:547-72.

[44] Ferrero-Miliani L, Nielsen OH, Andersen PS, Girardin SE. Chronic inflammation: importance of NOD2 and NALP3 in interleukin-1β generation. Clinical & Experimental Immunology 2007;147:227-35.

[45] Onat A, Hergenc G. Low-grade inflammation, and dysfunction of high-density lipoprotein and its apolipoproteins as a major driver of cardiometabolic risk. Metabolism;60:499-512.

[46] De Sutter J, Struyf S, Van de Veire NR, Philippe J, De Buyzere M, Van Damme J. Cardiovascular determinants and prognostic significance of CC Chemokine Ligand-18 (CCL18/PARC) in patients with stable coronary artery disease. J Mol Cell Cardiol 2010;49:894-6.

[47] Fried SK, Rao SP. Sugars, hypertriglyceridemia, and cardiovascular disease. Am J Clin Nutr 2003;78:873S-80S.

[48] Hochman JS, Tamis JE, Thompson TD, et al. Sex, clinical presentation, and outcome in patients with acute coronary syndromes. Global Use of Strategies to Open Occluded Coronary Arteries in Acute Coronary Syndromes IIb Investigators. N Engl J Med 1999;341:226-32.

[49] Elsaesser A, Hamm CW. Acute coronary syndrome: the risk of being female. Circulation 2004;109:565-7.

[50] Hasdai D, Porter A, Rosengren A, Behar S, Boyko V, Battler A. Effect of gender on outcomes of acute coronary syndromes. Am J Cardiol 2003;91:1466-9, A6.

[51] Friedlander Y, Arbogast P, Schwartz SM, et al. Family history as a risk factor for early onset myocardial infarction in young women. Atherosclerosis 2001;156:201-7.
[52] Austin MA, Hutter CM, Zimmern RL, Humphries SE. Genetic causes of monogenic heterozygous familial hypercholesterolemia: a HuGE prevalence review. Am J Epidemiol 2004;160:407-20.
[53] Abifadel M, Rabes JP, Devillers M, et al. Mutations and polymorphisms in the proprotein convertase subtilisin kexin 9 (PCSK9) gene in cholesterol metabolism and disease. Hum Mutat 2009;30:520-9.
[54] Damani SB, Topol EJ. Future use of genomics in coronary artery disease. J Am Coll Cardiol 2007;50:1933-40.
[55] Barbagallo CM, Emmanuele G, Cefalu AB, et al. Autosomal recessive hypercholesterolemia in a Sicilian kindred harboring the 432insA mutation of the ARH gene. Atherosclerosis 2003;166:395-400.
[56] Costet P, Krempf M, Cariou B. PCSK9 and LDL cholesterol: unravelling the target to design the bullet. Trends Biochem Sci 2008;33:426-34.
[57] Humphries SE, Norbury G, Leigh S, Hadfield SG, Nair D. What is the clinical utility of DNA testing in patients with familial hypercholesterolaemia? Curr Opin Lipidol 2008;19:362-8.
[58] Assmann G, Gotto AM, Jr. HDL cholesterol and protective factors in atherosclerosis. Circulation 2004;109:III8-14.
[59] Jaye M, Krawiec J. Endothelial lipase and HDL metabolism. Curr Opin Lipidol 2004;15:183-9.
[60] Naukkarinen J, Ehnholm C, Peltonen L. Genetics of familial combined hyperlipidemia. Curr Opin Lipidol 2006;17:285-90.
[61] Garg A, Simha V. Update on dyslipidemia. J Clin Endocrinol Metab 2007;92:1581-9.
[62] Enas EA, Chacko V, Senthilkumar A, Puthumana N, Mohan V. Elevated lipoprotein(a)--a genetic risk factor for premature vascular disease in people with and without standard risk factors: a review. Dis Mon 2006;52:5-50.
[63] Hooper AJ, van Bockxmeer FM, Burnett JR. Monogenic hypocholesterolaemic lipid disorders and apolipoprotein B metabolism. Crit Rev Clin Lab Sci 2005;42:515-45.
[64] Zambon A, Brown BG, Deeb SS, Brunzell JD. Genetics of apolipoprotein B and apolipoprotein AI and premature coronary artery disease. Journal of internal medicine 2006;259:473-80.
[65] Konopka A, Szperl M, Piotrowski W, Roszczynko M, Stepinska J. Influence of Renin-Angiotensin System Gene Polymorphisms on the Risk of ST-Segment-Elevation Myocardial Infarction and Association with Coronary Artery Disease Risk Factors. Mol Diagn Ther 2011;15:167-76.
[66] Dzimiri N, Muiya P, Mohamed G, et al. Haplotypes encompassing the PSMA6 and KIAA0391 Gene Cluster confer risk for Myocardial Infarction. FASEB J 2009; 23:573.1-.
[67] Inoue N, Kawashima S, Kanazawa K, Yamada S, Akita H, Yokoyama M. Polymorphism of the NADH/NADPH oxidase p22 phox gene in patients with coronary artery disease. Circulation 1998;97:135-7.

[68] Sethi AA, Nordestgaard BG, Tybjaerg-Hansen A. Angiotensinogen gene polymorphism, plasma angiotensinogen, and risk of hypertension and ischemic heart disease: a meta-analysis. Arteriosclerosis, thrombosis, and vascular biology 2003;23:1269-75.

[69] Sethi AA, Nordestgaard BG, Gronholdt ML, Steffensen R, Jensen G, Tybjaerg-Hansen A. Angiotensinogen single nucleotide polymorphisms, elevated blood pressure, and risk of cardiovascular disease. Hypertension 2003;41:1202-11.

[70] Sethi AA, Tybjaerg-Hansen A, Gronholdt ML, Steffensen R, Schnohr P, Nordestgaard BG. Angiotensinogen mutations and risk for ischemic heart disease, myocardial infarction, and ischemic cerebrovascular disease. Six case-control studies from the Copenhagen City Heart Study. Ann Intern Med 2001;134:941-54.

[71] Cha SH, Kim HT, Jang Y, et al. Association of alpha-adducin Gly460Trp polymorphism with coronary artery disease in a Korean population. J Hypertens 2007;25:2413-20.

[72] Zee RY, Cook NR, Cheng S, Erlich HA, Lindpaintner K, Ridker PM. Multi-locus candidate gene polymorphisms and risk of myocardial infarction: a population-based, prospective genetic analysis. Journal of thrombosis and haemostasis : JTH 2006;4:341-8.

[73] O'Donnell CJ, Lindpaintner K, Larson MG, et al. Evidence for association and genetic linkage of the angiotensin-converting enzyme locus with hypertension and blood pressure in men but not women in the Framingham Heart Study. Circulation 1998;97:1766-72.

[74] Raman VK, Lee YA, Lindpaintner K. The cardiac renin-angiotensin-aldosterone system and hypertensive cardiac hypertrophy. The American journal of cardiology 1995;76:18D-23D.

[75] Lindpaintner K. Genes, hypertension, and cardiac hypertrophy. N Engl J Med 1994;330:1678-9.

[76] Wang XL, Sim AS, Badenhop RF, McCredie RM, Wilcken DE. A smoking-dependent risk of coronary artery disease associated with a polymorphism of the endothelial nitric oxide synthase gene. Nat Med 1996;2:41-5.

[77] Klerk M, Verhoef P, Clarke R, Blom HJ, Kok FJ, Schouten EG. MTHFR 677C-->T polymorphism and risk of coronary heart disease: a meta-analysis. Jama 2002;288:2023-31.

[78] Stenina OI, Byzova TV, Adams JC, McCarthy JJ, Topol EJ, Plow EF. Coronary artery disease and the thrombospondin single nucleotide polymorphisms. Int J Biochem Cell Biol 2004;36:1013-30.

[79] Stenina OI, Desai SY, Krukovets I, et al. Thrombospondin-4 and its variants: expression and differential effects on endothelial cells. Circulation 2003;108:1514-9.

[80] Cui J, Randell E, Renouf J, et al. Thrombospondin-4 1186G>C (A387P) is a sex-dependent risk factor for myocardial infarction: a large replication study with increased sample size from the same population. American heart journal 2006;152:543 e1-5.

[81] Zwicker JI, Peyvandi F, Palla R, et al. The thrombospondin-1 N700S polymorphism is associated with early myocardial infarction without altering von Willebrand factor multimer size. Blood 2006;108:1280-3.

[82] Gao L, He GP, Dai J, et al. Association of thrombospondin-1 gene polymorphisms with myocardial infarction in a Chinese Han population. Chin Med J (Engl) 2008;121:78-81.

[83] Suriyaprom K, Phonrat B, Namjuntra P, Harnroongroj T, Tungtrongchitr R. The -11377C > G adiponectin gene polymorphism alters the adiponectin concentration and the susceptibility to type 2 diabetes in Thais. Int J Vitam Nutr Res;80:216-24.

[84] Siitonen N, Pulkkinen L, Lindstrom J, et al. Association of ADIPOQ gene variants with body weight, type 2 diabetes and serum adiponectin concentrations: the Finnish Diabetes Prevention Study. BMC Med Genet;12:5.

[85] Yang WS, Chuang LM. Human genetics of adiponectin in the metabolic syndrome. J Mol Med (Berl) 2006;84:112-21.

[86] Du W, Li Q, Lu Y, et al. Genetic variants in ADIPOQ gene and the risk of type 2 diabetes: a case-control study of Chinese Han population. Endocrine.

[87] Ikeda Y, Hama S, Kajimoto K, Okuno T, Tsuchiya H, Kogure K. Quantitative Comparison of Adipocytokine Gene Expression during Adipocyte Maturation in Non-obese and Obese Rats. Biol Pharm Bull;34:865-70.

[88] Galgani A, Valdes A, Erlich HA, et al. Homozygosity for the Ala allele of the PPARgamma2 Pro12Ala polymorphism is associated with reduced risk of coronary artery disease. Dis Markers 2010;29:259-64.

[89] Hetherington MM, Cecil JE. Gene-environment interactions in obesity. Forum of nutrition 2010;63:195-203.

[90] Ranjith N, Pegoraro RJ, Shanmugam R. Obesity-associated genetic variants in young Asian Indians with the metabolic syndrome and myocardial infarction. Cardiovasc J Afr;22:25-30.

[91] Nagi DK, Foy CA, Mohamed-Ali V, Yudkin JS, Grant PJ, Knowler WC. Angiotensin-1-converting enzyme (ACE) gene polymorphism, plasma ACE levels, and their association with the metabolic syndrome and electrocardiographic coronary artery disease in Pima Indians. Metabolism 1998;47:622-6.

[92] Assali A, Ghayour-Mobarhan M, Sahebkar A, et al. Association of angiotensin II type 1 receptor gene A1166C polymorphism with the presence of diabetes mellitus and metabolic syndrome in patients with documented coronary artery disease. Eur J Intern Med;22:254-61.

[93] Safranow K, Czyzycka E, Binczak-Kuleta A, et al. Association of C34T AMPD1 gene polymorphism with features of metabolic syndrome in patients with coronary artery disease or heart failure. Scand J Clin Lab Invest 2009;69:102-12.

[94] Muendlein A, Saely CH, Geller-Rhomberg S, et al. Single nucleotide polymorphisms of TCF7L2 are linked to diabetic coronary atherosclerosis. PLoS One 2011;6:e17978.

[95] Abu-Amero KK, Al-Mohanna F, Alboudairi O, Mohamed GH, Dzimiri N. The interactive role of diabetes mellitus type 2 and E-selectin S128R mutation on coronary heart disease manifestation. BMC Med Genet 2007;8:35.

[96] Zheng YY, Xie X, Ma YT, et al. Relationship between a Novel Polymorphism of the C5L2 Gene and Coronary Artery Disease. PLoS One 2011;6:e20984.

[97] Listi F, Candore G, Lio D, et al. Association between C1019T polymorphism of connexin37 and acute myocardial infarction: a study in patients from Sicily. Int J Cardiol 2005;102:269-71.

[98] Incalcaterra E, Caruso M, Balistreri CR, et al. Role of genetic polymorphisms in myocardial infarction at young age. Clin Hemorheol Microcirc;46:291-8.

[99] Incalcaterra E, Hoffmann E, Averna MR, Caimi G. Genetic risk factors in myocardial infarction at young age. Minerva Cardioangiol 2004;52:287-312.

[100] Frikke-Schmidt R, Nordestgaard BG, Stene MC, et al. Association of loss-of-function mutations in the ABCA1 gene with high-density lipoprotein cholesterol levels and risk of ischemic heart disease. Jama 2008;299:2524-32.

[101] Barlic J, Murphy PM. An oxidized lipid-peroxisome proliferator-activated receptor gamma-chemokine pathway in the regulation of macrophage-vascular smooth muscle cell adhesion. Trends Cardiovasc Med 2007;17:269-74.

[102] Hansson GK. Atherosclerosis--an immune disease: The Anitschkov Lecture 2007. Atherosclerosis 2009;202:2-10.

[103] Mackness MI, Mackness B, Durrington PN, Connelly PW, Hegele RA. Paraoxonase: biochemistry, genetics and relationship to plasma lipoproteins. Curr Opin Lipidol 1996;7:69-76.

[104] Kaplan M, Aviram M. Oxidized low density lipoprotein: atherogenic and proinflammatory characteristics during macrophage foam cell formation. An inhibitory role for nutritional antioxidants and serum paraoxonase. Clin Chem Lab Med 1999;37:777-87.

[105] Li HL, Liu DP, Liang CC. Paraoxonase gene polymorphisms, oxidative stress, and diseases. J Mol Med 2003;81:766-79.

[106] Grech ED, Dodd NJ, Jackson MJ, Morrison WL, Faragher EB, Ramsdale DR. Evidence for free radical generation after primary percutaneous transluminal coronary angioplasty recanalization in acute myocardial infarction. Am J Cardiol 1996;77:122-7.

[107] Goliasch G, Wiesbauer F, Grafl A, et al. The effect of p22-PHOX (CYBA) polymorphisms on premature coronary artery disease (</= 40 years of age). Thromb Haemost;105:529-34.

[108] Grove EL, Hvas AM, Kristensen SD. Immature platelets in patients with acute coronary syndromes. Thromb Haemost 2009;101:151-6.

[109] Kunicki TJ, Nugent DJ. The genetics of normal platelet reactivity. Blood 2010;116:2627-34.

[110] Karakas M, Zierer A, Herder C, et al. Leptin, adiponectin, their ratio and risk of Coronary Heart Disease: results from the MONICA/KORA Augsburg Study 1984-2002. Atherosclerosis 2010;209:220-5.

[111] A genome-wide association study in Europeans and South Asians identifies five new loci for coronary artery disease. Nat Genet 2011;43:339-44.

[112] Connelly JJ, Wang T, Cox JE, et al. GATA2 is associated with familial early-onset coronary artery disease. PLoS Genet 2006;2:e139.

[113] Elhawari S, Al-Boudari O, Muiya P, et al. A study of the role of the Myocyte-specific Enhancer Factor-2A gene in coronary artery disease. Atherosclerosis;209:152-4.

[114] Yuan H, Lu HW, Hu J, Chen SH, Yang GP, Huang ZJ. MEF2A gene and susceptibility to coronary artery disease in the Chinese people. Zhong Nan Da Xue Xue Bao Yi Xue Ban 2006;31:453-7.
[115] Bhagavatula MR, Fan C, Shen GQ, et al. Transcription factor MEF2A mutations in patients with coronary artery disease. Hum Mol Genet 2004;13:3181-8.
[116] Dzimiri N, Muiya P, Alsmadi O, et al. The KIAA0391 and PSMA6 gene cluster confers a risk factor for coronary artery disease. FASEB J 2009;23:573.2-.
[117] Hinohara K, Nakajima T, Sasaoka T, et al. Replication studies for the association of PSMA6 polymorphism with coronary artery disease in East Asian populations. J Hum Genet 2009;54:248-51.
[118] Linnemann AK, O'Geen H, Keles S, Farnham PJ, Bresnick EH. Genetic framework for GATA factor function in vascular biology. Proc Natl Acad Sci U S A 2011.
[119] Roberts R, Chen L, Wells GA, Stewart AF. Recent success in the discovery of coronary artery disease genes. Can J Physiol Pharmacol 2011.
[120] Tsai CT, Hwang JJ, Wu CK, et al. Polygenetic regression model of renin-angiotensin system genes and the risk of coronary artery disease in a large angiographic population. Clinica chimica acta; international journal of clinical chemistry 2011;412:619-24.
[121] Freitas AI, Mendonca I, Brion M, et al. RAS gene polymorphisms, classical risk factors and the advent of coronary artery disease in the Portuguese population. BMC Cardiovasc Disord 2008;8:15.
[122] Mendonca MI, Dos Reis RP, Freitas AI, et al. Interaction of paraoxonase-192 polymorphism with low HDL-cholesterol in coronary artery disease risk. Rev Port Cardiol;29:571-80.
[123] Mendonca MI, Dos Reis RP, Freitas AI, et al. Gene-gene interaction affects coronary artery disease risk. Rev Port Cardiol 2009;28:397-415.
[124] Benes P, Muzik J, Benedik J, et al. Single effects of apolipoprotein B, (a), and E polymorphisms and interaction between plasminogen activator inhibitor-1 and apolipoprotein(a) genotypes and the risk of coronary artery disease in Czech male caucasians. Molecular genetics and metabolism 2000;69:137-43.
[125] Peng DQ, Zhao SP, Nie S, Li J. Gene-gene interaction of PPARgamma and ApoE affects coronary heart disease risk. International journal of cardiology 2003;92:257-63.
[126] Wu CK, Luo JL, Wu XM, et al. A propensity score-based case-control study of renin-angiotensin system gene polymorphisms and diastolic heart failure. Atherosclerosis 2009;205:497-502.
[127] Tsai CT, Hwang JJ, Ritchie MD, et al. Renin-angiotensin system gene polymorphisms and coronary artery disease in a large angiographic cohort: detection of high order gene-gene interaction. Atherosclerosis 2007;195:172-80.
[128] Agirbasli D, Agirbasli M, Williams SM, Phillips JA, 3rd. Interaction among 5,10 methylenetetrahydrofolate reductase, plasminogen activator inhibitor and endothelial nitric oxide synthase gene polymorphisms predicts the severity of coronary artery disease in Turkish patients. Coronary artery disease 2006;17:413-7.

[129] Ye S, Dhillon S, Seear R, et al. Epistatic interaction between variations in the angiotensin I converting enzyme and angiotensin II type 1 receptor genes in relation to extent of coronary atherosclerosis. Heart 2003;89:1195-9.
[130] Corella D, Guillen M, Saiz C, et al. Associations of LPL and APOC3 gene polymorphisms on plasma lipids in a Mediterranean population: interaction with tobacco smoking and the APOE locus. Journal of lipid research 2002;43:416-27.
[131] Naber CK, Husing J, Wolfhard U, Erbel R, Siffert W. Interaction of the ACE D allele and the GNB3 825T allele in myocardial infarction. Hypertension 2000;36:986-9.
[132] Lopez-Miranda J, Williams C, Lairon D. Dietary, physiological, genetic and pathological influences on postprandial lipid metabolism. Br J Nutr 2007;98:458-73.
[133] Perez-Martinez P, Delgado-Lista J, Perez-Jimenez F, Lopez-Miranda J. Update on genetics of postprandial lipemia. Atheroscler Suppl;11:39-43.
[134] Harrap SB, Zammit KS, Wong ZY, et al. Genome-wide linkage analysis of the acute coronary syndrome suggests a locus on chromosome 2. Arteriosclerosis, thrombosis, and vascular biology 2002;22:874-8.
[135] Brscic E, Bergerone S, Gagnor A, et al. Acute myocardial infarction in young adults: prognostic role of angiotensin-converting enzyme, angiotensin II type I receptor, apolipoprotein E, endothelial constitutive nitric oxide synthase, and glycoprotein IIIa genetic polymorphisms at medium-term follow-up. American heart journal 2000;139:979-84.
[136] Isordia-Salas I, Mendoza-Valdez AL, Almeida-Gutierrez E, Borrayo-Sanchez G. Genetic factors of the hemostatic system in young patients with myocardial infarction. Cir Cir;78:93-7.
[137] Mannucci PM, Asselta R, Duga S, et al. The association of factor V Leiden with myocardial infarction is replicated in 1880 patients with premature disease. J Thromb Haemost;8:2116-21.
[138] Rallidis LS, Gialeraki A, Merkouri E, et al. Reduced carriership of 4G allele of plasminogen activator inhibitor-1 4G/5G polymorphism in very young survivors of myocardial infarction. J Thromb Thrombolysis;29:497-502.
[139] Pegoraro RJ, Ranjith N. Plasminogen activator inhibitor type 1 (PAI-1) and platelet glycoprotein IIIa (PGIIIa) polymorphisms in young Asian Indians with acute myocardial infarction. Cardiovasc J S Afr 2005;16:266-70.
[140] Pasalic D, Jurcic Z, Stipancic G, et al. Missense mutation W86R in exon 3 of the lipoprotein lipase gene in a boy with chylomicronemia. Clin Chim Acta 2004;343:179-84.
[141] Burzotta F, Paciaroni K, De Stefano V, et al. G20210A prothrombin gene polymorphism and coronary ischaemic syndromes: a phenotype-specific meta-analysis of 12 034 subjects. Heart 2004;90:82-6.
[142] Li YH, Chen JH, Tsai WC, et al. Synergistic effect of thrombomodulin promoter -33G/A polymorphism and smoking on the onset of acute myocardial infarction. Thromb Haemost 2002;87:86-91.
[143] Ranjith N, Pegoraro RJ, Rom L. Haemostatic gene polymorphisms in young indian asian subjects with acute myocardial infarction. Med Sci Monit 2003;9:CR417-21.

[144] Hubacek JA, Poledne R, Pitha J, Aschermann M, Skalicka H, Stanek V. Apolipoprotein E Arg136 --> Cys in individuals with premature myocardial infarction. Folia Biol (Praha) 2009;55:116-8.
[145] Liu PY, Chen JH, Li YH, Wu HL, Shi GY. Synergistic effect of stromelysin-1 (matrix metallo-proteinase-3) promoter 5A/6A polymorphism with smoking on the onset of young acute myocardial infarction. Thromb Haemost 2003;90:132-9.
[146] Gonzalez-Porras JR, Martin-Herrero F, Garcia-Sanz R, et al. Hyperhomocysteinemia is a risk factor of recurrent coronary event in young patients irrespective to the MTHFR C677T polymorphism. Thromb Res 2007;119:691-8.
[147] Biezeveld MH, Geissler J, Weverling GJ, et al. Polymorphisms in the mannose-binding lectin gene as determinants of age-defined risk of coronary artery lesions in Kawasaki disease. Arthritis Rheum 2006;54:369-76.
[148] Gonzalez-Conejero R, Corral J, Roldan V, et al. A common polymorphism in the annexin V Kozak sequence (-1C>T) increases translation efficiency and plasma levels of annexin V, and decreases the risk of myocardial infarction in young patients. Blood 2002;100:2081-6.
[149] Crobu F, Palumbo L, Franco E, et al. Role of TGF-beta1 haplotypes in the occurrence of myocardial infarction in young Italian patients. BMC Med Genet 2008;9:13.
[150] van Schie MC, de Maat MP, Isaacs A, et al. Variation in the von Willebrand factor gene is associated with von Willebrand factor levels and with the risk for cardiovascular disease. Blood;117:1393-9.
[151] Franco E, Palumbo L, Crobu F, et al. Renin-angiotensin-aldosterone system polymorphisms: a role or a hole in occurrence and long-term prognosis of acute myocardial infarction at young age. BMC Med Genet 2007;8:27.
[152] Yeh PS, Lin HJ, Li YH, et al. Prognosis of young ischemic stroke in Taiwan: impact of prothrombotic genetic polymorphisms. Thromb Haemost 2004;92:583-9.
[153] Neuvonen PJ. Drug interactions with HMG-CoA reductase inhibitors (statins): the importance of CYP enzymes, transporters and pharmacogenetics. Curr Opin Investig Drugs 2010;11:323-32.
[154] Sirtori CR, Mombelli G, Triolo M, Laaksonen R. Clinical response to statins: Mechanism(s) of variable activity and adverse effects. Ann Med 2011.
[155] Maggo SD, Kennedy MA, Clark DW. Clinical implications of pharmacogenetic variation on the effects of statins. Drug Saf 2011;34:1-19.
[156] Hubacek JA, Adamkova V, Prusikova M, et al. Impact of apolipoprotein A5 variants on statin treatment efficacy. Pharmacogenomics 2009;10:945-50.
[157] Regieli JJ, Jukema JW, Grobbee DE, et al. CETP genotype predicts increased mortality in statin-treated men with proven cardiovascular disease: an adverse pharmacogenetic interaction. Eur Heart J 2008;29:2792-9.
[158] Nieminen T, Kahonen M, Viiri LE, Gronroos P, Lehtimaki T. Pharmacogenetics of apolipoprotein E gene during lipid-lowering therapy: lipid levels and prevention of coronary heart disease. Pharmacogenomics 2008;9:1475-86.
[159] Niemi M. Transporter pharmacogenetics and statin toxicity. Clin Pharmacol Ther 2010;87:130-3.

[160] Peters BJ, Pett H, Klungel OH, et al. Genetic variability within the cholesterol lowering pathway and the effectiveness of statins in reducing the risk of MI. Atherosclerosis 2011;217:458-64.

[161] Abbasi F, Chu JW, McLaughlin T, Lamendola C, Leary ET, Reaven GM. Effect of metformin treatment on multiple cardiovascular disease risk factors in patients with type 2 diabetes mellitus. Metabolism 2004;53:159-64.

[162] Chien KL, Wang KC, Chen YC, et al. Common sequence variants in pharmacodynamic and pharmacokinetic pathway-related genes conferring LDL cholesterol response to statins. Pharmacogenomics 2010;11:309-17.

[163] Barber MJ, Mangravite LM, Hyde CL, et al. Genome-wide association of lipid-lowering response to statins in combined study populations. PLoS One 2010;5:e9763.

[164] Hu M, To KK, Mak VW, Tomlinson B. The ABCG2 transporter and its relations with the pharmacokinetics, drug interaction and lipid-lowering effects of statins. Expert Opin Drug Metab Toxicol 2011;7:49-62.

[165] Tiwari A, Bansal V, Chugh A, Mookhtiar K. Statins and myotoxicity: a therapeutic limitation. Expert Opin Drug Saf 2006;5:651-66.

[166] Voora D, Shah SH, Spasojevic I, et al. The SLCO1B1*5 genetic variant is associated with statin-induced side effects. J Am Coll Cardiol 2009;54:1609-16.

[167] Rowan C, Brinker AD, Nourjah P, et al. Rhabdomyolysis reports show interaction between simvastatin and CYP3A4 inhibitors. Pharmacoepidemiol Drug Saf 2009;18:301-9.

[168] Niemi M, Pasanen MK, Neuvonen PJ. Organic anion transporting polypeptide 1B1: a genetically polymorphic transporter of major importance for hepatic drug uptake. Pharmacol Rev 2011;63:157-81.

[169] Peters B, Maitland-van der Zee AH. Pharmacogenomic importance of pravastatin. Pharmacogenomics 2008;9:1207-10.

[170] Romaine SP, Bailey KM, Hall AS, Balmforth AJ. The influence of SLCO1B1 (OATP1B1) gene polymorphisms on response to statin therapy. Pharmacogenomics J;10:1-11.

[171] Mangravite LM, Medina MW, Cui J, et al. Combined influence of LDLR and HMGCR sequence variation on lipid-lowering response to simvastatin. Arteriosclerosis, thrombosis, and vascular biology 2010;30:1485-92.

[172] Shuldiner AR, O'Connell JR, Bliden KP, et al. Association of cytochrome P450 2C19 genotype with the antiplatelet effect and clinical efficacy of clopidogrel therapy. JAMA 2009;302:849-57.

[173] Xie HG, Zou JJ, Hu ZY, Zhang JJ, Ye F, Chen SL. Individual variability in the disposition of and response to clopidogrel: pharmacogenomics and beyond. Pharmacol Ther 2011;129:267-89.

[174] Gladding P, Webster M, Zeng I, et al. The pharmacogenetics and pharmacodynamics of clopidogrel response: an analysis from the PRINC (Plavix Response in Coronary Intervention) trial. JACC Cardiovasc Interv 2008;1:620-7.

[175] Beitelshees AL, Finck BN, Leone TC, et al. Interaction between the UCP2 -866 G>A polymorphism, diabetes, and beta-blocker use among patients with acute coronary syndromes. Pharmacogenet Genomics 2010;20:231-8.

[176] Donnelly LA, Doney AS, Tavendale R, et al. Common nonsynonymous substitutions in SLCO1B1 predispose to statin intolerance in routinely treated individuals with type 2 diabetes: a go-DARTS study. Clin Pharmacol Ther 2011;89:210-6.
[177] Peters BJ, Rodin AS, Klungel OH, et al. Pharmacogenetic interactions between ABCB1 and SLCO1B1 tagging SNPs and the effectiveness of statins in the prevention of myocardial infarction. Pharmacogenomics 2010;11:1065-76.
[178] Chasman DI, Posada D, Subrahmanyan L, Cook NR, Stanton VP, Jr., Ridker PM. Pharmacogenetic study of statin therapy and cholesterol reduction. Jama 2004;291:2821-7.

2

Lipoprotein(a) Oxidation, Autoimmune and Atherosclerosis

Jun-Jun Wang
Department of Laboratory, Jinling Hospital, Clinical School of Medicine College, Nanjing University, Nanjing, P. R. China

1. Introduction

Lipoprotein(a) [Lp(a)] is a plasma lipoprotein whose structure and composition closely resembles that of low density lipoprotein (LDL), but with one of additional molecule of apolipoprotein(a) [apo(a)], a large glycoprotein linked to apoB by a disulfide bond (Figure 1) [1, 2]. High Lp(a) levels have been established as an independent risk factor for atherocslerosis [3-5], and Lp(a) deposits have been found in atherosclerotic lesions but not in normal arterial walls [6-8].

Lp(a) can be modified by oxidation *in vitro*, and then be taken up by macrophages by means of scavenger receptors, where it promotes their transformation into foam cells within the arterial walls [9-13]. Oxidized Lp(a) [ox-Lp(a)] may also induce adhesion molecular expression on monocytes, promoting their recruitment and adhesion to the endothelium [14], and influence the responsiveness of platelets to various agonists [15]. Modified forms of Lp(a), some resembling oxidized Lp(a), have been identified in human atheromatous lesions [16]. In addition, ox-Lp(a) causes significant changes in apo(a) conformation, which could enhance the interaction of these particles with plasminogen binding sites as well as macrophage scavenger receptors, resulting in increased inhibitory effect on plasminogen activation and finally leading to attenuate fibrinolytic activity [17].

Ox-Lp(a) has been reported to play more potent role than native Lp(a) in atherosclerosis [10, 14, 17, 18], and autoantibodies against ox-Lp(a), Lp(a) immune complexes [Lp(a)-IC] have also been detected *in vivo* simultaneously [19, 20]. The present review article focuses specifically on the relationship between Lp(a) oxidation, autoimmune and atherosclerosis together with our recent work.

2. The pathogenic role of oxidized Lp(a)

Lp(a) contains a large specific glycoprotein called apo(a), attached by a single disulfide bridge to $apoB_{100}$ of LDL (Figure 1). The adverse cardiovascular qualities of Lp(a) have been related to both its LDL-like properties (i.e., formation of foam cells) and its presumed role in fibrinolysis.

3. Lp(a) oxidation

The structure, fatty acid composition, and antioxidant concentrations of Lp(a) and LDL are quite similar [21]. *In vitro* studies have shown that Lp(a) can be modified by oxidation (both chemical and cellular-mediated) in a fashion similar to LDL [22]. This modification, which involved lipid peroxidation measured as thiobarbituric acid-reactive substances (TBARS), caused marked changes in the structure and biological properties of Lp(a). Relative to native Lp(a), oxidized particles showed decreases of free amino groups and protein fragmentation, increased negative charge, and high aggregation ability. They were taken up and degraded readily by human monocyte/macrophages by means of scavenger receptors, a known pathway for clearance of ox-LDL in atheroma, inducing cholesteryl ester accumulation and promoting their transformation into foam cells within the arterial walls [9-13]. Similar to above-mentioned pathway, ox-Lp(a) might, in part, form aggregation and contribute to foam cell formation by additional macrophage uptake mechanism, like phagocytosis [9]. Ox-Lp(a) may also induce adhesion molecular expression on monocytes, promoting their recruitment and adhesion to the endothelium and stimulating intimal monocytes to differentiate into resident macrophages [14]. Moreover, subsequent to the induction of oxygen-derived radicals, oxidized Lp(a) may impair endothelium-dependent vasodilation [23].

4. Lp(a) and fibrinolysis

Besides above atherogenic potential, ox-Lp(a) might favor an impaired fibrinolytic activity as it has been shown through its inhibitory effect on plasminogen binding to monocyte-like cells and the induction of plasminogen activator inhibitor-1 (PAI-1) overproduction in cultured human umbilical vein endothelial cell. Several plausible mechanisms were proposed to explain the anti-fibrinolytic potential of Lp(a) [24]. A considerable part of the anti-fibrinolytic properties of apo(a) seemed to reside in its molecular similarity to plasminogen [25]. Lp(a) inhibited plasminogen binding and activation at the surface of stabilized fibrin, endothelial cells and platelets in a dose-dependent fashion [25].

Oxidative modification of Lp(a) causes significant changes in apo(a) conformation, resulting in enhanced interaction of these particles with plasminogen binding sites and macrophage scavenger receptors [17]. These findings were supported by some clinical studies. Pepin et al. [8] found that Lp(a) in atherosclerotic lesions was oxidized, and the oxidized Lp(a) could be a more tightly bound fraction than apoB. Two studies reported large variations in the lysine binding capacity of Lp(a) purified from different individuals [26, 27]. This heterogeneity appeared not to be associated with apo(a) isoforms. Wang et al. [28] developed an enzyme-linked sandwich immunosorbent assay (ELISA) to determine Lp(a)-associated plasminogen epitopes. The Lp(a)-associated plasminogen epitopes levels and this plasminogen epitopes to Lp(a) ratio have been found significantly increased in patients with hemodialysis, which may also be caused by the oxidative modification of Lp(a). In addition, Lp(a), especially in oxidized form, increases over two-fold the endothelial synthesis and secretion of PAI-1 *in vitro*, especially for the 2/2 PAI-1 genotype [29, 30].

5. Oxidized Lp(a) *in vivo* and autoantibody

The role of autoimmune-mediated pathways in the development of atherosclerosis has been the focus of much interest. Circulating ox-LDL and malondialdehyde (MDA) modified LDL

(MDA-LDL) have been reported to be useful markers for identifying coronary artery disease (CAD) [31-33]. Some studies support the relationship of increased levels of antibodies to ox-LDL with the severity of atherosclerosis and future development of myocardial infraction [34], although the pathogenic role of these antibodies in atherosclerosis is controversial.

Similarly, there is evidence supporting the presence of ox-Lp(a) *in vivo*. Thus, modified forms of Lp(a), some resembling ox-Lp(a) and some possibly degraded, have been identified in extracts of human advanced atherosclerotic plaques [16]. Romero et al. [35] reported the existence of autoantibodies against MDA-Lp(a) *in vivo*. Their study found the fact that most anti-MDA-Lp(a) also react against MDA-LDL and suggested the involvement of a common epitope in the reactivity of the majority of antibodies against these oxidatively modified lipoproteins, which might be caused by the existence of antibodies against modified apoB. While some patients were found seropositive for only one or the other autoantibodies against LDL or Lp(a), which supported the hypothesis of the existence of a separate antibody, which might be antibodies against modified apo(a).

Wang et al. [36] have isolated and identified the ox-Lp(a) autoantibodies by an affinity chromatographic column of Sepharose 4B coupled with ox-Lp(a) from healthy subjects. All the isolated antibodies, after being fully absorbed by the ox-LDL column, showed different low reactivity with ox-LDL, while some of them still appeared high reactivity with ox-Lp(a), which suggested that autoantibody against ox-apo(a) exist *in vivo* and the isolated human autoantibodies against ox-Lp(a), which can recognize both apo(a) and apoB epitopes of ox-Lp(a).

6. Oxidized Lp(a) assay

Apo(a) and apoB proteins of Lp(a) molecule can both be oxidatively modified *in vivo*. The degree of oxidized apo(a) or apoB protein of Lp(a) has been detected to estimate circulating ox-Lp(a) levels [37-40]. Yamada et al. [37] obtained a new 161E2 monoclonal antibody to react with oxidized Lp(a) but not with native Lp(a). The 161E2 monoclonal antibody was produced against synthetic peptide antigen, which was characterized as having various properties because its external exposure was induced as a result of oxidative modification. Using this antibody, they developed a ELISA to measure Lp(a) modified by oxidative stress, and found that hypertensive patients with complications showed a significantly higher level of oxidized Lp(a) in serum than did normotensive subjects, whereas there was no significant difference in native Lp(a) between normotensive and hypertensive subjects. Morishita R et al. [38] reported that ox-Lp(a) level in CAD patients with diabetes mellitus was significantly higher than in healthy volunteers. Moreover, serum ox-Lp(a) concentration showed a significant positive correlation with pulse wave velocity, an index of arteriosclerosis . Of importance, the deposition of oxidized Lp(a) was readily detected in calcified areas of coronary arteries in patients with myocardial infarction.

Podrez et al. [39] also found that oxidized apoB protein of plasma Lp(a) was a characteristic of the patients with end-stage renal disease undergoing continuous ambulatory peritoneal dialysis. Interestingly, from apolipoprotein E-receptor deficient mice, Tsimikas et al. [40] cloned the natural murine monoclonal IgM autoantibody E06, which could bind the cell-wall polysaccharide and prevent the uptake of oxidized LDL and apoptotic cells by scavenger receptors of macrophages. The plasma oxidized phospholipid was measured with the use of the murine monoclonal antibody E06, and the result showed that oxidized phospholipids presented on particles of apo B-100 and primarily on Lp(a) lipoprotein correlated with both the presence and extent of angiographically documented coronary artery disease. However, neither of the above methods can simultaneously detect apo(a) and apoB epitopes of ox-Lp(a).

Wang et al. [36] developed 2 "sandwich" ELISAs for measuring plasma ox-Lp(a) level, using human autoantibodies against ox-Lp(a) to capture ox-Lp(a) or polyclonal antibodies against ox-LDL to capture oxidized apoB of Lp(a), and then quantitating with monoclonal anti-apo(a) enzyme conjugate, respectively. A significantly positive relationship was found between ox-Lp(a) levels detected by 2 ELISAs. Compared to control, plasma ox-Lp(a) levels in patients with CAD detected by 2 ELISAs were both significantly increased.

7. The clinical value of circulating oxidized Lp(a)

The mean levels of Lp(a), ox-Lp(a) and Lp(a)-IC were found much lower in newborns than in children and increased rapidly to that in children after birth. No difference of their levels was found in each of the 13 year groups in the children (Figure 2) [41]. The fact that ox-Lp(a) and Lp(a)-IC were present in all the healthy children and especially in newborns was also supported by other studies [42-44], and anti-ox-LDL antibodies and LDL-IC were also easily detectable in asymptomatic young adults and children [45, 46], suggesting that the immune response to modified lipoproteins could appear very early in the process, perhaps play an initiating role in atherosclerotic process.

It is reported that ox-Lp(a) concentrations increased in CAD patients [36] and in rheumatoid arthritis patients with excessive cardiovascular events [47]. Moreover, the concentration of serum apo(a) epitope of ox-Lp(a) was reported to be significantly increased in hypertensive patients with complications and CAD patients with diabetes mellitus [37, 38]. ApoB protein of plasma Lp(a) was also found oxidized and was a characteristic of the patients with end-stage renal disease undergoing continuous ambulatory peritoneal dialysis [39]. Thus, it is noteworthy to investigate the causal role of ox-Lp(a) in atherosclerotic cardiovascular disease in a prospective study and to explore the exact pathogenic role of ox-Lp(a).

Several studies have found that ox-Lp(a) concentrations increased in both the ACS and stable CAD patients [48-50]. Interestingly, ox-Lp(a) concentrations and the ratios of ox-Lp(a)/Lp(a) were significantly higher in the ACS patients than those in the stable CAD patients as well as control, while they remained similar between the stable CAD and control, which suggested that the increased ox-Lp(a) concentrations might mainly be attributable to the occurrence of ACS. Furthermore, ox-Lp(a) levels were found to be associated with a graded increase in the extent of CAD in the patients with ACS, while not in the stable CAD [48]. In addition, Wang et al. [49] have evaluated clinical value of ox-Lp(a) levels detected by the 2 assays for measuring plasma ox-Lp(a) level using autoantibody against ox-Lp(a) [ox-Lp(a)1] or ox-LDL [ox-Lp(a)2] in ACS and stable CAD patients. A significantly positive relationship was found between ox-Lp(a) levels detected by 2 assays. Receiver-operating characteristic (ROC) curve analysis (Figure 3) confirmed that the performance of the association of ox-Lp(a) 1 with ACS was significantly superior to those of ox-Lp(a)2, Lp(a) and LDL cholesterol; while the performances of ox-Lp(a)2, Lp(a) and LDL cholesterol with ACS were similar. The performance of the association between ox-Lp(a)1 and stable CAD was also significantly superior to that between ox-Lp(a)2 and stable CAD. The ox-Lp(a) levels increased in CAD, especially in ACS, and might be one of the major contributing factors for the development of atherosclerosis. In addition, the autoantibody was isolated from human mix serum and can recognize both apo(a) and apoB epitopes of ox-Lp(a), the developed ELISA for ox-Lp(a) by using autoantibody may more accurately reflect the state of Lp(a) oxidation *in vivo*. It is concluded that ox-Lp(a) levels using antibodies against ox-Lp(a) might represent a better biochemical risk marker than those using antibodies against ox-LDL for ACS and stable CAD.

Wang et al. [50] have also studied plasma levels of Lp(a) and several ox-Lp(a) markers immediately before and serially up to 6 months after percutaneous coronary intervention (PCI). PCI resulted in acute elevations of native, oxidized Lp(a) and Lp(a)-IC levels in both ACS and stable CAD patients, and decrease of ox-Lp(a)-Ab (Figure 4). Interestingly, the change of ox-Lp(a) during PCI was found to correlate with the extent of angiographically documented disease only in ACS patients, while not in stable CAD. Tsimikas et al. [51] also reported that indirect and direct plasma markers of oxidized phospholipids (ox-PL) showed significant temporal elevations following ACS, but not in patients with stable CAD or in subjects without CAD. These observations indicate one possibility that ACS episode causes sustained rise of ox-Lp(a), and further support the hypothesis that ox-Lp(a) is present in ruptured or permeable plaques and is released into the circulation by PCI.

The above results are also supported by the studies about ox-PL, which have demonstrated convincingly that a key ox-PL is preferentially associated with Lp(a) [52] and correlates with both the presence and extent of angiographically documented CAD [40, 53], and their concentrations increase after ACS [51] and immediately after PCI [54].

8. The source of plasma ox-Lp(a)

Oxidized lipoprotein results from exposure of lipoprotein to oxidizing species, such as superoxide anion and hydrogen peroxide derived from all cells present in the artery wall, particularly macrophages, as well as enzymes such as lipoxygenases and products of myeloperoxidase, resulting in oxidation of the lipid and protein components [55].

The source of plasma ox-Lp(a) is unknown. Holvoet et al. [56] isolated ox-LDL from the plasma of patients with post-transplant CAD and analyzed its characteristics, which suggested that it did not originate from extensive metal ion-induced oxidation of LDL but that it might be generated by cell-associated oxidative enzymatic activity in the arterial wall. It was also demonstrated in animal models that the oxidation of LDL indeed occurs in the arterial wall and not in the blood [57].

Studies have shown that increased ox-Lp(a) level in stable CAD and especially in ACS is associate with the severity of angiographically documented disease in ACS, while not in stable CAD [48, 49]. Similarly, the extent of CAD was found related with the change of ox-Lp(a) levels before and after PCI in the ACS and stable CAD patients [50]. These above results suggested that ox-Lp(a) particles in the blood came from the arterial wall, such as directly released from ruptured or permeable plaques. It was also possible that oxidation-specific epitopes generated in the arterial intima, such as oxidized phospholipids, might have been transported by some mechanisms to Lp(a) acceptors, or might move between LDL and Lp(a).

Elevated Lp(a) level may also result in increased circulating ox-Lp(a). Ox-Lp(a) is found related with Lp(a), which shows that more Lp(a) in subjects with high Lp(a) has chance to be oxidized *in vivo*, resulting in strong immune response and leading to the formation of Lp(a)-IC [36, 47]. In addition, Lp(a) is known to act as an acute-phase reactant in patients with ACS. It has also been found increased Lp(a) and ox-Lp(a) levels are positively related with C-reactive protein in patients with rheumatoid arthritis [47], which suggests that inflammation promotes Lp(a) synthesis and its oxidation.

One of important problems remaining to be answered is whether the response to oxidized lipoprotein plays an initiating or a contributing role in the development of atherosclerosis. To answer this question through clinical studies, one major problem is the difficulty encountered in defining atherosclerosis-free individuals. The results that high levels of anti-ox-LDL antibodies and LDL-IC are present in individuals with confirmed atherosclerosis suggest that the immune response to ox-LDL may be a secondary phenomenon, possible contributing to the development of atherosclerosis. However, the studies have shown that ox-Lp(a) and Lp(a)-IC are present in all the healthy children and especially in newborns, and that anti-ox-LDL antibodies and LDL-IC are easily detectable in asymptomatic young adults and children [45, 46, 58], for early arterial lesions may not present in all the children, which suggest that the immune response to modified lipoproteins could appear very early in the process, perhaps being one of the initiating factors. In fact, oxidative stress has been reported to be present early in pregnancy and children, and to be associated with arterial dysfunction and enhanced intima-media thickness [43, 44]. In general, it has been accepted that lipoprotein traverses the subendothelial space where it becomes oxidized, and may induce endothelial dysfunction, one of the earliest manifestations of atherosclerosis. *In vitro* and *in vivo* studies have shown that ox-LDL promotes endothelial cell toxicity and vasoconstriction [59]. The above studies suggest that part of lipoproteins have been oxidized before they traverse the subendothelial space, prior to advanced lesion formation, and directly participating in the development of atherosclerosis.

9. Lp(a) immune complexes and β_2-glycoprotein I complexes with Lp(a)

It has been proposed that modified lipoproteins might contribute to atherogenesis by another mechanism-their ability to trigger an immune response leading to the production of autoantibodies and subsequently to the formation of IC. Some studies have shown that incubation of human monocyte-derived macrophages with insoluble or soluble LDL-IC induces foam cell formation *in vitro* more efficiently than any other known mechanism [60-62]. The pathogenic role of LDL-IC *in vivo* is also supported, and the studies have shown that plasma LDL-IC level increases in patients with CAD [63, 19] and that the cholesterol content of LDL-IC is a powerful discriminator for the presence of coronary atherosclerosis [20].

Lp(a) might also trigger an immune response leading to the production of autoantibodies and subsequently to the formation of IC. Interestingly, it has been found that Lp(a)-IC was present in both the plasma of patients with CAD and control, and Lp(a)-IC level increased in the CAD patients [64]. Furthermore, Wang et al. [65] studied the plasma Lp(a) and Lp(a)-IC levels in 232 subjects with various dyslipidemias. This study showed that both Lp(a) and Lp(a)-IC levels were different in various types of primary hyperlipidemia. Moreover, it was found that plasma Lp(a)-IC levels represented the similar distribution to that of Lp(a). In fact, both antibodies against oxidized apo(a) and apoB *in vivo* can form immune complexes with oxidative apo(a) or apoB of Lp(a). In addition, not a parallel increment between Lp(a)-IC and LDL-IC levels was found according to Lp(a) cutoff level (especially Lp(a)<300mg/l), which suggested that Lp(a)-IC level might act as an additional predictor of premature CAD [64]. Recently, Wang et al. have also found that incubation of human monocyte-derived macrophages with Lp(a)-IC induces foam cell formation by Fc γ receptor pathway *in vitro*.

It was reported that β_2-GPI was present in the sera of autoimmune diseases and was characterized by its ability to bind to negative charged molecules, including lipoproteins [66-69]. Recently, studies showed that β_2-GPI specifically interacted with LDL as well as ox-LDL, and formed complexes in the intima of atherosclerotic lesions, and then, these complexes were taken up by macrophages via anti-β_2-GPI autoantibody-mediated phagocytosis, contributing to the development of atherosclerosis [70]. *In vitro* studies also demonstrated that β_2-GPI bound Lp(a) with high affinity [71, 72], suggesting that β_2-GPI might bind Lp(a) to form complexes of β_2-GPI with Lp(a) [β_2-GPI-Lp(a)] *in vivo*. Furthermore, preliminary data suggest that additional ox-PL are present in the lipid phase of Lp(a) (Figure 5) [73].

Our studies have found that β_2-GPI-Lp(a) indeed existed in serum samples, and that β_2-GPI-Lp(a) as well as ox-Lp(a) concentrations were significantly elevated in systemic lupus erythematosus (SLE) patients with excessive cardiovascular events [74], and in active rheumatoid arthritis (RA) patients [75]. Furthermore, β_2-GPI-Lp(a) levels were found increased in both the patients with ACS and stable CAD. The logistic regression analysis of risk factors revealed that the presence of β_2-GPI-Lp(a) as well as ox-Lp(a) or Lp(a) was a strong risk factor for stable CAD, and especially for ACS, suggesting that the β_2-GPI-Lp(a) complexes might act as an additional predictor of atherosclerosis [76].

An important role in the accumulation of ox-PL on Lp(a) may also be played by β_2-GPI, which binds to the kringle IV domain of apo(a) [71], as well as to anionic phospholipids and ox-PL [77]. Importantly, high β_2-GPI levels were also found on the Lp(a) of CAD patients, whereas removal of apo(a) from the Lp(a) particles of these patients led to reduction of the β_2-GPI levels and to increase in the lipoprotein-associated phospholipase A_2 (Lp-PLA_2) catalytic efficiency. Substrates for Lp-PLA_2 contain oxidatively fragmented residues at the *sn-2* position (ox-PL). Thus, the higher amounts of β_2-GPI on the Lp(a) of CAD patients could contribute to the sequestration of ox-PL on the surface of Lp(a) [78].

10. Conclusions

In summary, Lp(a) might be oxidatively modified *in vivo*, which causes marked changes in the structure and biological properties of Lp(a). Oxidatively modified Lp(a) has more pathogenicity in both formation of foam cells and fibrinolysis. Elevated plasma concentrations of ox-Lp(a) reflect the presence and extent of angiographically documented CAD, especially clinically expressed in ACS. The elevated plasma concentrations of ox-Lp(a) suggest plaque instability and may be useful for the identification of patients with ACS. The assay of ox-Lp(a) may provide a new approach to investigate the causal role of ox-Lp(a) in atherosclerotic cardiovascular disease in a prospective study and to explore the exact pathogenic role of ox-Lp(a).

11. Annex

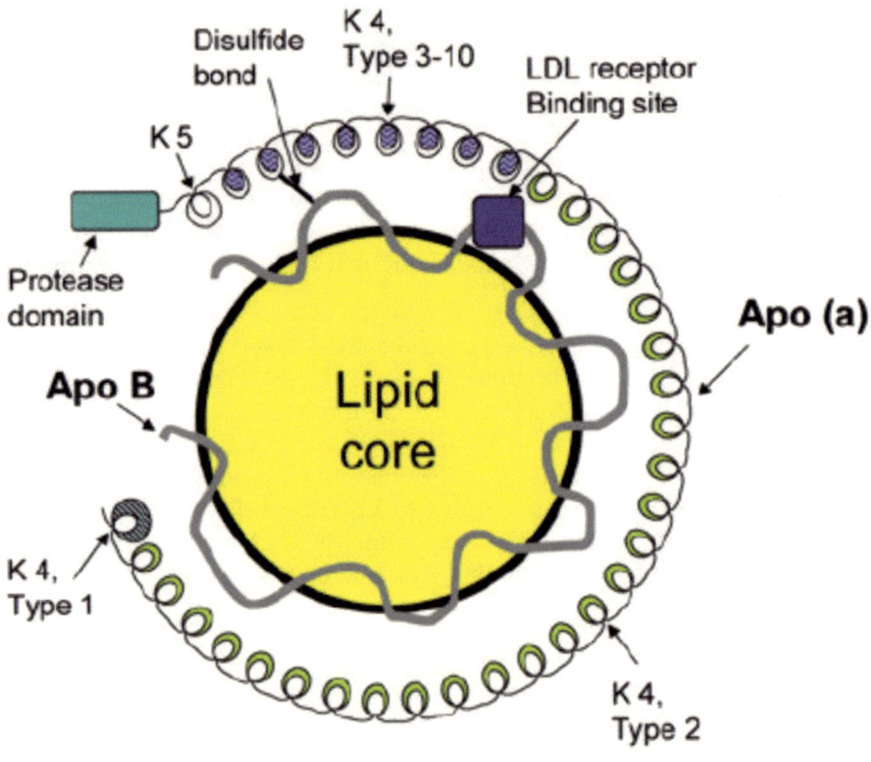

Lp(a) is an LDL-like particle composed of a lipid core (cholesteryl esters; triglycerides) encapsulated by a surface layer (phospholipid; free cholesterol). As with LDL, Lp(a) contains one molecule of apoB, linked to the apo(a) by a single disulfide bond. The apo(a) moiety consists of a single copy of kringles (K) 4, types 1 and 3 through 10, kringle 5, and a protease domain analogous to the structure of plasminogen. Lp(a) always has multiple copies of kringle 4, type 2 contributing to the abundant heterogeneity of the molecule.

Fig. 1. Schematic Model of Lp(a) Structure.

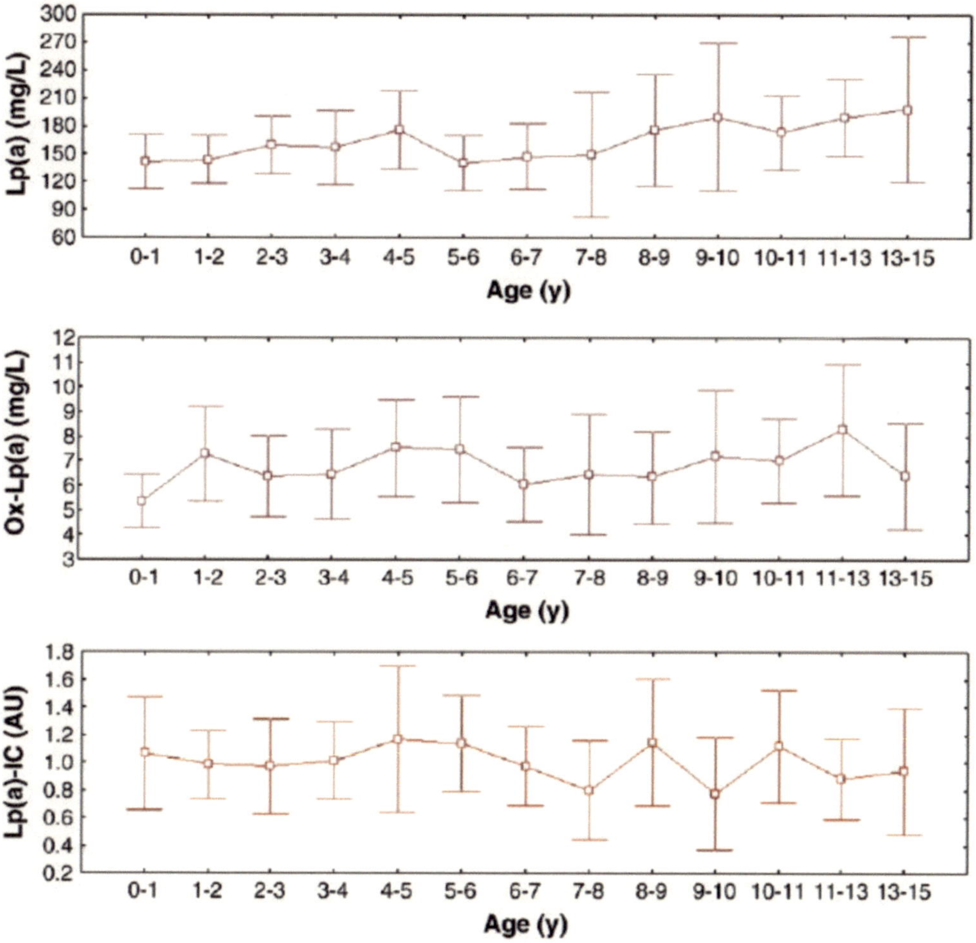

No difference of their levels was found among the age groups.

Fig. 2. Mean levels of Lp(a), ox-Lp(a) and Lp(a)-IC in each of the 13 year groups in the 747 children.

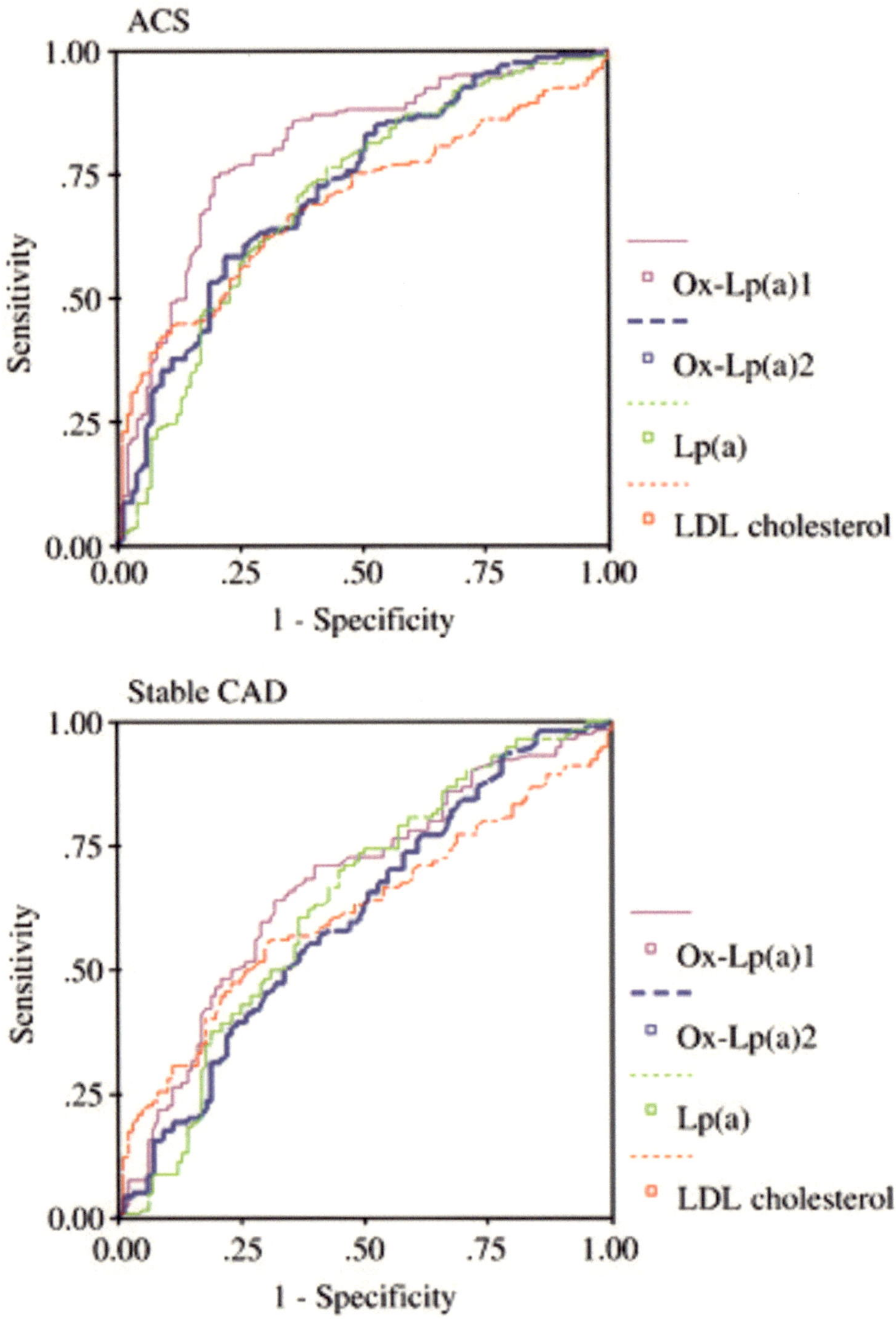

Ox-Lp(a)1: detected by anti-ox-Lp(a); ox-Lp(a)2: detected by anti-ox-LDL.

Fig. 3. Receiver-operating characteristic curve analysis of ox-Lp(a) and Lp(a) levels in patients with ACS and stable CAD.

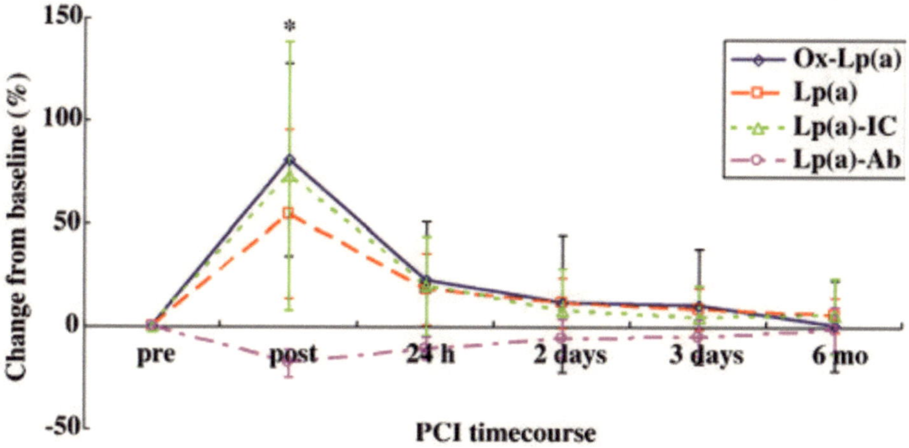

The change is expressed as mean percent change from pre-PCI levels. * P<0.001 by ANOVA. Lp(a): P<0.001 compared with before and 6-month time points; P<0.05 compared with 2- and 3-day time points. Ox-Lp(a): P<0.001 compared with before, 3-day, and 6-month time point; P<0.01 compared with 2-day time point. Lp(a)-IC: P<0.05 compared with before, 3-day, and 6-month time point. Ox-Lp(a)-Ab: P<0.001 compared with before and 6-month time points; P<0.01 compared with 2- and 3-day time points.

Fig. 4. Changes of Lp(a), ox-Lp(a), Lp(a)-IC, and ox-Lp(a)-Ab levels after PCI.

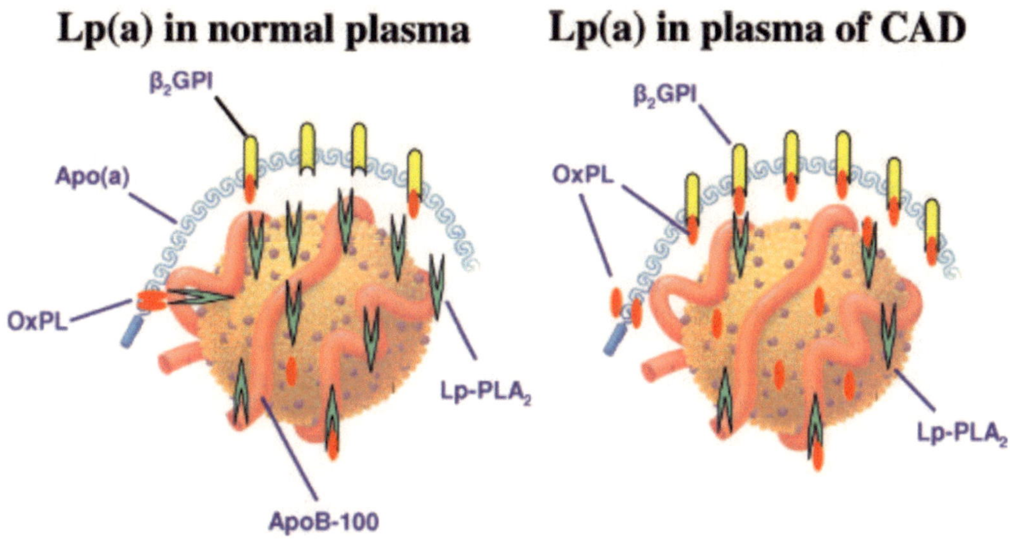

Lp(a) of CAD patients contains higher levels of β2-GPI and ox-PL and significantly less amount of Lp-PLA2 mass compared with Lp(a) from normal plasma.

Fig. 5. Association of Lp-PLA2 and ox-PL with Lp(a) in normal plasma as well as in plasma of patients with CAD.

12. References

[1] Scanu AM, Lawn RM, Berg K. Lipoprotein(a) and atherosclerosis. Ann Intern Med 1991, 115(3): 209-218.

[2] Uterman G. The mysteries of lipoprotein(a). Science 1989, 246(4932): 904-910.

[3] Dahlen G, Guyton JR, Attar M, Farmer JA, Kautz JA, Gotto AM. Association of levels of lipoprotein(a), plasma lipids, and other lipoproteins with coronary artery disease documented by angiography. Circulation 1986, 74(4): 758-765.

[4] Scanu AM, Fless GM. Lipoprotein(a): Heterogeneity and biological relevance. J Clin Invest 1990, 85(6): 1705-1715.

[5] Zhuang YY, Li JJ, Wang JJ. Apolipoprotein(a) phenotypes in cardio-cerebrovasculor diseases. Chem Phys Lipids, 1994, 67-68: 291-297.

[6] Rath M, Niendorf A, Reblin T, Dietel M, Krebber HJ, Beisiegel U. Detection and quantification of lipoprotein(a) in the arterial wall of 107 coronary bypass patients. Atherosclerosis 1989, 9(5): 579-592.

[7] Cushing GL, Gaubatz JW, Nava ML, et al. Quantitation and localization of apolipoproteins (a) and B in coronary artery bypass vein grafts resected at re-operation. Atherosclerosis 1989, 9(5): 593-603.

[8] Pepin JM, O'Neil JA, Hoff HF. Quantification of apo(a) and apoB in human atherosclerotic lesion. J Lipid Res 1991, 32(2): 317-327.

[9] Naruszewicz M, Selinger E, Davignon J. Oxidative modification of lipoprotein(a) and the effect of β-carotene. Metabolism 1992, 41(11): 1215-1224.

[10] Haberland ME, Fless GM, Scanu AM, Fogelman AM. Malondialdehyde modification of lipoprotein(a) produces avid uptake by human monocyte-macrophages. J Biol Chem 1992, 267(6): 4143-4151.

[11] Jialal I. Evolving lipoprotein risk factors: lipoprotein(a) and oxidized low-density lipoprotein. Clin Chem 1998, 44(8 Pt 2):1827-1832.

[12] Schaefer EJ, Lamon Fava S, Jenner JL, et al. Lipoprotein(a) levels and risk of coronary heart disease in men. The lipid Research Clinics Coronary Primary Prevention Trial. JAMA 1994, 271(13): 999-1003.

[13] Serdar Z, Sarandol E, Dirican M, Yesilbursa D, Serdar A, Tokullugil A. Relation between lipoprotein(a) and in vitro oxidation of apolipoprotein B-containing lipoproteins. Clin Biochem 2000, 33(4): 303-309.

[14] Ragab MS, Selvarag P, Sgoutas DS. Oxidized lipoprotein(a) induces cell adhesion molecule Mac-1 (CD 11b) and enhances adhesion of the monocytie cell line U937 to cultured endothelial cells. Atherosclerosis 1996, 123(1-2): 103-113.

[15] Rand ML, Sangrar W, Hancock MA, Taylor DM, Marcovina SM, Packham MA, Koschinsky ML. Apolipoprotein(a) enhances platelet response to the thrombin receptor-activating peptide SFLLRN. Arterioscler Thromb Vasc Biol, 1998; 18(9): 1393-1399.

[16] Hoff HF, O'Neil J, Yashiro A. Partial characterization of lipoproteins containing apo(a) in human atherosclerotic lesions. J Lipid Res 1993, 34(5): 789-798.

[17] Naruszewicze M, Giroux LM, Davignon J. Oxidative modification of Lp(a) causes changes in the structure and biological properties of apo(a). Chem phys Lipids 1994, 67-68: 167-174.

[18] Zioncheck TF, Powell LM, Rice GC, Eaton DL, Lawn RM. Interaction of recombinant apolipoprotein(a) and lipoprotein(a) with macrophages. J Clin Invest 1991, 87(3): 767-771.

[19] Tertov VV, Orekhov AN, Kacharava AG, Sobenin LA, Perova NV, Smirnov VN. Low density lipoprotein-containing circulating immune complexes and coronary atherosclerosis. Exp Mol Path 1990, 52(3): 300-308.
[20] Orekhov AN, Kalenich OS, Tertov VV, Novikov ID. Lipoprotein immune complexes as markers of atherosclerosis. Int J Tissue React 1991, 13(5): 233-236.
[21] Sattler W, Kostner GM, Waeg G, Esterbauer H. Oxidation of lipoprotein Lp(a): a comparison with low-density lipoprotein. Biochim Biophs Acta 1991, 1081(1): 65-74.
[22] Kleinveld HA, Duif PF, Van Rijin IIJ. Oxidation of lipoprotein (a) and low density lipoprotein containing density gradient ultracentrifugation fractions. Biochim Biophs Acta 1996, 1303(1): 15-21.
[23] Galle J, Bengen J, Schollmeyer P, Wanner C. Impairment of endothelium-dependent dilation in rabbit renal arteries by oxidized lipoprotein(a). Role of oxygen-derived radicals. Circulation, 1995, 92(6): 1582-1589.
[24] Edelberg J, Pizzo SV. Lipoprotein (a) regulates plasmin generation and inhibition. Chem Phys Lipids 1994, 67-68: 363-368.
[25] McLean JW, Tomlinson JE, Kuang WJ, et al. cDNA sequence of human apolipoprotein(a) is homologous to plasminogen. Nature 1987, 330(6144): 132-137.
[26] Armstrong VW, Harrach B, Robenek H, Helmhold M, Walli AK, Seidel D. Heterogeneity of human lipoprotein Lp(a): cytochemical and biochemical studies on the interaction of two Lp(a) species with the LDL receptor. J Lipid Res 1990, 31(3): 429-441.
[27] Bas Leerink C, Duif PF, Gimpel JA, Kortlandt W, Bouma BN, van Rijn HJ. Lysine-binding heterogeneity of Lp(a): consequences for fibrin binding and inhibition of plasminogen activation. Thromb Hemostas 1992, 68(2): 185-188.
[28] Wang JJ, Zhuang YY, Yao XD. Quantitation of plasminogen epitopes of serum Lipoprotein(a) by sandwich enzyme linked immunosorbent assay. Clin Chim Acta 1997, 265(1): 121-130.
[29] Li XN, Grenett HE, Benza RL, et al. Genotype-specific transcriptional regulation of PAI-1 expression by hypertriglyceridemic VLDL and Lp(a) in cultured human endothelial cells. Arterioscler Thromb Vasc Biol 1997, 17(11): 3215-3223.
[30] Ren S, Man RY, Angel A, Shen GX. Oxidative modification enhances lipoprotein(a)-induced overproduction of plasminogen activator inhibitor-1 in cultured vascular endothelial cells. Atherosclerosis 1997, 128(1):1-10.
[31] Holvoet P, Vanhaecke J, Janssens S, Van de Werf F, Collen D. Oxidized LDL and malondialdehyde-modified LDL in patients with acute coronary syndromes and stable coronary artery disease. Circulation 1998, 98(15): 1487-1494.
[32] Vanhaecke J, Stassen JM, VanCleemput J, Collen D, Holvoet P. Correlation between oxidized low density lipoproteins and coronary artery disease in heart transplant patients. J Am Coll Cardiol 1997, 29(2): 8081-8081.
[33] Holvoet P, Collen D, van de Werf F. Malondialdehyde-modified LDL as a marker of acute coronary syndromes. JAMA 1999, 281(18): 1718-1721.
[34] Salonen JT, Yla-Herttuala S, Yamamoto R, Butler S, Korpela H, Salonen R, Nyyssonen K, Palinski W, Witztum JL. Autoantibody to oxidized LDL and progression of carotid atherosclerosis. Lancet 1992, 339(8798): 883-887.
[35] Romero FI, Atsumi T, Tinahones FJ, Gomez-zumaquero JM, Amengual O, Khamashta MA, Hughes GRV. Autoantibodies against malondialdehyde-modified lipoprotein(a) in antiphospholipid syndrome. Arthritis Rheumatism 1999, 42(12): 2606-2611.

[36] Wang JJ, Zhang CN, Gong JB, Zhu YH, Fu Li, Wang XD, Li K. Development of new ELISA for oxidized lipoprotein(a) by using purified human oxidized lipoprotein(a) autoantibodies as capture antibody. Clin Chim Acta, 2007, 385(1-2): 73-78.
[37] Yamada S, Morishita R, Nakamura S, et al. Development of antibody against epitope of lipoprotein(a) modified by oxidation: evaluation of new enzyme-linked immunosorbent assay for oxidized lipoprotein(a). Circulation 2000, 102(14): 1639-1644.
[38] Morishita R, Ishii J, Kusumi Y, Yamada S, Komai N, Ohishi M, Nomura M, Hishida H, Niihashi M, Mitsumata M: Association of serum oxidized lipoprotein(a) concentration with coronary artery disease: potential role of oxidized lipoprotein(a) in the vasucular wall. J Atheroscler Thromb, 2009, 16(4): 410-418.
[39] Podrez EA, O'Neil J, Salomon RG, Schreiber MJ, Hoff HF. Measurement of oxidation in plasma Lp(a) in CAPD patients using a novel ELISA. Kidney Int 1998, 54(2): 637-645.
[40] Tsimikas S, Brilakis ES, Miller ER, et al. Oxidized phospholipids, Lp(a) lipoprotein, and coronary artery disease. N Engl J Med 2005, 353(1): 46-57.
[41] Wang JJ, Niu DM, Meng Y, Han AZ, Li K, Zhang CN. Plasma oxidized lipoprotein(a) and its immune complexes are present in newborns and children. Clin Chim Acta 2009, 407(1-2): 1-5.
[42] Abe A, Maeda S, Makino K, Seishima M, Shimokawa K, Noma A, Kawade M. Enzyme-linked immunosorbent assay of lipoprotein(a) in serum and cord blood. Clin Chim Acta 1988, 177(1): 31-40.
[43] Peter Stein T, Scholl TO, Schluter MD, Leskiw MJ, Chen X, Spur BW, Rodriguez A. Oxidative stress early in pregnancy and pregnancy outcome. Free Radic Res 2008, 42(10): 841-848.
[44] Martino F, Loffredo L, Carnevale R, et al. Oxidative stress is associated with arterial dysfunction and enhanced intima-media thickness in children with hypercholesterolemia: the potential role of nicotinamide–adenine dinucleotide phosphate oxidase. Pediatrics 2008, 122(3): 648-655.
[45] Tinahones FJ, Gómez-Zumaquero JM, Garrido-Sánchez L, et al. Influence of age and sex on levels of anti-oxidized LDL antibodies and anti-LDL immune complexes in the general population. J Lipid Res 2005, 46(3): 452-457.
[46] Islam S, Gutin B, Treiber F, Hobbs G, Kamboh I, Lopes-Virella M. Association of apolipoprotein(a) phenotypes and oxidized low-density lipoprotein immune complexes in children. Arch Pediatr Adolesc Med 1999, 153(1): 57-62.
[47] Wang JJ, Hu B, Kong LT, Cai H, Zhang CN. Native, oxidized lipoprotein(a) and lipoprotein(a) immune complex in patients with active and inactive rheumatoid arthritis: plasma concentrations and relationship to inflammation. Clin Chim Acta 2008, 390(1-2): 67-71.
[48] Wang JJ, Zhang CN, Meng Y, Han AZ, Gong JB, Li K. Elevated levels of oxidized lipoprotein(a) are associated with the presence and severity of acute coronary syndromes. Clin Chim Acta 2009, 408(1-2): 79-82.
[49] Wang JJ, Han AZ, Meng Y, Gong JB, Zhang CN, Li K. Measurement of oxidized lipoprotein (a) in patients with acute coronary syndromes and stable coronary artery disease by 2 ELISAs: using different capture antibody against oxidized lipoprotein (a) or oxidized LDL. Clin Biochem 2010, 43(6): 571-575.

[50] Wang JJ, Zhang CN, Han AZ, Gong JB, Li K. Percutaneous coronary intervention results in acute increases in native and oxidized lipoprotein(a) in patients with acute coronary syndrome and stable coronary artery disease. Clinical Biochemistry 2010; 43(13-14): 1107-1111.
[51] Tsimikas S, Bergmark C, Beyer RW, et al. Temporal increases in plasma markers of oxidized low-density lipoprotein strongly reflect the presence of acute coronary syndromes. J Am Coll Cardiol 2003, 41(3): 360-370.
[52] Edelstein C, Pfaffinger D, Hinman J, et al. Lysine-phosphatidylcholine adducts in kringle V impart unique immunological and potential proinflammatory properties to human apolipoprotein (a). J Biol Chem 2003, 278(52): 841-847.
[53] Tsimikas S, Kiechl S, Willeit J, et al. Oxidized phospholipids predict the presence and progression of carotid and femoral atherosclerosis and symptomatic cardiovascular disease. Five-year prospective results from the Bruneck study. J Am Coll Cardiol 2006, 47(11): 2219-2228.
[54] Tsimikas S, Lau HK, Han KR, et al. Percutaneous coronary intervention results in acute increases in oxidized phospholipids and lipoprotein(a). Short-term and long-term immunologic responses to oxidized low-density lipoprotein. Circula-tion 2004, 109(25): 3164-3170.
[55] Tsimikas S. Oxidative biomarkers in the diagnosis and prognosis of cardiovascular disease. Am J Cardiol 2006, 98(11A): 9-17.
[56] Holvoet P, Stassen JM, Van Cleemput J, Collen D, Vanhaecke J. Oxidized low density lipoproteins in patients with transplant-associated coronary artery disease. Arterioscler Thromb Vasc Biol 1998, 18(1): 100-107.
[57] Holvoet P, Theilmeier G, Shivalkar B, Flameng W, Collen D. LDL hypercholesterolemia is associated with accumulation of oxidized LDL, atherosclerotic plaque growth, and compensatory vessel enlargement in coronary arteries of miniature pigs. Arterioscler Thromb Vasc Biol 1998, 18(3): 415-422.
[58] Virella G, Virella I, Lemain RB, Preyor MB, Lopes-Virella MF. Antioxidized low density lipoprotein antibodies in patients with coronary disease and normal healthy volunteers. Int J Clin Lab Res 1993, 23(2): 95-101.
[59] Navab M, Ananthramaiah GM, Reddy ST, et al. Thematic review series: the pathogenesis of atherosclerosis: the oxidation hypothesis of atherogenesis: the role of oxidized phospholipids and HDL. J Lipid Res 2004, 45(6): 993-1007.
[60] Lopes-Virella MF, Griffith RL, Shunk KA, Virella GT. Enhanced uptake and impaired intracellular metabolism of low density lipoprotein complexes with anti- low density lipoprotein antibodies. Arterioscler Thromb 1991, 11(5): 1356-1367.
[61] Griffith RL, Virella GT, Stevenson HC, Lopes-Virella MF. LDL metabolism by macrophages activated with LDL immune complexes: a possible mechanism of foam cell formation. J Exp Med 1986, 168(3): 1041-1059.
[62] Gisinger C, Virella GT, Lopes-Virella MF. Erythrocyte-bound low density lipoprotein immune complexes lead to cholesterol ester accumulation in human monocyte-derived macrophages. Clin Immunol Immunopathol 1991, 59(1): 37-51.
[63] Tertov VV, Orekhov AN, Sayadyan KS, Serebrennikov SG, Kacharava AG, Lyakishev AA, Smirnov VN. Correlation between cholesterol content and circulating immune complexes and atherogenic properties of CHD patients' serum manifested in cell culture. Atherosclerosis 1990, 81(3): 183-189.

[64] Wang JJ, Qiang HJ, Zhang CN, Liu XC, Chen DN, Wang SM. Detection of IgG bound Lp(a) immune complexes in patients with coronary heart disease. Clin Chim Acta, 2003, 327(1-2): 115-122.

[65] Wang JJ, Zhang CN, Chen DN, Liu XC, Feng XM. Lipoprotein (a) and its immune complexes concentrations in dyslipidemic subjects. Clin Biochem, 2004, 37(8): 710-713.

[66] Nimpf J, Bevers EM, Bomans PH, Till U, Wurm H, Kostner GM, Zwaal RF. Prothrombinase activity of human platelets is inhibited by β2-glycoprotein I. Biophys Acta 1986, 884(1): 142-149.

[67] George J, Harats D, Gilburd B, et al. Immunolocalization of β2-glycoprotein I (apolipoprotein H) to human atherosclerotic plaques: potential implications for lesion progression. Circulation 1999, 99(17): 2227-2230.

[68] Polz E, Kostner GM. The binding of β2-glycoprotein I to human serum lipoprotein: distribution among density fraction. FEBS Lett 1979, 102(1): 183-186.

[69] Schousboe I. β2-glycoprotein I: a plasma inhibitor of the contact activation of the intrinsic blood coagulation pathway. Blood 1985, 66(5): 1086-1091.

[70] Matsuura E, Kobayashi K, Koike T, Shoenfeld Y, Khamashtab MA, Hughes GRV. Atherogenic autoantigen-oxidized LDL complexes with β2-glycoprotein I. Immunobiology 2003, 207(1): 17-22.

[71] Kochl S, Fresser F, Lobentanz E, Baier G, Utermann G. Novel interaction of apolipoprotein(a) with β2-glycoprotein I mediated by the Kringle IV domain. Blood 1997, 90(4): 1482-1489.

[72] Lopez-Lira F, Rosales Leon L, Martinez VM, Ruiz-Ordaz BH. The role of beta2-glycoprotein I (beta(2)GPI) in the activation of plasminogen. Biochim Biophys Acta 2006, 1764(4): 815-823.

[73] Tsimikas S, Tsironis LD, Tselepis AD. New insights into the role of lipoprotein(a)-associated lipoprotein-associated phospholipase A2 in atherosclerosis and cardiovascular disease. Arterioscler Thromb Vasc Biol 2007, 27(10): 2094-2099.

[74] Zhang CN, Li K, Shi BL, Wang XD, Liu XZ, Qin WS, Han AZ, Wang JJ. Detection of serum beta(2)-GPI-Lp(a) complexes in patients with systemic lupus erythematosus. Clin Chim Acta, 2010, 411(5-6): 395-399.

[75] Zhang CN, Li XJ, Niu DM, et al. Increased serum levels of β2-GPI-Lp(a) complexes and their association with premature atherosclerosis in patients with rheumatoid arthritis. Clinica Chimica Acta 2011, 412(15-16): 1332-1336.

[76] Wang JJ, Gong JB, Li HQ, Niu DM, HanAZ, Wu J, Zhang CN. Lipoprotein(a) complexes with beta2-glycoprotein I in patients with coronary artery disease. J Atheroscler Thromb, 2011(in press).

[77] McNeil PH, Simpson RJ, Chesterman CN, Krilis SA: Anti-phospholipid antibodies are directed against a complex antigen that includes a lipidbinding inhibitor of coagulation: beta 2-glycoprotein I (apolipoprotein H). Proc Natl Acad Sci U S A, 1990; 87(11): 4120-4124.

[78] Tsironis LD, Katsouras CS, Lourida ES, Mitsios JV, Goudevenos J, Elisaf M, Tselepis AD: Reduced PAF-acetylhydrolase activity associated with Lp (a) in patients with coronary artery disease. Atherosclerosis, 2004; 177(1): 193-201.

3

ICAM-1: Contribution to Vascular Inflammation and Early Atherosclerosis

Sabine I. Wolf and Charlotte Lawson
Dept of Veterinary Basic Sciences, Royal Veterinary College
United Kingdom

1. Introduction

Atherosclerosis is a progressive chronic inflammatory disease characterised by the accumulation of lipids and fibrous elements in large arteries and increasingly threatens human health worldwide. Atherosclerotic lesion formation is a complex process which can proceed over decades. A number of different factors contribute to the formation of atherosclerotic lesions including the accumulation of lipids, activation of T-cells, transformation of macrophages into foam cells and proliferation of smooth muscle cells. The earliest events that lead to lesion formation are still very much under investigation. A number of risk factors have been identified that contribute to the pathogenesis of atherosclerosis, including hypertension, smoking, increased concentrations of plasma cholesterol, diabetes, obesity, age and male gender. All these risk factors can influence endothelial cell function resulting in increased permeability, increased adhesion of leukocytes and the expression of procoagulant molecules.

Intercellular adhesion molecule-1 (ICAM-1, CD54) is an immunoglobulin (Ig)-like cell adhesion molecule expressed by several cell types including leukocytes and endothelial cells. It is constitutively expressed at low levels on endothelial cells and leukocytes and up-regulated following exposure to pro-inflammatory stimuli. ICAM-1 is important for the firm arrest and transmigration of leukocytes out of blood vessels and into tissue, as well as immunological synapse formation during T cell activation. It is present in atherosclerotic lesions and is involved in the progression of atherosclerotic lesions. We and others have shown that crosslinking of ICAM-1 on the cell surface leads to "outside in" signal transduction and to result in the initiation of several pro-inflammatory signalling cascades and rearrangement of actin cytoskeleton, leading to speculation that ICAM-1 "is more than just glue".

A soluble ICAM-1 molecule has been identified in serum, consisting of all five extracellular Ig-domains of membrane-bound ICAM-1-molecule, but lacking the transmembrane and cytoplasmic domains. sICAM-1 is present in normal human serum, whilst elevated sICAM-1 have been found in serum from patients with cardiovascular disease, cancer, autoimmune disease and several studies have correlated serum levels of sICAM-1 with severity of disease. Several studies have shown that sICAM-1 is able to bind to ligands of ICAM-1 and a yet unknown receptor and is able to instigate signalling cascades. Here, we present our recent data which suggests that sICAM-1 acts as a pro-inflammatory agent when endothelial cells are subjected to prolonged arterial shear forces, including initiation of cytokine and chemokine expression, which could lead to monocyte attraction to inflamed regions of the vasculature.

2. Atherosclerosis

Atherosclerosis is a protracted, complex process, which takes place over several decades. The main contributing factors are lipid accumulation, activation of T-cells, transformation of macrophages into foam cells and the proliferation of underlying smooth muscle cells (Ross 1999; Lusis 2000).

Many theories have been discussed over the years about the initiation phase of atherosclerosis. William and Tabas suggested that a loss of endothelial cells within the blood vessel wall allowed increased permeability of leukocytes and lipoproteins into the subendothelial space and caused plaque formation (Williams and Tabas 1995). However, studies showing the presence of an intact endothelial cell layer at the site of plaque formation rejected the "endothelial cell denudation" theory. The theory was replaced by the "response to injury" hypothesis by Ross (Ross and Glomset 1974; Ross 1999). Ross suggested that injury of the endothelium lead to endothelial cell dysfunction and altered smooth muscle cell behaviour. Currently, more evidence points towards the "response to retention" hypothesis, which identified atherogenic lipoproteins as a key initiation step (Schwenke and Carew 1989; Schwenke and Carew 1989). The direct binding of these lipoproteins to the endothelium and the subsequent accumulation within the subendothelial space is thought to trigger endothelial cell activation, which is followed by an inflammatory response (Williams and Tabas 1995).

Apart from lipid there are a number of other factors that have been associated with accelerated cardiovascular disease and could contribute to vascular inflammation. It is widely appreciated that there is a greatly increased risk of cardiovascular disease with increase in body mass index independent of serum cholesterol (Lavie , Milani et al. 2009), and that patients with type II diabetes, chronic renal disease (Karalliedde, and Viberti 2004), and autoimmune disorders such as rheumatoid arthritis or lupus (Frostegård 2011) are far more likely to develop atherosclerosis independent of cholesterol and other traditional risk factors. A number of chronically infectious agents have also been linked to atherosclerosis including *Chlamydia pneumoniae* (Laurila, Bloigu et al. 1997) and *Helicobacter pylori* (Hoffmeister, Rothenbacher et al. 2001). These associations are likely to be due to an increase in systemic inflammation, characterised by chronically elevated levels of CRP and pro-inflammatory cytokines such as TNF-α, IL-1, IL-6. These circulating factors are all known to contribute to endothelial activation *in vitro* and to the expression of genes involved in vascular inflammation and atherosclerosis progression *in vivo* (Hansson 2009).

The earliest event visible within the blood vessel wall is the appearance of a "fatty lesion". These lesions can be found at branches, bifurcations and curvations of the arterial blood vessel walls (Lusis 2000). At these locations a disturbed flow pattern of the blood can be detected compared with the parallel (laminar) flow seen at "tubular" blood vessel sections. The disturbed shear stress at curved blood vessel locations activates endothelial cells and results in accumulation of lipoproteins (LDL), and activated macrophages within the subendothelial spaces. Skalen *et al.* (Skålén, Gustafsson et al. 2002) showed that lipoproteins initially bind to negatively charged sulphate groups on proteoglycans in the artery wall before translocating to the subendothelial space. The significance has been demonstrated in mice deficient in proteoglycans, which develop a reduced number of atherosclerotic lesions (Skålén, Gustafsson et al. 2002). Native LDL contributes to the inflammation at lesion site by undergoing modification by oxidation, lipolysis or proteolysis before being taken up by macrophages (reviewed by (Lusis 2000)). The uptake and accumulation of modified lipoproteins transforms the macrophages into foam cells, which are retained within the fatty streak.

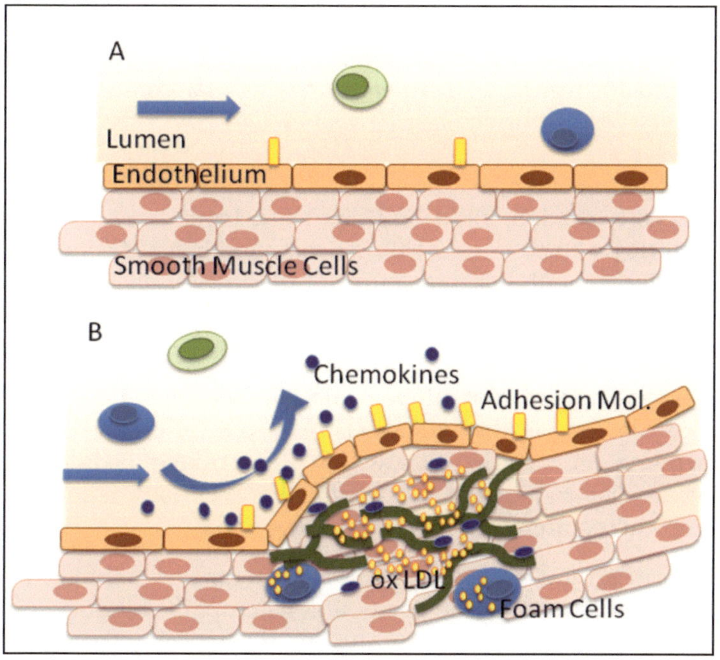

Fig. 1. Schematic cartoons showing healthy, tubular blood vessel (A) and curved blood vessel with plaque formation in process (B).

Oxidised LDL also contributes to the progression of the early lesion by itself stimulating endothelial cells to produce pro-inflammatory molecules, which leads to the recruitment of further immune cells. One important molecule released is the chemokine CCL-2 (MCP-1), which is responsible for recruiting monocytes to the lesion site (Gerszten, Garcia-Zepeda et al. 1999). Activated endothelial cells upregulate adhesion molecules including ICAM-1 on their cell surface facilitating transmigration of further leukocytes. The inflammatory environment within the lesion leads to the migration and proliferation of smooth muscle cells, infiltration of immune cells including B-cells, dendritic cells, mast cells and T-cells as well as elaboration of a collagen-rich matrix (Hansson and Libby 2006). The advanced lesion consists of a core containing foam cells, lipids and necrotic debris, which is surrounded by smooth muscle cells. The growth is asymmetrical protruding into the lumen and resulting in further blood flow changes. The exact composition of the plaque dictates the stability of the plaque. The fibrous cap, which is produced by smooth muscle cells and influenced by immune cells, prevents the contact between blood components and pro-thrombotic material within the lesion. Thrombus formation occurs once the fibrous cap raptures and coagulation factors come into contact with contents of the lesion (Hansson and Libby 2006).

2.1 Role of endothelium

All large blood vessels, including the vessels of the arterial tree, are made up of several distinct tissue layers: the intima, media and adventitia. The intima is the inner lining and is formed of a single continuous layer of endothelial cells on the luminal side with a specialised subendothelial basement membrane and the internal elastic lamina. Beneath this vascular smooth muscle cells, elastic and collagen fibres, together with the external elastic lamina, make up the media. A connective tissue sheath, which may be vascularised with vasa vasorum, forms the outer layer, the adventitia.

The vascular endothelium, located on the luminal side of the intima, functions as a highly selective barrier, and its restrictive permeability is a vital component in healthy blood vessels. However, studies during the last 20 years have shown that the endothelium does not act as a passive barrier as previously thought, but is highly dynamic and controls a variety of functions. It is involved in the regulation of vessel tone, coagulation and fibrinolysis, leukocyte adhesion, fluid and solute exchange and the control of smooth muscle cell growth (Ross 1999; Lusis 2000). Indeed endothelial dysfunction contributes to many cardiovascular conditions including atherosclerosis, hypertension, stroke, inflammation, vasospastic disorders, diabetic microangiopathy, autoimmune disease, hypercholesterolemia, thrombosis and tumour growth (reviewed by (Lusis 2000)).

Endothelial cells react to a number of different stimuli, they are not only exposed to humoral factors from the circulation, but they are also subject to a variety of biomechanical stimuli. They differ depending on their location within the vascular beds and exhibit varying phenotypes. They are responsive to the environment of their local tissue and change barrier function accordingly to requirement of the underlying tissue.

Endothelial cells form a tight monolayer with well organised cell-to-cell junctions. These junctions are held together strongly by homo- and heterophilic binding of a number of key adhesion molecules expressed on neighbouring endothelial cells. The junctions play a vital role not only in permeability control, but also regulate leukocyte trans-endothelial migration and endothelial cell growth. The most important molecules involved in the cell-to-cell junction are considered to be PECAM-1 and VE-Cadherin.

2.2 Importance of flow

Cyclic stretch, fluid shear stress and hydrostatic pressure are the three main hemodynamic forces present within the blood vessel (Gimbrone, Topper et al. 2000). The importance of each force varies between the different cell types within the blood vessel wall. Smooth muscle cells mainly respond to cyclic stretch, whereas shear stress is the major force experienced by endothelial cells (Li, Haga et al. 2005). Shear stress acts parallel to the vessel wall within the lumen. It has a uniform, laminar pattern in "linear", unbranched areas of the vasculature. Depending on the location and type of the blood vessel, the (positive) shear stress values range between 10-40 dynes/cm^2 in the arterial network, and 1-20 dynes/cm^2 in the venular microcirculation (Surapisitchat, Hoefen et al. 2001; Lehoux, Castier et al. 2006). Endothelial cells exposed to prolonged laminar shear stress align and elongate in the direction of flow by reorientating their actin cytoskeleton, microtubules and intermediate filaments (Resnick, Yahav et al. 2003). This arrangement reduces the mechanical load experienced by endothelial cells and induces a quiescent state in which apoptotic, inflammatory and atherogenic genes are suppressed (Resnick, Yahav et al. 2003). Endothelial cells themselves secrete a number of factors which contribute to this quiescent state, including the vasodilator nitric oxide (NO) and the vasorelaxant PGI_2. NO is released into the lumen of the blood vessel where it acts to inhibit the attachment of platelets and leukocytes onto the luminal surface of endothelial cells. NO is also secreted into the basal side and prevents growth of smooth muscles cells underneath the endothelium. NO has also been reported to suppress the activation of transcription factors for adhesion molecules including ICAM-1 (De Caterina, Libby et al. 1995; Lindemann, Sharafi et al. 2000). The lack of expressed adhesion molecules on the endothelium prevents vascular inflammation and irregular cell proliferation (Figure 2a).

Sites exposed to steady laminar flow with high shear stress are atheroprotective (Gimbrone, Topper et al. 2000). At bifurcations and bends in the vasculature the laminar flow pattern becomes disrupted and creates sites with recirculating blood flow. The shear stress values vary from negative, to zero to positive values (Resnick, Yahav et al. 2003). Sites experiencing turbulent and disturbed flow are prone to develop atherosclerosis (Figure 2b) (Gimbrone, Topper et al. 2000).

Endothelial cells have been shown to possess a variety of mechanoreceptors, which not only sense shear stress but are able to react to changes by influencing gene expression. Several different molecules have been identified on endothelial cells as mechanoreceptors including two members of the integrin family, $\alpha_v\beta_3$ (Tzima, del Pozo et al. 2001) and $\alpha_5\beta_1$ (Chen, Li et al. 1999). Changes in shear stress lead to integrin clustering, thereby triggering the recruitment of shc to their cytoplasmic tails. This results in the initiation of signal cascades, which leads to phosphorylation of MAPK-kinases ERK and JNK (reviewed by (Shyy and Chien 2002)). One important example of a receptor tyrosine kinase acting as a mechanosensor on the endothelium is VEGFR-2 (Chen, Li et al. 1999). Rapid and transient phosphorylation of the tyrosine residues within the cytoplasmic tail of VEGFR-2 and the association with shc has been observed upon exposure to shear stress (Chen, Li et al. 1999). Another important group of mechanoreceptors are G-proteins and /or G-protein coupled receptors. Gudi and colleagues (Gudi, Clark et al. 1996) reported that G-protein activation takes place immediately upon exposure. In addition, several ion channels that are sensitive to shear stress have been identified. Studies have shown that K^+ channels induce NO when exposed to shear stress in bovine aortic endothelial cells (Ohno, Cooke et al. 1995; Helmlinger, Berk et al. 1996; Yamamoto, Korenaga et al. 2000). The glycoprotein PECAM-1 (CD31), which is involved in endothelial cell to cell adhesion, has also been shown to be sensitive to changes in shear stress. It is thought that fluid shear stress disrupts the conformation of the cytoplasmic tail revealing two tyrosine residues and enabling signal transduction (Fujiwara, Masuda et al. 2001; Osawa, Masuda et al. 2002). Recently, monocilia on endothelial cells in chick embryos and primary cilia on human vascular endothelial cells have been found in regions exposed to low or oscillatory shear stress. These have been proposed to contribute to endothelial activation and dysfunction (Van der Heiden, Groenendijk et al. 2006; Van der Heiden, Hierck et al. 2008). Caveolae have also been suggested to act as mechanoreceptors. Caveolae are plasma membrane invaginations, rich in cholesterol and identified by the protein marker caveolin-1. It is thought that signalling is initiated by the shear stress- induced movements of these rigid structures, which contain G-coupled receptors, Ca^{2+} channels, VEGFR-2 and eNOS (Frank and Lisanti 2006). Another possible mechanosensitive structure on the luminal surface of endothelial cells may be the polysaccharide network that makes up the glycocalyx. The glycocalyx is known to act as a selectively permeable barrier for macromolecules based on their size and charge. However, it is also thought to sense mechanical forces and transduce the signals into intracellular responses (Florian, Kosky et al. 2003; Thi, Tarbell et al. 2004).

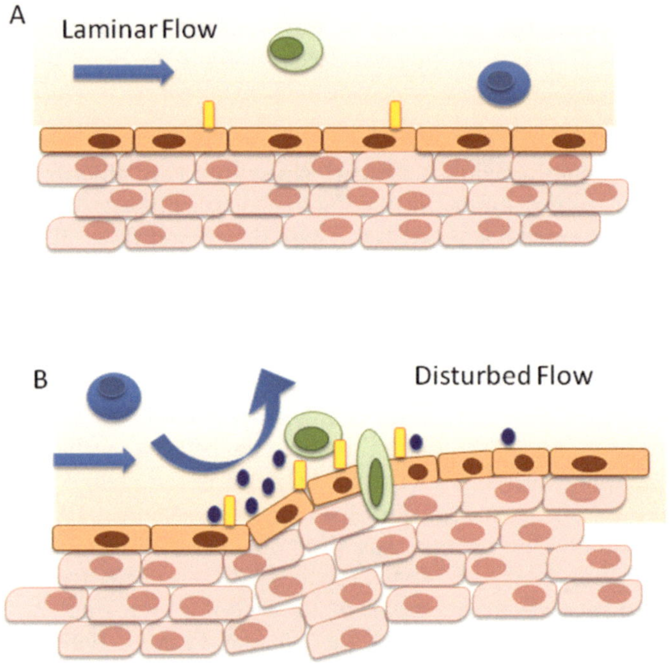

Fig. 2. Cartoon showing the different flow patterns experienced by endothelial cells. Parallel, laminar shear stress is present in unbranched, tubular parts of the blood vessel (A). Disturbed shear stress can be found at bends or bifurcation of blood vessels (B).

Depending on the type of blood vessel and the nature and strength of shear stress that the endothelium is subjected to in different locations in the vasculature, it is likely that a range of different mechanoreceptors are involved in mechanosensing and signal transduction. More research is required to identify the exact roles of each mechanosensor, the signalling pathways they activate and their contribution to endothelial activation or quiescence.

2.3 Endothelial cell inflammatory responses

There are a number of features of endothelial cell dysfunction including changes on the cell surface such as upregulation of adhesion molecules, exposure of pro-coagulant molecules, loss of highly selective barrier function and changes in vascular tone (reviewed by (Malyszko 2010)).

In quiescent, non-inflamed endothelial cells, NO prevents many responses leading to dysfunction and inflammation. However, once NO production is disrupted the brakes are removed from many of these harmful pathways. Oxidative stress within the endothelium has been reported as one of the key consequences of disrupted NO production, due to the formation of reactive oxygen species (ROS) and peroxynitrites. These harmful metabolic by-products can initiate pro-inflammatory signalling cascades, leading to upregulation of adhesion molecules including ICAM-1 and VCAM-1, chemokine and cytokine secretion. This contributes to increased monocyte adhesion and trans-endothelial migration. In addition ROS are responsible for oxidation of circulating lipoproteins. Together these events are very important for initiation of fatty streak formation in early atherosclerosis (reviewed by (Collins and Tzima 2011)).

3. ICAM-1

3.1 Structure of ICAM-1

Intracellular adhesion molecule 1 (ICAM-1, CD54) is a type I transmembrane glycoprotein, which belongs to the immunoglobin (Ig)-superfamily. It is constitutively expressed at basal levels on endothelial cells and leukocytes, but is upregulated by inflammatory stimulators such as TNF-α (Pober, Gimbrone et al. 1986), IFN-γ (Dustin, Rothlein et al. 1986), IL-1 (Dustin, Rothlein et al. 1986) and LPS (Sampath, Kukielka et al. 1995) as well as shear stress (Nagel, Resnick et al. 1994). Upregulation of ICAM-1 is inhibited by glucocorticoids (Cronstein, Kimmel et al. 1992) and by IL-4 (Renkonen, Mattila et al. 1992).

ICAM-1 is encoded on seven exons with exon 1 encoding the signal sequence, exon 2 to 6 each extracellular Ig-domain and exon 7 the transmembrane and intracellular domains. The molecular weight ranges between 80-114kDa as the level of glycosylation varies heavily between different cell types. The ICAM-1 extracellular domain consists of 453 mainly hydrophobic amino acids, which form five Ig-domains with β-sheet structure, each Ig-domain stabilised by disulfide bonds (Figure 3). The Ig-domains are followed by a single hydrophobic transmembrane region and a short 28 amino acid cytoplasmic domain, which is lacking any conventional signalling motifs. Tyrosine residues within the cytoplasmic tail have been shown to be important for intracellular ICAM-1 signalling (Tsakadze, Sen et al. 2004).

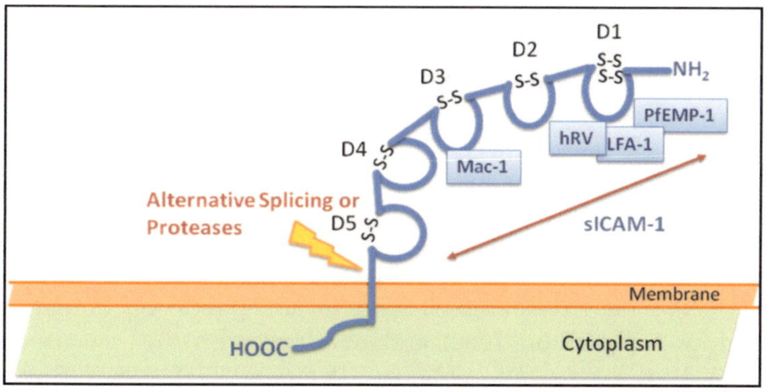

Fig. 3. Cartoon showing membrane bound ICAM-1 with its five Ig-domains (D1 - D5) and ligands LAF-1, mac-1, *plasmodium falciparum* erythrocyte membrane protein-1 (PfEMP-1) and human rhinovirus (hRV). Arrow indicates membrane region, which becomes cleaved off by proteases or alternative splicing releasing solube ICAM-1 (sICAM-1). (Adapted from Lawson and Wolf 2009 and Van de Stolpe and Van der Saag 1996).

Studies by Kirchhausen *et al.* (Kirchhausen, Staunton et al. 1993) have shown that ICAM-1 has a characteristic 140° bend between domain 3 and domain 4. This bend enables formation of homo dimers and multimers resulting in a "YYYY" configuration. The dimerisation is not required for ligand binding but increases binding avidity. The resulting stronger and prolonged interaction with its ligands is especially beneficial during antigen presentation and leukocyte transmigration.

3.2 Ligands for ICAM-1

ICAM-1 has several ligands including the membrane-bound β2 integrin receptors CD11a/CD18 (LFA-1) and CD11b/CD18 (mac-1) present on leukocytes (Marlin and Springer 1987; Staunton, Marlin et al. 1988; Smith, Marlin et al. 1989) and fibrinogen (Languino, Plescia et al. 1993; Languino, Duperray et al. 1995; van de Stolpe and van der Saag 1996). A major group of human rhinovirus (Greve, Davis et al. 1989; Staunton, Merluzzi et al. 1989) and erythrocytes infected with *plasmodium falciparum* (Ockenhouse, Ho et al. 1991; Ockenhouse, Tegoshi et al. 1992) are also able to bind to ICAM-1.

The integrin ligands of ICAM-1 are members of the type I transmembrane heterodimeric glycoprotein family and consist of two non-convalently linked chains. LFA-1 and mac-1 possess the same β_2-integrin subunit (CD18) but different α-chains namely α_L (CD11a) for LFA-1 and α_M (CD11b) for mac-1. Both integrins bind via an "inserted" (I) domain on the respective α-chain to an acidic residue on ICAM-1. LFA-1 binds to glutamic acid (residue 34) on ICAM-1 in the presence of magnesium and calcium ions. The ligand binding results in a reorientation of glutamic acid positioned within the third domain (residue 241) and the formation of a critical salt bridge with lysine (residue 39). The binding site for integrin mac-1 is located within the third domain of ICAM-1 and is dependent on the glycosylation level. High levels of N-linked oligosaccharides sterically and electrostatically hinder access to the binding site. As the level of glycosylation is dependent on cell type, different cell types will allow a diverse ligand binding pattern. Activation of the integrins is required before binding of LFA-1 or mac-1 to ICAM-1 can occur. On resting cells, integrins exhibit a low affinity conformation for ligand binding. Following "inside-out" signalling, a conformational change takes places exposing a high affinity ligand binding site. Integrins play an important role in the immune system as demonstrated in patients with type I leukocyte adhesion deficiency (LAD), a rare autosomal recessive disorder, which causes a complete lack of β_2 – integrins. This deficiency causes severe defects in the inflammatory immune system and leads to multiple, chronic and life-threatening bacterial infections (Blankenberg 2003).

In addition to activated integrins, the majority of rhinovirus family (91 serotypes) and some members of the coxsackie virus A family bind ICAM-1 (Greve, Davis et al. 1989; Staunton, Merluzzi et al. 1989). The virus families bind to an epitope on domain one which lies directly next to LFA-1 (Staunton 1990) and overlaps with the one used by *plasmodium falciparum* infected erythrocytes (Ockenhouse, Betageri et al. 1992). Binding to ICAM-1 initiates the entry of the virus into the host cell (Bella and Rossmann 1999).

Another ligand, which has been shown to bind to ICAM-1 is fibrinogen (Altieri, Duperray et al. 1995). The plasma glycoprotein is involved in blood coagulation, inflammation and tissue repair (Tsakadze, Zhao et al. 2002). Its binding to ICAM-1 enables the adhesion of circulating platelets and inflammatory cells to the endothelium and fibrinogen deposition, which can lead to increased leukocyte transmigration, endothelial cell survival and vasocontriction (Tsakadze, Zhao et al. 2002).

3.3 Function of ICAM-1

The main function of ICAM-1 is to provide firm adhesion, a characteristic which is pivotal in leukocyte transendothelial migration and antigen presentation.

The leukocyte transmigration process, which is also called diapedesis, can be divided into four sequential, but overlapping steps as summarised in Figure 4 (Springer 1994):

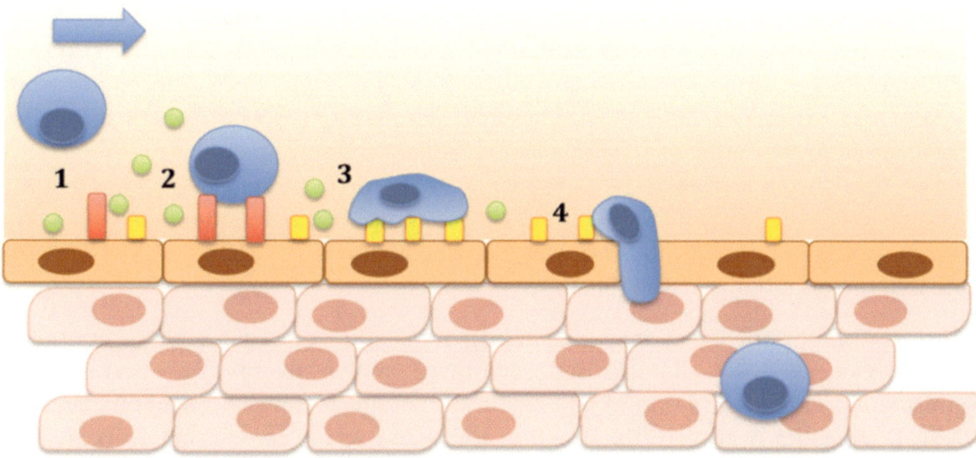

Fig. 4. Cartoon showing four subsequent transmigration steps: rolling (1), tethering (2), adhesion (3) and transmigration (4). (Adapted from Springer 1994).

The first transmigration step is mediated by selectin binding. Selectins from one cell interact with sialylated carbohydrates on the other, opposing cell. E- and P-Selectin present on endothelial cells loosely bind to sialyl Lewis^X related carbohydrates on leukocytes and P-selectin glycoprotein ligand-1 (PSGL-1). L-selectin is present on all circulating leukocytes and binds to CD34, PSGL-1 and sialyl Lewis^X on endothelial cells. Loose binding of leukocytes to endothelial cells allows the cells to slow down and "roll" along the endothelium. It also facilitates the exposure to chemokines such as CCL-2, CXCL-8, CCL-5 and CCL-3. Patients with LAD II lack biosynthesis of fucose, which plays a pivotal role for carbohydrate ligand binding. LAD II is a milder form of LAD, but underlines the importance of selectin binding within the immune system (Blankenberg, Barbaux et al. 2003).

Chemokines play a pivotal role in the second transmigration step. Slow rolling leukocytes are directed by a chemokine gradient towards the dysfunctional endothelial site. The chemokine exposure triggers outside-in signalling events within leukocytes, which leads to integrin activation. Chemokines involved in leukocyte attraction and activation include CXCL-8 (neutrophils) and CCL-2 (monocytes).

The activated integrins on the surface of leukocyte are now able to firmly bind to the adhesion molecules present on the inflamed endothelium. Strong adhesion is facilitated by the binding of ICAM-1 to LFA-1, VCAM-1 to VLA-4 and MADCAM-1 to $\alpha_4\beta_7$. The binding allows leukocytes to spread and slowly migrate over the endothelial cell monolayer in search of transmigration opportunities. The importance of ICAM-1 within the third transmigration step has been demonstrated in studies using anti-ICAM-1 blocking antibodies or endothelial cells lacking ICAM-1 (Greenwood, Wang et al. 1995; Reiss and Engelhardt 1999; Lehmann, Jablonski-Westrich et al. 2003).

The junction proteins PECAM-1, VE-cadherin, junctional adhesion molecules (JAMs) and CD99 are found in endothelial junctions. Their homophilic (PECAM-1, CD99 and JAMs) and heterophilic binding (JAMs with integrins) allow the formation of a tightly packed endothelial cell layer with very selective permeability (Ley, Laudanna et al. 2007). When leukocytes are firmly attached to the endothelium, they develop microvilli-like projections called podosomes, with which they probe the endothelial surface (Barreiro, Yanez-Mo et al. 2002). These docking stations are rich in ICAM-1 and VCAM-1 and F-actin. Integrin binding initiates signalling events in endothelial cells, which is thought to lead to endothelial cell contraction and weakening of junctional bonds (reviewed by (van Buul and Hordijk 2004)). Studies using ICAM-1 deficient cells show reduced transmigration events, but not complete inhibition. This shows that ICAM-1 is involved in the final leukocyte transmigration step but not essential, similar to CD18 (Sligh, Ballantyne et al. 1993; Lehmann, Jablonski-Westrich et al. 2003). Once the junctional adhesion molecule bonds are released leukocytes are able to migrate into the underlying tissue (Springer 1994).

Another very important event in which ICAM-1 plays a vital role is the immunological synapse. This event is characterised by three major events: junction formation, reorganisation and the formation of a stable immunological complex (Grakoui, Bromley et al. 1999). During the first step, the junction formation, close contact between an antigen presenting cell (APC) and T-cell is facilitated with the help of ICAM-1 and LFA-1. The binding of ICAM-1 to its ligand overcomes the steric hindrance from glycoproteins CD45 and CD43 present on the cell surface for the T-cell receptor (TCR) complex and enables interaction with MHC-peptide present on APCs. In the event of low affinity between the TCR and MHC-peptide complex, the interactions between the two cells stops here. If the TCR and MHC-peptide complex show high affinity towards each other, a signal cascade is triggered, which leads to reorganisation of the molecules involved. TCR and MHC-peptide complexes move inwards towards the centre with the outwards moving LFA-1/ICAM-1 molecules forming a tight circle around them. This reorganisation step allows the formation of a stable immunological complex. During this reorganisation and ring formation process, ICAM-1 polymerises, thereby exhibiting higher affinity binding to LFA-1. In addition, concentrating TCR-MHC-peptide complexes within the ring centre facilitates optimal communication between the cells and signalling cascade (Grakoui, Bromley et al. 1999).

ICAM-1 has also been reported to act as costimulatory ligand during MHC I and MHC II restricted antigen presentation (Gaglia, Greenfield et al. 2000).

ICAM-1 has been shown to be present in atherosclerotic lesions (Poston, Haskard et al. 1992) and involved in the progression of atherosclerotic lesions. The involvement of ICAM-1 in atherosclerosis has been demonstrated in apoE $^{-/-}$ mice deficient in ICAM-1, which had reduced lesion size (Nageh, Sandberg et al. 1997). Time course analysis revealed that ICAM-1 is not only involved in the initial plaque formation but also in subsequent progression in mice (Bourdillon, Poston et al. 2000; Kitagawa, Matsumoto et al. 2002). These data were supported by results obtained in apoE $^{-/-}$ mice treated with anti-ICAM-1 neutralising antibodies (Patel, Thiagarajan et al. 1998).

3.4 Signalling via ICAM-1

The Outside-in signalling event triggered by ICAM-1 multimerisation was discovered several years ago (Durieu-Trautmann, Chaverot et al. 1994; Rothlein, Kishimoto et al. 1994). Experimental methods to identify the mechanism underlying the signalling cascade include co-cultures of endothelial cells with leukocytes, immobilised fibrinogen and antibody-crosslinking of ICAM-1 on the cell surface. The cytoplasmic tail of ICAM-1 does not contain any conventional intrinsic kinase activity or known protein-protein interaction domains, that could contribute to signalling cascades, but does contain a high number of positively charged amino acids and one tyrosine site (Lyck, Reiss et al. 2003). Adapter molecules, which have been linked to the signalling cascade depend partly on the vascular bed from which endothelial cells originate and the experimental *in vitro* model used. Molecules which have been associated with ICAM-1 include: alpha-actinin (Carpén, Pallai et al. 1992), ERM-proteins (Wójciak-Stothard, Williams et al. 1999), cortactin (Durieu-Trautmann, Chaverot et al. 1994), beta-tubulin and glyceraldehyde-3-phsophate dehydrogenase (Federici, Camoin et al. 1996). The Src-homology domain 2 has been shown to bind in a phosphotyrosine dependent manner following the activation of ICAM-1 by fibrinogen (Pluskota, Chen et al. 2000; Pluskota and D'Souza 2000). These findings were opposed by Lyck et al (Lyck, Reiss et al. 2003), who showed that brain EC lacking the phosphotyrosine within ICAM-1's cytoplasmic tail are still capable of facilitating transmigration of T-cells. Activation of src-kinase family members p53/p65lyn have been reported in B-cells following crosslinking of ICAM-1 (Holland and Owens 1997).

The small GTPase rho, has been proposed as another important molecule in the ICAM-signalling cascade and the resulting rearrangement of the actin cytoskeleton (Etienne, Adamson et al. 1998; Adamson, Etienne et al. 1999; Wójciak-Stothard, Williams et al. 1999; Thompson, Randi et al. 2002). Mutagenesis of a five amino acid fragment within the cytoplasmic tail identified RKIKK as an important sequence, which seemed to be involved in rho activation following ICAM-1 crosslinking by antibodies on the cell surface (Oh, Lee et al. 2007). Activation of rho has been shown to trigger phosphorylation of focal adhesion kinase, paxillin and p130 as well as activation of JNK (Etienne, Adamson et al. 1998).

Production of reactive oxygen species, which is required for activation of src tyrosine kinase has been observed when crosslinking ICAM-1 on pulmonary microvascular EC (Wang, Pfeiffer et al. 2003). Activation of src kinase is required for initiating ERM-molecule ezrin and p38 MAPK kinase pathway. Further signalling components initiated by ICAM-1 crosslinking on brain microvascular EC are intracellular calcium release and activation of protein kinase C, which are thought to lead to phosphorylation of cortactin (Etienne-Manneville, Manneville et al. 2000).

MAPK-kinase pathways ERK-1/2 and/or JNK have been shown to the triggered depending on experimental design and cell type (Etienne, Adamson et al. 1998; Sano, Nakagawa et al. 1998; Lawson, Ainsworth et al. 1999; Lawson, Ainsworth et al. 2001). We have demonstrated that AP-1 activation is the result of ERK-1 activation (Lawson, Ainsworth et al. 1999), together with the ERK-dependent production and secretion of IL-8 and RANTES (Sano, Nakagawa et al. 1998) as well as upregulation of VCAM-1 on the cell surface (Lawson, Ainsworth et al. 1999; Lawson, Ainsworth et al. 2001). Recently we have also shown that patient auto-reactive antibodies against ICAM-1 can also cause endothelial cell signalling (Lawson, Holder et al. 2005).

3.5 Importance of ICAM-1 polymorphism in different vascular diseases

Two single-base pair polymorphisms of ICAM-1 have been described, which are located in exon 4 and exon 6. The first modification in exon 4 substitutes the amino acid glycine with arginine at codon 241 within the third Ig-domain. The second polymorphic change is located within the 5th domain at codon 469 and replaces glutamic acid with lysine. Domain four and five do not bind any ligands, but are involved in the protein stability and therefore might affect ligand binding. The polymorphic substitution has been associated with coronary heart disease, myocardial infarction (Jiang, Klein et al. 2002) and peripheral artery disease (Gaetani, Flex et al. 2002) but larger studies are required to confirm the association. We have shown an increase in cell surface expression of both endogenous and transfected ICAM-1 G241/E469 genotype, which may account for some of the genetic associations that have been reported (Holder 2008).

4. Soluble ICAM-1

A circulating form of ICAM-1 consisting of only the five extracellular Ig-domains has been identified. Soluble ICAM-1 (sICAM-1) lacks the transmembrane region and cytoplasmic tail of membrane bound ICAM-1.

sICAM-1 has been detected in various body fluids including serum (Rothlein, Mainolfi et al. 1991; Seth, Raymond et al. 1991), cerebrospinal fluid (Tsukada, Matsuda et al. 1993), synovial fluid (Mason, Kapahi et al. 1993), sputum (Chihara, Yamamoto et al. 1994), urine (Teppo, von Willebrand et al. 2001) and bronchoalveolar fluid (Shijubo, Imai et al. 1994). sICAM-1 is present in normal human serum at concentrations between 100-450 ng/ml (Gearing and Newman 1993), whilst elevated sICAM-1 has been found in serum from patients with cardiovascular disease, cancer, autoimmune disease and several studies have correlated serum levels of sICAM-1 with severity of disease (for review see (Witkowska and Borawska 2004)).

The molecular weight of monomeric sICAM-1 varies between 80-110kDa depending on the level of glycosylation induced by the originating cell (Rothlein, Mainolfi et al. 1991). Studies have demonstrated that sICAM-1 is present in serum not only as monomer but also forms homo- and hetero-multimers with isoforms ranging from 240, 340 and over 500kDa (Rothlein, Mainolfi et al. 1991; Seth, Raymond et al. 1991).

A variety of cells have been shown to express sICAM-1 including primary endothelial cells, human aortic smooth muscle cells, melanoma cells and hematopoietic cell lines, but no expression mechanism has been identified. Alternative splicing has been suggested as one mechanistic pathway for the production of sICAM-1 (Wakatsuki, Kimura et al. 1995). The inflammatory cytokines TNF-α, IL-1α and IFN-γ have been reported to induce shedding of sICAM-1 from the cell surface of different primary cells and cell lines (Becker, Dummer et al. 1991; Leeuwenberg, Smeets et al. 1992; Pigott, Dillon et al. 1992; Fonsatti, Altomonte et al. 1997; Leung 1999). Furthermore, several proteases including matrix metalloproteases (MMP) (Lyons and Benveniste 1998); Tarín, Gomez, et al. 2009), human leukocyte elastase (Champagne, Tremblay et al. 1998) and TNF-α converting enzyme (TACE) (Tsakadze, Sithu et al. 2006) have been demonstrated to cleave sICAM-1 from the cell surface. The cleavage site on ICAM-1 seems to vary depending on cell type, glycosylation pattern and therefore also on the proteases involved. Further analysis showed that cleavage of membrane bound ICAM-1 by MMP-13 is dependent on NO and might be part of NO-mediated atheroprotection (Tarín, Gomez et al. 2009).

4.1 sICAM-1 as a biomarker in vascular disease

Increased levels of sICAM-1 have been found in patients with cardiovascular disease, cancer, autoimmune disease. Studies investigating the involvement of sICAM-1 in tumour surveillance by interfering with T-cell and tumour interaction have demonstrated that levels of sICAM-1 correlated with tumour progression in melanoma (Giavazzi 1992) and colorectal cancer (Alexiou 2001). Increased levels of sICAM-1 have also been linked to progression of atherosclerotic lesions in apoE $^{-/-}$ mice (Kitagawa, Matsumoto et al. 2002). These findings were supported in clinical studies with patients suffering from coronary heart disease (Hwang, Ballantyne et al. 1997; Ridker, Hennekens et al. 1998). Investigation between different risk factors associated with atherosclerosis showed a link between intake of saturated fatty acids and elevated levels of sICAM-1 (Bemelmans, Lefrandt et al. 2002). Increased levels of sICAM-1 were also found in type 2 diabetic patients (Becker, van Hinsbergh et al. 2002). Serum levels of sICAM-1 in cardiovascular patients treated with statins were confirmed to be lower in some groups (Romano, Mezzetti et al. 2000; Blann, Gurney et al. 2001; Bickel, Rupprecht et al. 2002), whereas some studies could not find a significant reduction (Rauch, Osende et al. 2000; Jilma, Joukhadar et al. 2003).

The use of sICAM-1 as a biomarker has lead to several studies with a range of different cardiovascular disease profiles and varying patient numbers. A significant correlation between future coronary artery disease events and elevated levels of sICAM-1 has been noted by several groups (Hwang, Ballantyne et al. 1997; Ridker, Hennekens et al. 1998; Malik, Danesh et al. 2001) but opposed by other studies (Ridker, Buring et al. 2001). Using sICAM-1 levels as biomarker for future secondary cardiovascular diseases in patients with coronary artery diseases again showed varying results with Blankenberg et al. (Blankenberg, Rupprecht et al. 2001) finding no significant correlation, a finding contradicted by others showing its potential as independent biomarker (Wallén, Held et al. 1999; Haim, Tanne et al. 2002).

Several genome studies have found a significant link on chromosome 19 close to the location of the ICAM-1 gene which might be responsible for elevated sICAM-1 levels (Kent, Mahaney et al. 2007; Bielinski, Pankow et al. 2008; Barbalic, Dupuis et al. 2010). Furthermore, Kent and colleagues (Kent, Mahaney et al. 2007) suggested the presence of SNPs within ICAM-1 to be involved in regulation of protein expression, function and its potential for cleavage. Several studies have examined the association of the SNPs within the ICAM-1 gene and sICAM-1 with atherosclerosis but have so far proved inconclusive (Tang, Pankow et al. 2007; Bielinski, Pankow et al. 2008; Bielinski, Reiner et al. 2011). Further clinical studies with larger patient numbers are required to clarify the situation.

4.2 Pro-inflammatory signalling cascades initiated by sICAM-1

Studies have reported that sICAM-1 binds competitively to ligands of membrane bound ICAM-1 such as LFA-1, mac-1 and human rhinovirus (Marlin, Staunton et al. 1990; Martin, Martin et al. 1993) and may therefore have potential as a therapeutic to block leukocyte:endothelial interactions when administered at high concentrations. However, a number of studies have also shown that addition of sICAM-1 at a physiologically relevant concentration activates proinflammatory cascades and causes angiogenesis in different *in vitro* and *in vivo* models. Incubation of murine brain microvascular EC or astrocytes with sICAM-1 lead to the increased secretion of the proinflammatory chemokine MIP-2 via activation of src tyrosine kinase and Erk phosphorylation (Otto, Heinzel-Pleines et al. 2000; Otto, Gloor et al. 2002). Gho and colleagues investigated the effects of sICAM-1 on EC angiogenesis. They demonstrated that sICAM-1 stimulated chemotactic EC migration, EC tube formation on Matrigel and sprouting in an aortic ring assay (Gho, Kleinman et al. 1999) and stimulates tumor growth in vivo (Gho, Kim et al. 2001). These data suggest that sICAM-1 could contribute to the progression of atherosclerosis and other chronic inflammatory diseases.

4.3 sICAM-1 contributes to monocyte recruitment by endothelial cells under laminar flow

Whilst the effect of sICAM-1 interaction with endothelium has been documented during static culture conditions, it is pertinent to investigate the biological effects of these interactions using a model of arterial flow to replicate the forces applied to EC under physiological conditions. We have used a parallel plate chamber and flow loop (see Macey, Wolf et al. 2009; Macey, Wolf et al. 2010; Lawson, Rose et al. 2010) to examine sICAM-1 mediated pro-inflammatory effects on human umbilical vein EC (HUVEC) acclimatised to arterial flow conditions. These may provide useful insights into the initiation of endothelial dysfunction and inflammatory activation that is a feature of atheroma progression.

We subjected HUVEC to laminar flow of 10dyn/cm^2 for 8h and analysed the cells for changes in Erk-1/-2 phosphorylation (phospho-Erk) as an indication of HUVEC activation after exposure of cells to flow for different times. As shown in Figure 5A the level of phospho-Erk was reduced to 42±7% after exposure to 10dyn/cm^2 flow for 8h compared to HUVEC in static culture ($p<0.001$). Levels of phospho-Erk in HUVEC subjected to flow remained below phospho-Erk in equivalent static cultures for at least a further 24h (data not shown). sICAM-1 has been shown to induce phospho-Erk in mouse astrocytes in static culture (Otto, Gloor et al. 2002), we therefore examined the effect of sICAM-1 in HUVEC pre-exposed to 10dyn/cm^2 flow. As seen in Figure 5B in HUVEC pre-exposed to flow for 8hr followed by sICAM-1 incubation caused a transient elevation of phospho-Erk after 15min (Figure 5B 292±28% of untreated flowed HUVEC $p<0.01$).

In static cell culture, sICAM-1 at physiologically relevant concentrations has been reported to induce expression of pro-inflammatory mediators (Otto, Heinzel-Pleines et al. 2000; Otto, Gloor et al. 2002). mRNA levels of IL-8 and MCP-1 were significantly increased 1hr after exposure to sICAM-1 in HUVECs (figure 6A and B). However, we observed no significant effect of sICAM-1 on secretion of MCP-1 and IL-8 in HUVEC cultured under static conditions (Figure 6C and D). Secretion of both chemokines were significantly reduced in EC exposed to 10dyn/cm^2 shear forces for 24h compared to static cultures (Figure 6C and D) after acclimatisation to shear stress as would be expected from previous reports (Metallo, Vodyanik et al. 2008). Addition of sICAM-1 to the culture media of HUVEC pre-exposed to shear and with continued exposure to shear lead to a three fold increase in MCP-1 secretion (Figure 6C), but did not induce any changes in IL-8 levels (figure 6D). To determine whether sICAM-1 mediated phosphorylation of Erk-1/-2 is involved in the upregulation of MCP-1 secretion, 1μM of the MEK inhibitor U0126 or its inactive analogue U0124 was added to HUVEC pre-exposed to flow and prior to addition of sICAM-1 to the flow medium. As seen in Figure 6E, there was no significant effect of U0124 on this (1949±123pg/ml sICAM-1 induced secretion vs 1645±73.58 pg/ml in the presence of 1μM U0124 and sICAM-1 p=0.1348 ns). In contrast, a significant reduction in secretion of MCP-1 was observed in cells pre-treated with 1μM U0126 prior to addition of sICAM-1 (1141±128.4pg/ml, p=0.0177 compared to cells treated with sICAM-1 alone; p=0.0039 compared to cells treated with 1μM U0124 before sICAM-1 (Figure 6E)).

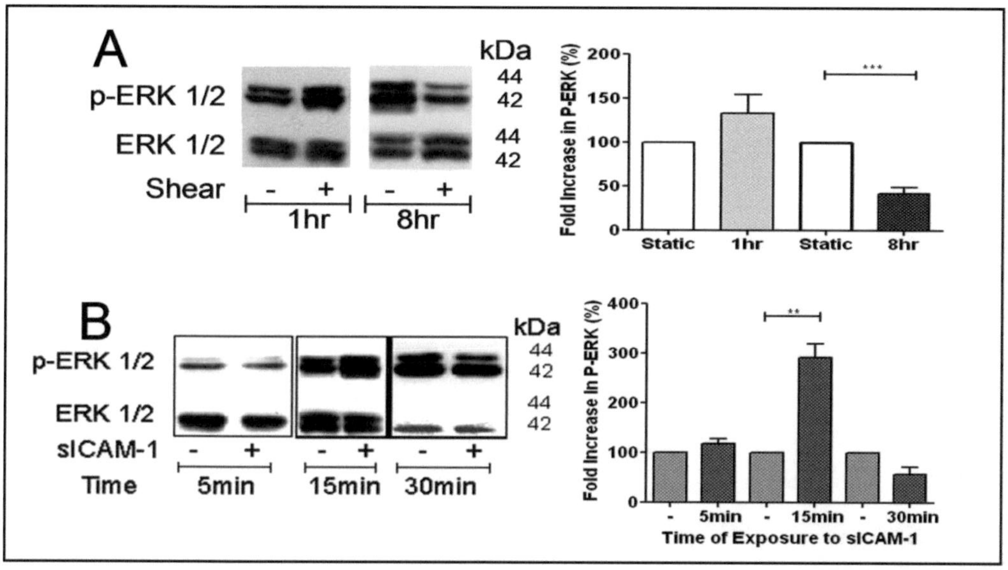

Fig. 5. sICAM-1 mediated Erk-1/-2 phosphorylation in HUVEC. A. HUVEC were subjected to laminar shear forces of 10dyn/cm^2 for 8h in a parallel plate flow chamber and recirculating flow loop, or cells from the same isolate were maintained in static culture. Protein was harvested and phospho-Erk was measured by western blotting and immunodetection (anti-phospho-Erk-1/-2 antibody from Cell Signaling Inc.), followed by stripping of blots and detection of total Erk expression (anti-total-Erk-1/-2 antibody from Cell Signaling Inc.). Representative blots shown. Stimulation index was calculated from densitometry measured for each replicate and pooled from n=3 sets of replicates for each time point. B. HUVEC were subjected to laminar shear forces of 10dyn/cm^2 for 8h in duplicate, before 100ng/ml sICAM-1 was added to one culture from each duplicate for indicated times. Protein was harvested and phospho-Erk was measured by western blotting and immunodetection followed by stripping of blots and detection of total Erk expression. Representative blots shown. Stimulation index calculated from densitometry measured for each replicate and pooled from n=3 sets of replicates for each time point. Pooled stimulation index data was used for paired T tests calculated using Prism. **p<0.01, ***p<0.001.

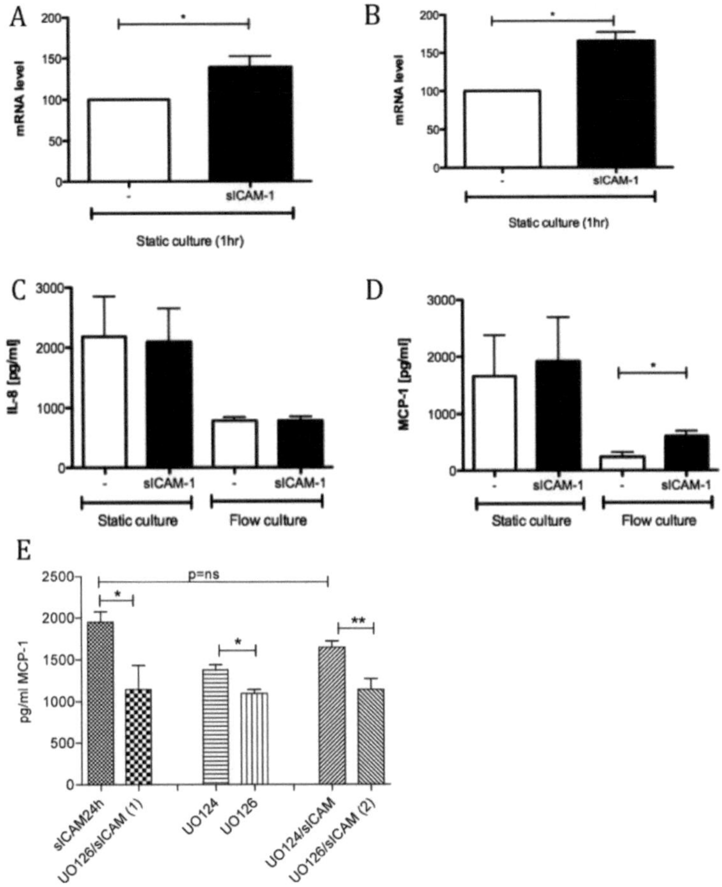

Fig. 6. Effect of sICAM-1 and shear stress on IL-8 and MCP-1 secretion in HUVEC. (A, B) mRNA for MCP-1 and IL-8 were measured in HUVEC in static culture following exposure to 100ng/ml sICAM-1 for 1hr. (C, D) HUVEC were grown in static culture or subjected to laminar shear forces of 10dyn/cm^2 in a parallel plate flow chamber and recirculating flow loop for 16h to acclimatise before addition of 100ng/ml sICAM-1 for a further 24h. Secretion of MCP-1 and IL-8 were measured by ELISA. (E) HUVEC were acclimatised to shear stress for 16hr before addition of MEK inhibitor U0126 (1µM) or the inactive analogue U0124 (1µM) followed by 100ng/ml sICAM-1 for 24hr. Secretion of MCP-1 and IL-8 were measured by ELISA. n=3 separate isolates for each pair of conditions. *$p<0.05$ and **$p<0.01$.

5. Conclusions

Our data suggest that the MEK-Erk pathway plays a role in sICAM-1 mediated MCP-1 production in HUVEC pre-exposed to laminar flow, and therefore that cleavage of ICAM-1 from the cell surface has a two fold effect; on the one hand providing a negative feedback mechanism to limit leukocyte adhesion and diapedesis, but on the other enhancing monocyte chemotaxis towards the endothelium. Thus sICAM-1 released into the circulation may be considered a pro-inflammatory mediator in the context of vascular inflammation and atherosclerosis progression.

At this time, no receptor has been identified for sICAM-1 and none of the common ligands for ICAM-1, such as LFA-1 and Mac-1, are present on HUVEC either in the activated or resting state. Two potential candidates for receptors have been suggested so far, namely the homophilic binding to membrane bound ICAM-1, or an unknown receptor of 49kD (Gho, Kleinman *et al.* 1999; Otto, Gloor et al. 2002). Otto et al showed that sICAM-1 did not bind to cell surface ICAM-1 using ICAM-1 deficient murine astrocytes but identified the involvement of an unidentified receptor (Otto, Gloor et al. 2002). It is possible that the level of expression of this unknown receptor on the cell surface could vary under different flow conditions, for example the receptor could be regulated through activation of a shear stress response element (SSRE) and therefore result in different expression levels on EC depending on the kinetics and/or type of shear stress to which the cells have been exposed. Since prolonged exposure to flow increases ICAM-1 expression (Nagel, Resnick et al. 1994; Chiu, Wung et al. 1997) and an SSRE has been identified in the promoter for ICAM-1 (Nagel, Resnick et al. 1994) we speculate that cell surface ICAM-1 could act as a receptor for sICAM-1 in the experiments presented here. Further experiments are necessary using blocking FAb fragments to ICAM-1 to determine this.

Experimental data obtained *in vitro* or in animal models together with data obtained from clinical samples indicates an important role for sICAM-1 within cardiovascular disease. More experimental studies are required to characterise the precise role of sICAM-1. By understanding the pathways and mechanisms involved in shedding sICAM-1 into the lumen and its role within the inflammation site, new potential methods to interfere with disease progression might become possible. In addition, larger clinical studies are also required to determine the potential use of sICAM-1 as non-invasive diagnostic biomarker for cardiovascular disease.

6. Acknowledgements

S.I.W was funded by a project grant from the British Heart Foundation.

7. References

Adamson, P., S. Etienne, et al. (1999). "Lymphocyte migration through brain endothelial cell monolayers involves signaling through endothelial ICAM-1 via a rho-dependent pathway." *J Immunol* 162(5): 2964-73.

Altieri, D. C., A. Duperray, et al. (1995). "Structural recognition of a novel fibrinogen gamma chain sequence (117-133) by intercellular adhesion molecule-1 mediates leukocyte-endothelium interaction." *J Biol Chem* 270(2): 696-9.

Barbalic, M., J. Dupuis, et al. (2010). "Large-scale genomic studies reveal central role of ABO in sP-selectin and sICAM-1 levels." *Hum Mol Genet* 19(9): 1863-72.

Barreiro, O., M. Yanez-Mo, et al. (2002). "Dynamic interaction of VCAM-1 and ICAM-1 with moesin and ezrin in a novel endothelial docking structure for adherent leukocytes." *J Cell Biol* 157(7): 1233-45.

Becker, A., V. W. van Hinsbergh, et al. (2002). "Why is soluble intercellular adhesion molecule-1 related to cardiovascular mortality?" *Eur J Clin Invest* 32(1): 1-8.

Becker, J. C., R. Dummer, et al. (1991). "Shedding of ICAM-1 from human melanoma cell lines induced by IFN-gamma and tumor necrosis factor-alpha. Functional consequences on cell-mediated cytotoxicity." *J Immunol* 147(12): 4398-401.

Bella, J. and M. G. Rossmann (1999). "Review: rhinoviruses and their ICAM receptors." *J Struct Biol* 128(1): 69-74.

Bemelmans, W. J., J. D. Lefrandt, et al. (2002). "Change in saturated fat intake is associated with progression of carotid and femoral intima-media thickness, and with levels of soluble intercellular adhesion molecule-1." *Atherosclerosis* 163(1): 113-20.

Bickel, C., H. J. Rupprecht, et al. (2002). "Influence of HMG-CoA reductase inhibitors on markers of coagulation, systemic inflammation and soluble cell adhesion." *Int J Cardiol* 82(1): 25-31.

Bielinski, S. J., J. S. Pankow, et al. (2008). "Circulating soluble ICAM-1 levels shows linkage to ICAM gene cluster region on chromosome 19: the NHLBI Family Heart Study follow-up examination." *Atherosclerosis* 199(1): 172-8.

Bielinski, S. J., J. S. Pankow, et al. (2008). "ICAM1 and VCAM1 polymorphisms, coronary artery calcium, and circulating levels of soluble ICAM-1: the multi-ethnic study of atherosclerosis (MESA)." *Atherosclerosis* 201(2): 339-44.

Bielinski, S. J., A. P. Reiner, et al. (2011). "Polymorphisms in the ICAM1 gene predict circulating soluble intercellular adhesion molecule-1(sICAM-1)." *Atherosclerosis* 216(2): 390-4.

Blankenberg, S., S. Barbaux, et al. (2003). "Adhesion molecules and atherosclerosis." Atherosclerosis 170(2): 191-203.

Blankenberg, S., H. J. Rupprecht, et al. (2001). "Circulating cell adhesion molecules and death in patients with coronary artery disease." *Circulation* 104(12): 1336-42.

Blann, A. D., D. Gurney, et al. (2001). "Influence of pravastatin on lipoproteins, and on endothelial, platelet, and inflammatory markers in subjects with peripheral artery disease." *Am J Cardiol* 88(1): A7-8, 89-92.

Bourdillon, M. C., R. N. Poston, et al. (2000). "ICAM-1 deficiency reduces atherosclerotic lesions in double-knockout mice (ApoE(-/-)/ICAM-1(-/-)) fed a fat or a chow diet." *Arterioscler Thromb Vasc Biol* 20(12): 2630-5.

Carpén, O., P. Pallai, et al. (1992). "Association of intercellular adhesion molecule-1 (ICAM-1) with actin-containing cytoskeleton and alpha-actinin." *J Cell Biol* 118(5): 1223-34.

Champagne, B., P. Tremblay, et al. (1998). "Proteolytic cleavage of ICAM-1 by human neutrophil elastase." *J Immunol* 161(11): 6398-405.

Chen, K. D., Y. S. Li, et al. (1999). "Mechanotransduction in response to shear stress. Roles of receptor tyrosine kinases, integrins, and Shc." *J Biol Chem* 274(26): 18393-400.

Chihara, J., T. Yamamoto, et al. (1994). "Soluble ICAM-1 in sputum of patients with bronchial asthma." *Lancet* 343(8905): 1108.

Chiu, J. J., B. S. Wung, et al. (1997). "Reactive oxygen species are involved in shear stress-induced intercellular adhesion molecule-1 expression in endothelial cells." *Arterioscler Thromb Vasc Biol* 17(12): 3570-7.

Collins, C. and E. Tzima (2011). "Hemodynamic forces in endothelial dysfunction and vascular aging." *Exp Gerontol* 46(2-3): 185-8.

Cronstein, B. N., S. C. Kimmel, et al. (1992). "A mechanism for the antiinflammatory effects of corticosteroids: the glucocorticoid receptor regulates leukocyte adhesion to endothelial cells and expression of endothelial-leukocyte adhesion molecule 1 and intercellular adhesion molecule 1." *Proc Natl Acad Sci U S A* 89(21): 9991-5.

De Caterina, R., P. Libby, et al. (1995). "Nitric oxide decreases cytokine-induced endothelial activation. Nitric oxide selectively reduces endothelial expression of adhesion molecules and proinflammatory cytokines." *J Clin Invest* 96(1): 60-8.

Durieu-Trautmann, O., N. Chaverot, et al. (1994). "Intercellular adhesion molecule 1 activation induces tyrosine phosphorylation of the cytoskeleton-associated protein cortactin in brain microvessel endothelial cells." *J Biol Chem* 269(17): 12536-40.

Dustin, M. L., R. Rothlein, et al. (1986). "Induction by IL 1 and interferon-gamma: tissue distribution, biochemistry, and function of a natural adherence molecule (ICAM-1)." *J Immunol* 137(1): 245-54.

Etienne-Manneville, S., J. B. Manneville, et al. (2000). "ICAM-1-coupled cytoskeletal rearrangements and transendothelial lymphocyte migration involve intracellular calcium signaling in brain endothelial cell lines." J Immunol 165(6): 3375-83.

Etienne, S., P. Adamson, et al. (1998). "ICAM-1 signaling pathways associated with Rho activation in microvascular brain endothelial cells." *J Immunol* 161(10): 5755-61.

Federici, C., L. Camoin, et al. (1996). "Association of the cytoplasmic domain of intercellular-adhesion molecule-1 with glyceraldehyde-3-phosphate dehydrogenase and beta-tubulin." *Eur J Biochem* 238(1): 173-80.

Florian, J. A., J. R. Kosky, et al. (2003). "Heparan sulfate proteoglycan is a mechanosensor on endothelial cells." *Circ Res* 93(10): e136-42.

Fonsatti, E., M. Altomonte, et al. (1997). "Tumour-derived interleukin 1alpha (IL-1alpha) up-regulates the release of soluble intercellular adhesion molecule-1 (sICAM-1) by endothelial cells." *Br J Cancer* 76(10): 1255-61.

Frank, P. G. and M. P. Lisanti (2006). "Role of caveolin-1 in the regulation of the vascular shear stress response." *J Clin Invest* 116(5): 1222-5.

Frostegård J. (2011). "Cardiovascular co-morbidity in patients with rheumatic diseases." *Arthritis Res Ther.* 13(3):225.

Fujiwara, K., M. Masuda, et al. (2001). "Is PECAM-1 a mechanoresponsive molecule?" *Cell Struct Funct* 26(1): 11-7.

Gaetani, E., A. Flex, et al. (2002). "The K469E polymorphism of the ICAM-1 gene is a risk factor for peripheral arterial occlusive disease." *Blood Coagul Fibrinolysis* 13(6): 483-8.

Gaglia, J. L., E. A. Greenfield, et al. (2000). "Intercellular adhesion molecule 1 is critical for activation of CD28-deficient T cells." *J Immunol* 165(11): 6091-8.

Gearing, A. J. and W. Newman (1993). "Circulating adhesion molecules in disease." *Immunol Today* 14(10): 506-12.

Gerszten, R. E., E. A. Garcia-Zepeda, et al. (1999). "MCP-1 and IL-8 trigger firm adhesion of monocytes to vascular endothelium under flow conditions." *Nature* 398(6729): 718-23.

Gho, Y. S., P. N. Kim, et al. (2001). "Stimulation of tumor growth by human soluble intercellular adhesion molecule-1." *Cancer Res* 61(10): 4253-7.

Gho, Y. S., H. K. Kleinman, et al. (1999). "Angiogenic activity of human soluble intercellular adhesion molecule-1." *Cancer Res* 59(20): 5128-32.

Gimbrone, M. A., J. N. Topper, et al. (2000). "Endothelial dysfunction, hemodynamic forces, and atherogenesis." *Ann N Y Acad Sci* 902: 230-9; discussion 239-40.

Grakoui, A., S. K. Bromley, et al. (1999). "The immunological synapse: a molecular machine controlling T cell activation." *Science* 285(5425): 221-7.

Greenwood, J., Y. Wang, et al. (1995). "Lymphocyte adhesion and transendothelial migration in the central nervous system: the role of LFA-1, ICAM-1, VLA-4 and VCAM-1. off." *Immunology* 86(3): 408-15.

Greve, J. M., G. Davis, et al. (1989). "The major human rhinovirus receptor is ICAM-1." *Cell* 56(5): 839-47.

Gudi, S. R., C. B. Clark, et al. (1996). "Fluid flow rapidly activates G proteins in human endothelial cells. Involvement of G proteins in mechanochemical signal transduction." *Circ Res* 79(4): 834-9.

Haim, M., D. Tanne, et al. (2002). "Soluble intercellular adhesion molecule-1 and long-term risk of acute coronary events in patients with chronic coronary heart disease. Data from the Bezafibrate Infarction Prevention (BIP) Study." *J Am Coll Cardiol* 39(7): 1133-8.

Hansson, G. K. and P. Libby (2006). "The immune response in atherosclerosis: a double-edged sword." *Nat Rev Immunol* 6(7): 508-19.

Hansson G.K. (2009). "Inflammatory mechanisms in atherosclerosis." *J Thromb Haemost.* 7 Suppl 1:328-31

Helmlinger, G., B. C. Berk, et al. (1996). "Pulsatile and steady flow-induced calcium oscillations in single cultured endothelial cells." *J Vasc Res* 33(5): 360-9.

Hoffmeister A, Rothenbacher D, et al. (2001). "Current infection with Helicobacter pylori, but not seropositivity to Chlamydia pneumoniae or cytomegalovirus, is associated with an atherogenic, modified lipid profile." *Arterioscler Thromb Vasc Biol.* 21(3):427-32.

Holder A.L., S. Wolf, et al (2008) "Expression of endothelial intercellular adhesion molecule-1 is determined by genotype: effects on efficiency of leukocyte adhesion to human endothelial cells." *Hum Immunol.* 69:71-8

Holland, J. and T. Owens (1997). "Signaling through intercellular adhesion molecule 1 (ICAM-1) in a B cell lymphoma line. The activation of Lyn tyrosine kinase and the mitogen-activated protein kinase pathway." *J Biol Chem* 272(14): 9108-12.

Hwang, S. J., C. M. Ballantyne, et al. (1997). "Circulating adhesion molecules VCAM-1, ICAM-1, and E-selectin in carotid atherosclerosis and incident coronary heart disease cases: the Atherosclerosis Risk In Communities (ARIC) study." *Circulation* 96(12): 4219-25.

Jiang, H., R. M. Klein, et al. (2002). "C/T polymorphism of the intercellular adhesion molecule-1 gene (exon 6, codon 469). A risk factor for coronary heart disease and myocardial infarction." *Int J Cardiol* 84(2-3): 171-7.

Jilma, B., C. Joukhadar, et al. (2003). "Levels of adhesion molecules do not decrease after 3 months of statin therapy in moderate hypercholesterolaemia." *Clin Sci (Lond)* 104(2): 189-93.

Karalliedde J., and G. Viberti (2004)."Microalbuminuria and cardiovascular risk." *Am J Hypertens.* 17(10):986-93.

Kent, J. W., M. C. Mahaney, et al. (2007). "Quantitative trait locus on Chromosome 19 for circulating levels of intercellular adhesion molecule-1 in Mexican Americans." *Atherosclerosis* 195(2): 367-73.

Kirchhausen, T., D. E. Staunton, et al. (1993). "Location of the domains of ICAM-1 by immunolabeling and single-molecule electron microscopy." *J Leukoc Biol* 53(3): 342-6.

Kitagawa, K., M. Matsumoto, et al. (2002). "Involvement of ICAM-1 in the progression of atherosclerosis in APOE-knockout mice." *Atherosclerosis* 160(2): 305-10.

Languino, L. R., A. Duperray, et al. (1995). "Regulation of leukocyte-endothelium interaction and leukocyte transendothelial migration by intercellular adhesion molecule 1-fibrinogen recognition." *Proc Natl Acad Sci U S A* 92(5): 1505-9.

Languino, L. R., J. Plescia, et al. (1993). "Fibrinogen mediates leukocyte adhesion to vascular endothelium through an ICAM-1-dependent pathway." *Cell* 73(7): 1423-34.

Lavie C.J., R.V. Milani, H.O. Ventura. (2009). Obesity and cardiovascular disease: risk factor, paradox, and impact of weight loss. *J Am Coll Cardiol.* 53(21):1925-32.

Laurila A, Bloigu A, et al. (1997). "Chronic Chlamydia pneumoniae infection is associated with a serum lipid profile known to be a risk factor for atherosclerosis." *Arterioscler Thromb Vasc Biol.* 17(11):2910-3.

Lawson, C., M. Ainsworth, et al. (1999). "Ligation of ICAM-1 on endothelial cells leads to expression of VCAM-1 via a nuclear factor-kappaB-independent mechanism." *J Immunol* 162(5): 2990-6.

Lawson, C., M. E. Ainsworth, et al. (2001). "Effects of cross-linking ICAM-1 on the surface of human vascular smooth muscle cells: induction of VCAM-1 but no proliferation." *Cardiovasc Res* 50(3): 547-55.

Lawson, C., A. L. Holder, et al. (2005). "Anti-intercellular adhesion molecule-1 antibodies in sera of heart transplant recipients: a role in endothelial cell activation." *Transplantation* 80(2): 264-71.

Lawson, C. and S.I. Wolf. (2009). "ICAM-1 signaling in endothelial cells." *Pharmacol Rep.* 61(1):22-32.

Lawson C, M. Rose and S. Wolf. (2010) Leucocyte adhesion under haemodynamic flow conditions. *Methods Mol Biol.* 616:31-47.

Leeuwenberg, J. F., E. F. Smeets, et al. (1992). "E-selectin and intercellular adhesion molecule-1 are released by activated human endothelial cells in vitro." *Immunology* 77(4): 543-9.

Lehmann, J. C., D. Jablonski-Westrich, et al. (2003). "Overlapping and selective roles of endothelial intercellular adhesion molecule-1 (ICAM-1) and ICAM-2 in lymphocyte trafficking." *J Immunol* 171(5): 2588-93.

Lehoux, S., Y. Castier, et al. (2006). "Molecular mechanisms of the vascular responses to haemodynamic forces." *J Intern Med* 259(4): 381-92.

Leung, K. H. (1999). "Release of soluble ICAM-1 from human lung fibroblasts, aortic smooth muscle cells, dermal microvascular endothelial cells, bronchial epithelial cells, and keratinocytes." *Biochem Biophys Res Commun* 260(3): 734-9.

Ley, K., C. Laudanna, et al. (2007). "Getting to the site of inflammation: the leukocyte adhesion cascade updated." *Nat Rev Immunol* 7(9): 678-89.

Li, Y. S., J. H. Haga, et al. (2005). "Molecular basis of the effects of shear stress on vascular endothelial cells." *J Biomech* 38(10): 1949-71.

Lindemann, S., M. Sharafi, et al. (2000). "NO reduces PMN adhesion to human vascular endothelial cells due to downregulation of ICAM-1 mRNA and surface expression." *Thromb Res* 97(3): 113-23.

Lusis, A. J. (2000). "Atherosclerosis." *Nature* 407(6801): 233-41.

Lyck, R., Y. Reiss, et al. (2003). "T-cell interaction with ICAM-1/ICAM-2 double-deficient brain endothelium in vitro: the cytoplasmic tail of endothelial ICAM-1 is necessary for transendothelial migration of T cells." *Blood* 102(10): 3675-83.

Lyons, P. D. and E. N. Benveniste (1998). "Cleavage of membrane-associated ICAM-1 from astrocytes: involvement of a metalloprotease." *Glia* 22(2): 103-12.

Macey M.G., S.I. Wolf, C.P. Wheeler-Jones and C. Lawson. (2009) "Expression of blood coagulation factors on monocytes after exposure to TNF-treated endothelium in a novel whole blood model of arterial flow." *J Immunol Methods.* 350(1-2):133-41.

Macey M.G., S.I. Wolf, C. Lawson (2010). "Microparticle formation after exposure of blood to activated endothelium under flow." *Cytometry A.* 77(8):761-8.

Malik, I., J. Danesh, et al. (2001). "Soluble adhesion molecules and prediction of coronary heart disease: a prospective study and meta-analysis." *Lancet* 358(9286): 971-6.

Malyszko, J. (2010). "Mechanism of endothelial dysfunction in chronic kidney disease." *Clin Chim Acta* 411(19-20): 1412-20.

Marlin, S. D. and T. A. Springer (1987). "Purified intercellular adhesion molecule-1 (ICAM-1) is a ligand for lymphocyte function-associated antigen 1 (LFA-1)." *Cell* 51(5): 813-9.

Marlin, S. D., D. E. Staunton, et al. (1990). "A soluble form of intercellular adhesion molecule-1 inhibits rhinovirus infection." *Nature* 344(6261): 70-2.

Martin, S., A. Martin, et al. (1993). "Functional studies of truncated soluble intercellular adhesion molecule 1 expressed in Escherichia coli." *Antimicrob Agents Chemother* 37(6): 1278-84.

Mason, J. C., P. Kapahi, et al. (1993). "Detection of increased levels of circulating intercellular adhesion molecule 1 in some patients with rheumatoid arthritis but not in patients with systemic lupus erythematosus. Lack of correlation with levels of circulating vascular cell adhesion molecule 1." *Arthritis Rheum* 36(4): 519-27.

Metallo, C. M., M. A. Vodyanik, et al. (2008). "The response of human embryonic stem cell-derived endothelial cells to shear stress." *Biotechnol Bioeng* 100(4): 830-7.

Nageh, M. F., E. T. Sandberg, et al. (1997). "Deficiency of inflammatory cell adhesion molecules protects against atherosclerosis in mice." *Arterioscler Thromb Vasc Biol* 17(8): 1517-20.

Nagel, T., N. Resnick, et al. (1994). "Shear stress selectively upregulates intercellular adhesion molecule-1 expression in cultured human vascular endothelial cells." *J Clin Invest* 94(2): 885-91.

Ockenhouse, C. F., R. Betageri, et al. (1992). "Plasmodium falciparum-infected erythrocytes bind ICAM-1 at a site distinct from LFA-1, Mac-1, and human rhinovirus." *Cell* 68(1): 63-9.

Ockenhouse, C. F., M. Ho, et al. (1991). "Molecular basis of sequestration in severe and uncomplicated Plasmodium falciparum malaria: differential adhesion of infected erythrocytes to CD36 and ICAM-1." *J Infect Dis* 164(1): 163-9.

Ockenhouse, C. F., T. Tegoshi, et al. (1992). "Human vascular endothelial cell adhesion receptors for Plasmodium falciparum-infected erythrocytes: roles for endothelial leukocyte adhesion molecule 1 and vascular cell adhesion molecule 1." *J Exp Med* 176(4): 1183-9.

Oh, H. M., S. Lee, et al. (2007). "RKIKK motif in the intracellular domain is critical for spatial and dynamic organization of ICAM-1: functional implication for the leukocyte adhesion and transmigration." *Mol Biol Cell* 18(6): 2322-35.

Ohno, M., J. P. Cooke, et al. (1995). "Fluid shear stress induces endothelial transforming growth factor beta-1 transcription and production. Modulation by potassium channel blockade." *J Clin Invest* 95(3): 1363-9.

Osawa, M., M. Masuda, et al. (2002). "Evidence for a role of platelet endothelial cell adhesion molecule-1 in endothelial cell mechanosignal transduction: is it a mechanoresponsive molecule?" *J Cell Biol* 158(4): 773-85.

Otto, V. I., S. M. Gloor, et al. (2002). "The production of macrophage inflammatory protein-2 induced by soluble intercellular adhesion molecule-1 in mouse astrocytes is mediated by src tyrosine kinases and p42/44 mitogen-activated protein kinase." *J Neurochem* 80(5): 824-34.

Otto, V. I., U. E. Heinzel-Pleines, et al. (2000). "sICAM-1 and TNF-alpha induce MIP-2 with distinct kinetics in astrocytes and brain microvascular endothelial cells." *J Neurosci Res* 60(6): 733-42.

Patel, S. S., R. Thiagarajan, et al. (1998). "Inhibition of alpha4 integrin and ICAM-1 markedly attenuate macrophage homing to atherosclerotic plaques in ApoE-deficient mice." *Circulation* 97(1): 75-81.

Pigott, R., L. P. Dillon, et al. (1992). "Soluble forms of E-selectin, ICAM-1 and VCAM-1 are present in the supernatants of cytokine activated cultured endothelial cells." *Biochem Biophys Res Commun* 187(2): 584-9.

Pluskota, E., Y. Chen, et al. (2000). "Src homology domain 2-containing tyrosine phosphatase 2 associates with intercellular adhesion molecule 1 to regulate cell survival." *J Biol Chem* 275(39): 30029-36.

Pluskota, E. and S. E. D'Souza (2000). "Fibrinogen interactions with ICAM-1 (CD54) regulate endothelial cell survival." *Eur J Biochem* 267(15): 4693-704.

Pober, J. S., M. A. Gimbrone, et al. (1986). "Overlapping patterns of activation of human endothelial cells by interleukin 1, tumor necrosis factor, and immune interferon." *J Immunol* 137(6): 1893-6.

Poston, R. N., D. O. Haskard, et al. (1992). "Expression of intercellular adhesion molecule-1 in atherosclerotic plaques." *Am J Pathol* 140(3): 665-73.

Rauch, U., J. I. Osende, et al. (2000). "Statins and cardiovascular diseases: the multiple effects of lipid-lowering therapy by statins." *Atherosclerosis* 153(1): 181-9.

Reiss, Y. and B. Engelhardt (1999). "T cell interaction with ICAM-1-deficient endothelium in vitro: transendothelial migration of different T cell populations is mediated by endothelial ICAM-1 and ICAM-2." *Int Immunol* 11(9): 1527-39.

Renkonen, R., P. Mattila, et al. (1992). "IL-4 decreases IFN-gamma-induced endothelial ICAM-1 expression by a transcriptional mechanism." *Scand J Immunol* 35(5): 525-30.

Resnick, N., H. Yahav, et al. (2003). "Fluid shear stress and the vascular endothelium: for better and for worse." *Prog Biophys Mol Biol* 81(3): 177-99.

Ridker, P. M., J. E. Buring, et al. (2001). "Soluble P-selectin and the risk of future cardiovascular events." *Circulation* 103(4): 491-5.

Ridker, P. M., C. H. Hennekens, et al. (1998). "Plasma concentration of soluble intercellular adhesion molecule 1 and risks of future myocardial infarction in apparently healthy men." *Lancet* 351(9096): 88-92.

Romano, M., A. Mezzetti, et al. (2000). "Fluvastatin reduces soluble P-selectin and ICAM-1 levels in hypercholesterolemic patients: role of nitric oxide." *J Investig Med* 48(3): 183-9.

Ross, R. (1999). "Atherosclerosis--an inflammatory disease." *N Engl J Med* 340(2): 115-26.

Ross, R. and J. Glomset (1974). "Studies of primate arterial smooth muscle cells in relation to atherosclerosis." *Adv Exp Med Biol* 43(0): 265-79.

Rothlein, R., T. K. Kishimoto, et al. (1994). "Cross-linking of ICAM-1 induces co-signaling of an oxidative burst from mononuclear leukocytes." *J Immunol* 152(5): 2488-95.

Rothlein, R., E. A. Mainolfi, et al. (1991). "A form of circulating ICAM-1 in human serum." *J Immunol* 147(11): 3788-93.

Sampath, R., G. L. Kukielka, et al. (1995). "Shear stress-mediated changes in the expression of leukocyte adhesion receptors on human umbilical vein endothelial cells in vitro." *Ann Biomed Eng* 23(3): 247-56.

Sano, H., N. Nakagawa, et al. (1998). "Cross-linking of intercellular adhesion molecule-1 induces interleukin-8 and RANTES production through the activation of MAP kinases in human vascular endothelial cells." *Biochem Biophys Res Commun* 250(3): 694-8.

Schwenke, D. C. and T. E. Carew (1989a). "Initiation of atherosclerotic lesions in cholesterol-fed rabbits. I. Focal increases in arterial LDL concentration precede development of fatty streak lesions." *Arteriosclerosis* 9(6): 895-907.

Schwenke, D. C. and T. E. Carew (1989b). "Initiation of atherosclerotic lesions in cholesterol-fed rabbits. II. Selective retention of LDL vs. selective increases in LDL permeability in susceptible sites of arteries." *Arteriosclerosis* 9(6): 908-18.

Seth, R., F. D. Raymond, et al. (1991). "Circulating ICAM-1 isoforms: diagnostic prospects for inflammatory and immune disorders." *Lancet* 338(8759): 83-4.

Shijubo, N., K. Imai, et al. (1994). "Soluble intercellular adhesion molecule-1 (ICAM-1) in sera and bronchoalveolar lavage fluid of patients with idiopathic pulmonary fibrosis and pulmonary sarcoidosis." *Clin Exp Immunol* 95(1): 156-61.

Shyy, J. Y. and S. Chien (2002). "Role of integrins in endothelial mechanosensing of shear stress." *Circ Res* 91(9): 769-75.

Skålén, K., M. Gustafsson, et al. (2002). "Subendothelial retention of atherogenic lipoproteins in early atherosclerosis." *Nature* 417(6890): 750-4.

Sligh, J. E., C. M. Ballantyne, et al. (1993). "Inflammatory and immune responses are impaired in mice deficient in intercellular adhesion molecule 1." *Proc Natl Acad Sci U S A* 90(18): 8529-33.

Smith, C. W., S. D. Marlin, et al. (1989). "Cooperative interactions of LFA-1 and Mac-1 with intercellular adhesion molecule-1 in facilitating adherence and transendothelial migration of human neutrophils in vitro." *J Clin Invest* 83(6): 2008-17.

Springer, T. A. (1994). "Traffic signals for lymphocyte recirculation and leukocyte emigration: the multistep paradigm." *Cell* 76(2): 301-14.

Staunton, D. E., S. D. Marlin, et al. (1988). "Primary structure of ICAM-1 demonstrates interaction between members of the immunoglobulin and integrin supergene families." Cell 52(6): 925-33.

Staunton, D. E., V. J. Merluzzi, et al. (1989). "A cell adhesion molecule, ICAM-1, is the major surface receptor for rhinoviruses." *Cell* 56(5): 849-53.

Surapisitchat, J., R. J. Hoefen, et al. (2001). "Fluid shear stress inhibits TNF-alpha activation of JNK but not ERK1/2 or p38 in human umbilical vein endothelial cells: Inhibitory crosstalk among MAPK family members." *Proc Natl Acad Sci U S A* 98(11): 6476-81.

Tang, W., J. S. Pankow, et al. (2007). "Association of sICAM-1 and MCP-1 with coronary artery calcification in families enriched for coronary heart disease or hypertension: the NHLBI Family Heart Study." BMC *Cardiovasc Disord* 7: 30.

Tarín, C., M. Gomez, et al. (2009). "Endothelial nitric oxide deficiency reduces MMP-13-mediated cleavage of ICAM-1 in vascular endothelium: a role in atherosclerosis." *Arterioscler Thromb Vasc Biol* 29(1): 27-32.

Teppo, A. M., E. von Willebrand, et al. (2001). "Soluble intercellular adhesion molecule-1 (sICAM-1) after kidney transplantation: the origin and role of urinary sICAM-1?" *Transplantation* 71(8): 1113-9.

Thi, M. M., J. M. Tarbell, et al. (2004). "The role of the glycocalyx in reorganization of the actin cytoskeleton under fluid shear stress: a "bumper-car" model." *Proc Natl Acad Sci U S A* 101(47): 16483-8.

Thompson, P. W., A. M. Randi, et al. (2002). "Intercellular adhesion molecule (ICAM)-1, but not ICAM-2, activates RhoA and stimulates c-fos and rhoA transcription in endothelial cells." *J Immunol* 169(2): 1007-13.

Tsakadze, N. L., U. Sen, et al. (2004). "Signals mediating cleavage of intercellular adhesion molecule-1." *Am J Physiol Cell Physiol* 287(1): C55-63.

Tsakadze, N. L., S. D. Sithu, et al. (2006). "Tumor necrosis factor-alpha-converting enzyme (TACE/ADAM-17) mediates the ectodomain cleavage of intercellular adhesion molecule-1 (ICAM-1)." *J Biol Chem* 281(6): 3157-64.

Tsakadze, N. L., Z. Zhao, et al. (2002). "Interactions of intercellular adhesion molecule-1 with fibrinogen." *Trends Cardiovasc Med* 12(3): 101-8.

Tsukada, N., M. Matsuda, et al. (1993). "Increased levels of intercellular adhesion molecule-1 (ICAM-1) and tumor necrosis factor receptor in the cerebrospinal fluid of patients with multiple sclerosis." *Neurology* 43(12): 2679-82.

Tzima, E., M. A. del Pozo, et al. (2001). "Activation of integrins in endothelial cells by fluid shear stress mediates Rho-dependent cytoskeletal alignment." *EMBO J* 20(17): 4639-47.

van Buul, J. D. and P. L. Hordijk (2004). "Signaling in leukocyte transendothelial migration." *Arterioscler Thromb Vasc Biol* 24(5): 824-33.

van de Stolpe, A. and P. T. van der Saag (1996). "Intercellular adhesion molecule-1." *J Mol Med* 74(1): 13-33.

Van der Heiden, K., B. C. Groenendijk, et al. (2006). "Monocilia on chicken embryonic endocardium in low shear stress areas." *Dev Dyn* 235(1): 19-28.

Van der Heiden, K., B. P. Hierck, et al. (2008). "Endothelial primary cilia in areas of disturbed flow are at the base of atherosclerosis." *Atherosclerosis* 196(2): 542-50.

Wakatsuki, T., K. Kimura, et al. (1995). "A distinct mRNA encoding a soluble form of ICAM-1 molecule expressed in human tissues." *Cell Adhes Commun* 3(4): 283-92.

Wallén, N. H., C. Held, et al. (1999). "Elevated serum intercellular adhesion molecule-1 and vascular adhesion molecule-1 among patients with stable angina pectoris who suffer cardiovascular death or non-fatal myocardial infarction." *Eur Heart J* 20(14): 1039-43.

Wang, Q., G. R. Pfeiffer, et al. (2003). "Activation of SRC tyrosine kinases in response to ICAM-1 ligation in pulmonary microvascular endothelial cells." *J Biol Chem* 278(48): 47731-43.

Williams, K. J. and I. Tabas (1995). "The response-to-retention hypothesis of early atherogenesis." *Arterioscler Thromb Vasc Biol* 15(5): 551-61.

Witkowska, A. M. and M. H. Borawska (2004). "Soluble intercellular adhesion molecule-1 (sICAM-1): an overview." *Eur Cytokine Netw* 15(2): 91-8.

Wójciak-Stothard, B., L. Williams, et al. (1999). "Monocyte adhesion and spreading on human endothelial cells is dependent on Rho-regulated receptor clustering." *J Cell Biol* 145(6): 1293-307.

Yamamoto, K., R. Korenaga, et al. (2000). "Fluid shear stress activates Ca(2+) influx into human endothelial cells via P2X4 purinoceptors." *Circ Res* 87(5): 385-91.

4

Molecular and Cellular Aspects of Atherosclerosis: Emerging Roles of TRPC Channels

Guillermo Vazquez, Kathryn Smedlund, Jean-Yves K. Tano and Robert Lee
Department of Physiology and Pharmacology, University of Toledo Health Science Campus, Toledo, OH, USA

1. Introduction

1.1 Endothelial inflammatory signaling and monocyte recruitment

Recruitment of circulating monocytes to activated areas of the endothelium and their migration to the subintimal inflammatory foci represents one of the earliest events in atherogenesis (Linton and Fazio 2003; Hansson 2005). Importantly, monocyte recruitment can be recognized throughout all lesional stages including advanced lesions, where plaque infiltration and neovascularization occur. Indeed, available experimental evidence supports the notion that in advanced stages monocyte infiltration contributes to plaque instability and rupture (Virmani, Burke et al. 2006). Monocyte recruitment to the subendothelial milieu implies a sequence of events that begin with monocyte rolling along and tethering to the endothelial surface, firm adhesion and activation, and ultimately migration to the subintima. At the molecular level, the entire sequence entails interaction of integrins on the monocyte surface with cell adhesion molecules (CAMs) expressed on the endothelial cell. Monocyte rolling and tethering is mainly mediated by CAMs from the selectin group (v.g., E-selectin) while firm adhesion and migration are mostly mediated by CAMs from the immunoglobulin (Ig) superfamily, such as intercellular cell adhesion molecule-1 (ICAM-1) and vascular cell adhesion molecule-1 (VCAM-1). Compelling evidence accumulated over the last decade has clearly established that VCAM-1 (CD106) has a prominent role in mediating attachment and migration of monocytes (the Cluster of Differentiation nomenclature (Zola, Swart et al. 2005) is given for reference, but "VCAM-1" will be used throughout the text).

1.1.1 VCAM-1 expression and atherosclerosis

Although other adhesion molecules, such as ICAM-1 (CD54) or E-selectin, also contribute to adhesion of monocytes to endothelial cells, VCAM-1 is unique in that its expression level and pattern are highly sensitive to the action of several pro-inflammatory/pro-atherogenic stimuli. While other CAMs are constitutively expressed in non-activated endothelium, VCAM-1 is virtually absent, but its markedly upregulated when endothelium is exposed to atherorelevant stimuli (Galkina and Ley 2007). For example, in hypercholesterolemic animals both ICAM-1 and VCAM-1 are induced in early lesions. However, VCAM-1 expression is largely restricted to lesions, or to sites prone to lesion formation, and can also be detected even before the onset of visible fatty streaks, while ICAM-1 also extends into uninvolved aorta and lesion-protected regions (Iiyama, Hajra et al. 1999). This dissimilar pattern immediately suggested different functions for ICAM-1 and VCAM-1, at least in lesion initiation. A more direct comparison of VCAM-1 and ICAM-1 in atherosclerosis was possible through generation of mice homozygous for a VCAM-1 molecule lacking the Ig-like extracellular domain 4 ($Vcam1^{D4D/D4D}$) which partially circumvents the embryonic lethality of *Vcam-1*$^{-/-}$ mice. Using such mouse model it was possible to show that whereas both ICAM-1 and VCAM-1 are upregulated in lesions, VCAM-1 has a dominant role in early lesion formation (Cybulsky, Iiyama et al. 2001; Dansky, Barlow et al. 2001). Atherorelevant stimuli such as tumor necrosis factor-α (TNFα), locally released nucleotides, vascular endothelial growth factor (VEGF) or oxidized low density lipoprotein (oxLDL), are potent inducers of VCAM-1 expression (Galkina and Ley 2007). Depending on the stimulus and/or the regional location of the endothelial cell along the vascular bed, VCAM-1 expression is regulated through Nuclear Factor κappaB (NFκB), Nuclear Factor of Activated T cells (NFAT) or both (Armesilla, Lorenzo et al. 1999; Kim, Moon et al. 2001; Yao and Duh 2004).

1.1.2 VCAM-1 structure and function

Human VCAM-1 is a single transmembrane protein with seven Ig-like extracellular domains (1-7) but can also be expressed as a form with only domains 1-3 and 5-7 (Chuluyan, Osborn et al. 1995). The extracellular domains 1 and 4 mediate specific binding to the integrin $\alpha_4\beta_1$ (Very Late Antigen 4, VLA-4) on the monocyte facilitating firm adhesion to the endothelium. The cytoplasmic domain is only 19 amino acids long, and has a PDZ-binding motif, but specific interactions or functional relevance remain unknown. Interaction of VCAM-1 with $\alpha_4\beta_1$ conveys a conformational message through the transmembrane domain towards the cytosolic region, triggering intracellular signaling events. Importantly, VCAM-1-dependent signaling is a prerequisite for successful migration of bound monocytes (Matheny, Deem et al. 2000; Deem, Abdala-Valencia et al. 2007). Some salient features within this signaling are the recruitment and activation of the Rho-family GTPase Rac-1, Rac-1 dependent stimulation of NADPH oxidase and production of hydrogen peroxide (H_2O_2) (van Wetering, van den Berk et al. 2003). VCAM-1-dependent release of H_2O_2 to the extracellular milieu is thought to contribute to activation of matrix metalloproteases and the increased endothelial permeability observed during atherogenesis. This may be particularly important in advanced lesions by creating additional endothelial damage and plaque instability (Virmani, Burke et al. 2006). Calcium (Ca^{2+}) release and influx subsequent to VCAM-1-$\alpha_4\beta_1$ interaction or antibody-induced VCAM-1 crosslinking have also been related to the signaling required for monocyte migration (Isabelle Ricard 1997; Cook-Mills 2002; Cook-Mills, Johnson et al. 2004). However, neither the nature of the channels involved nor the underlying mechanism/s are yet known. In coronary artery endothelial cells of human origin (HCAECs) activation of VCAM-1 by antibody-induced crosslinking results in approximately three-fold increase in the rate of cation influx compared to non-treated cells (Smedlund and Vazquez, unpublished observations). Such increase in cation influx occurs over the existing constitutive influx, and thus is possible that both constitutive and regulated activity of cation channels play a role. Because TRPC3 accounts for most of the constitutive cation entry in HCAECs and also significantly contributes to regulated influx (Vazquez and Putney 2006; Smedlund and Vazquez 2008) it is likely that TRPC3 represents a component of the signaling underlying VCAM-1-dependent monocyte transmigration.

1.2 Role of macrophage survival and apoptosis in lesion development

As mentioned above, monocyte recruitment to the subintima is a fundamental event in atherogenesis (Linton and Fazio 2003). Transmigration of the monocyte to the subendothelial milieu is followed by its differentiation into macrophage, which is now recognized as a key cell component in determining lesion progression and fate. Lesional macrophages engulf modified lipoproteins, mostly oxLDL, becoming lipid-laden macrophages; this results in a lipid overload of the macrophage which imposes a significant stress to the endoplasmic reticulum (ER), mostly due to accumulation of free cholesterol. Consequently, an irreversible ER-stress response is triggered leading to macrophage apoptosis. Indeed, the majority of apoptotic lesional cells are macrophages (Linton and Fazio 2003; Tabas 2010). Clearance of apoptotic cells is conducted by resident phagocytes, which phagocytose the apoptotic macrophage and exit the lesion site through lymphatic circulation or by migrating back to the blood stream. This clearing process, known as efferocytosis, is crucial in preventing the apoptotic cells from dying in situ which would otherwise lead to post-apoptotic necrosis and the subsequent exacerbation of the inflammatory response. Notably, the balance between production of apoptotic macrophages and their clearance by efferocytosis constitutes a defining factor in lesion formation, remodeling and progression ((Tabas 2010) and references therein). For instance, macrophage apoptosis in early lesions is beneficial in that reduces lesion cellularity and size and plaque progression (Arai, Shelton et al. 2005; Liu, Thewke et al. 2005; Babaev, Chew et al. 2008; Wang, Liu et al. 2008) while increased apoptosis in advanced plaques enlarges the necrotic core and promotes plaque instability (Linton, Babaev et al. 1999; Seimon, Wang et al. 2009; Yancey, Blakemore et al. 2010). Thus, altered expression and/or deregulation of signaling proteins directly or indirectly involved in macrophage survival/apoptosis can have a significant impact on lesion progression.

2. TRPC channels

2.1 Structure, function and role in cardiovascular disease

Calcium influx has long been recognized as an essential component of physiological and pathophysiological events. Changes in intracellular Ca^{2+} concentration that follow Ca^{2+} influx through plasma membrane Ca^{2+} channels not only modulate a myriad of Ca^{2+}-dependent signaling pathways but also affect the driving force for other ions by modifying the membrane potential. Ca^{2+} influx is of particular importance in vascular function and cardiovascular disease, where the effects of Ca^{2+} influx can be seen throughout the entire cardiovascular system, in smooth muscle and endothelial cells, cardiomyocytes, lymphocytes, monocytes, macrophages, among other cell types. Of the many Ca^{2+} channels identified in the last half century, Transient Receptor Potential Canonical (TRPC) channels are recognized as major contributors to Ca^{2+} influx and play a role in various physiological and pathological states. The TRPC family belongs to the TRP superfamily of ion channel forming proteins, and are the most closely related to the founding member *Drosophila* TRP protein (Vazquez, Wedel et al. 2004). TRPC proteins can be grouped into four subgroups, TRPC1, TRPC2 (a pseudogene in humans), TRPC3/6/7 and TRPC4/5 (Trebak, Vazquez et al. 2003; Vazquez, Wedel et al. 2004).

Despite some structural variation across the subgroups of the TRPC family, there are several structural motifs which are conserved throughout members. The cytoplasmic N- and C-termini are separated by six transmembrane domains (TM1-TM6), with a re-entry loop between TM5 and TM6 which is thought to line the wall of the channel pore ((Vazquez, Wedel et al. 2004) and references therein). Other shared structural motifs of TRPCs include ankyrin repeats and a putative caveolin binding site on the N-terminus, and on the C-terminus the so called TRP signature motif (EWKFAR), a proline-rich motif and a calmodulin/IP_3 receptor binding (CIRB) site; predicted coiled-coil regions are present on both N- and C-termini, and in TRPC4 and 5, an extended C-terminus includes a PDZ binding motif (Vazquez, Wedel et al. 2004). An examination of the function of the TRPC cytoplasmic motifs hints at mechanisms of channel activation and signaling pathways. For instance, ankyrin repeats form specialized structures with the repeated units stacking against one another to form a protein-binding interface; this allows for interaction with other proteins and seems to play a role in channel trafficking to the plasma membrane. Coiled-coil regions are commonly associated with oligomerization and may contribute to formation of specific homo- and heterotetramers of TRPCs or association with other proteins containing coiled-coil motifs (Vazquez, Wedel et al. 2004). The proline-rich motif and CIRB region have also been associated to interactions with different signaling molecules, with variations existing throughout individual TRPC members. The mechanisms underlying activation and regulation of TRPC channels has been matter of extensive research and debate, with efforts mostly centered at elucidating whether they form store-operated (activated by mere depletion of internal Ca^{2+} stores) or non-store-operated channels (discussed in (Trebak, Vazquez et al. 2003; Vazquez, Wedel et al. 2004; Smyth, DeHaven et al. 2006). Whereas some properties of TRPC channels observed in heterologus expression systems correlate well with those of TRPCs expressed under native conditions, many others do not. It is imperative to elucidate the mechanism/s underlying regulation of TRPC channels in their native environment, as this would greatly contribute to assign definitive roles to individual TRPC members. Nevertheless, equally important to comprehend their role in cardiovascular physiology and disease is to identify cellular and molecular events which, directly or indirectly, may rely upon appropriate TRPC function.

TRPC proteins are ubiquitously expressed throughout the cardiovascular system and hematopoietic cells and all members have been implicated not only in physiological cardiovascular functions but most importantly, in the pathogenesis of cardiovascular disease. Indeed, TRPCs have been implicated in a variety of processes known to be critical in cardiovascular pathology such as endothelial dysfunction, vascular relaxation, oxidative stress, and angiogenesis among others. This has recently been reviewed by us (Tano, Smedlund et al. 2010) and others (Abramowitz and Birnbaumer 2009) and the reader is referred to those for further details. The following sections focus on recent findings that specifically point to a potential role of TRPC3 in atherorelevant processes.

3. Participation of TRPC3 in atherorelevant molecular/cellular processes

3.1 TRPC3 and regulated expression of VCAM-1

Calcium signaling is an important component of the mechanism by which several inflammatory factors induce VCAM-1 expression. For instance, changes in intracellular Ca^{2+} associated to Ca^{2+} release from internal stores have been linked to the ability of Substance P to induce VCAM-1 subsequent to Ca^{2+}-dependent activation of NFAT and NFκB in microvascular endothelium (Quinlan, Naik et al. 1999), and of β_2-microglobulin to induce VCAM-1 expression in synovial fibroblasts (Chen, O'Neill et al. 2002). In the human coronary endothelial cells HCAEC, Ca^{2+} mobilization contributes to lipoprotein A- and ATP-dependent VCAM-1 expression (Allen, Khan et al. 1998; Seye, Yu et al. 2003). Nevertheless, the specific role of Ca^{2+} influx in VCAM-1 expression was never directly examined before. In recent work we specifically explored the impact of Ca^{2+} influx in regulated expression of VCAM-1 in HCAECs (Vazquez and Putney 2006; Smedlund and Vazquez 2008). Our studies demonstrated that, whereas HCAECs express all members of the TRPC family, only TRPC3 forms, or is part of, endogenous Ca^{2+}-permeable channels that contribute to ATP stimulated Ca^{2+} influx. Such mechanism occurs downstream ATP-dependent activation of purinergic $P2Y_2$ receptors and results in upregulation of VCAM-1 total and plasma membrane associated levels with subsequent increase in monocyte adhesion (Smedlund and Vazquez 2008). This represented the first direct indication that Ca^{2+} influx plays a role in the signaling driving VCAM-1 expression and that TRPC3 forms native Ca^{2+}-permeable channels whose activity is fundamental within the signaling underlying VCAM-1 expression and monocyte recruitment. Because TRPC3 is the only TRPC member whose high constitutive, non-regulated activity has been shown to operate under either heterologous or native expression conditions (Trebak, Vazquez et al. 2003) those findings raised the question whether TRPC3 contributes to expression of VCAM-1 through regulated activity, constitutive activity, or both. In a follow up study using TNFα to induce VCAM-1 expression and a combination of real-time fluorescence and silencing RNA approaches, we conclusively showed that it is the constitutive function of TRPC3 which mediates most of the Ca^{2+} influx required for regulated expression of VCAM-1 in HCAECs (Smedlund and Vazquez 2008).

In most endothelial cells VCAM-1 expression is regulated, at the transcriptional level, by nuclear factor kappa B (NFkB)(Zhang 2008) and we have shown that this is also the case in HCAECs. NFkB activation involves its release from the inhibitory protein IkBα and then the subsequent translocation of NFkB to the nucleus where it modulates transcriptional activity of target genes. Release of NFkB from IkBα is preceded by phosphorylation of IkBα by IkBα kinases (IKKs) followed by its ubiquitination and proteasomal degradation (Tergaonkar 2006). Because in most cells types examined so far NFkB activation depends, directly or indirectly, on Ca^{2+} influx, and TNFα-induced VCAM-1 requires constitutive Ca^{2+} influx (Smedlund, Tano et al. 2010), we examined whether TRPC3, through its constitutive function, contributes to the mechanism by which NFkB modulates VCAM-1 expression in HCAECs. Interestingly, our studies showed that knockdown of TRPC3 in HCAECs drastically reduced the ability of TNFα to induce phosphorylation of IkBα and its upstream regulator IKKβ (Smedlund, Tano et al. 2010), and this correlated with an inhibition of IkBα degradation. These findings indicated for the first time that TRPC3 constitutive function is an obligatory component in the signaling driving TNFα-dependent activation of NFkB. In addition, we showed that TRPC3-mediated Ca^{2+} entry is fundamental to activate the calmodulin (CAM)/calmodulin kinase II (CAMKII) axis in a NADPH oxidase-dependent manner, and this signaling axis in turn activates NFkB (Smedlund, Tano et al. 2010). Importantly, our studies brought about a conceptually novel perspective on the role of TRPCs in cardiovascular disease, as they underscored for the first time, the potential pathological impact of upregulated expression of a TRPC channel endowed with high constitutive activity and how this may relate with pathological Ca^{2+}-dependent signaling, independently of the canonical pathway driven by receptor stimulation. This is of particular interest to the field, as in those instances where TRPCs participate in mechanisms associated to inflammatory vascular disease (reviewed by us in (Tano, Smedlund et al. 2010)) their contribution relates to regulated, or receptor-dependent channel function, rather than constitutive activity. In vivo studies are underway using mouse models of atherosclerosis with genetically manipulated levels of endothelial TRPC3 in order to determine the potential impact of TRPC3 expression and constitutive function in the context of the molecular and cellular events that lead to atherosclerotic lesion development in the intact vessel.

3.2 TRPC3 and macrophage survival

As stated earlier (section 2.2) the balance between apoptotic macrophages and their clearance by resident phagocytes at the lesion site is determinant in the progression of the atherosclerotic lesion. Within this context, signaling events that modulate the survival rate of the macrophage have a tremendous impact on such balance, provided efferocytic properties of resident phagocytes remain unaffected. Recent studies in our laboratory have implicated non-regulated, constitutive Ca^{2+} influx in the signaling associated with macrophage survival. Two major pathways are essential for the survival of macrophages in the atherosclerotic lesions: the phosphatidylinositol-3-kinase (PI3K)/AKT axis and the NFkB route. In the PI3K/AKT pathway, macrophage survival signals (v.g., insulin-like growth factor, prostaglandin E2) acting through either receptor tyrosine kinases or G-protein coupled receptors induce activation of PI3K in the plasma membrane and the subsequent generation of 3′-phosphorylated phosphoinositides such as phosphatidylinositol 3, 4 bisphosphate/3,4,5 trisphosphate. These phosphoinositides allow for recruitment and activation of PDK-1 which then leads to full activation of AKT kinase. One of the major mechanisms of AKT-dependent survival takes place through AKT-mediated phosphorylation of the pro-apoptotic protein BAD, a member of the Bcl-2 family. Upon AKT-mediated phosphorylation, BAD releases the anti-apoptotic proteins Bcl-2 and Bcl-x, preventing mitochondrial release of cytochrome c and thus progression of the mitochondrial apoptotic pathway (Datta, Brunet et al. 1999). As for macrophage survival through the transcription factor NFκB, it is known that activation of NFkB exquisitely regulates the transcriptional status of several survival genes. Both of the survival pathways described above are highly active in THP-1 derived macrophages (TDMs) upon exposure to the atherorelevant cytokine TNFα (Tano and Vazquez 2011). Notably, maneuvers that prevent constitutive Ca^{2+} entry through Ca^{2+} permeable channels drastically reduce the phosphorylation of IkBα, AKT and its downstream target BAD, with the subsequent increase in macrophage apoptotic rate (Tano and Vazquez 2011). In addition, when TDMs are pre-treated with pharmacological inhibitors of CAM and CAMKII, activation of survival signaling is prevented as efficiently as blockade of constitutive Ca^{2+} influx does. These findings indicated for the first time that activation of macrophage survival pathways depends, to a significant extent, on constitutive Ca^{2+} influx presumably through a mechanism involving the CAM/CAMKII axis (Tano and Vazquez 2011). A particularly interesting observation derived from those studies was that inhibition of PI3K function completely abrogated TNFα-dependent NFkB activation suggesting that the PI3K/AKT axis exerts a regulatory action on the NFkB pathway. Operation of such crosstalk has been demonstrated in cell types other than macrophages, where AKT-dependent transactivation of NFkB acts as an alternative AKT-dependent anti-apoptotic route independently of the AKT/BAD axis (Romashkova and Makarov 1999; Madrid, Wang et al. 2000; Bai, Ueno et al. 2009). In summary, our studies suggest that in human macrophages a CAM/CAMKII axis links constitutive Ca^{2+} influx to activation of AKT, which then serves as a signaling node to promote survival through NFκB and/or phosphorylation of BAD.

Macrophages from both human and mouse origin express TRPC3, and TRPC3 constitutive function has been shown to be operational in different cell types from these two mammalian species. These attributes make TRPC3 a great candidate to mediate the constitutive Ca^{2+} influx that supports the macrophage survival mechanisms described above. We indeed examined this possibility in recent studies that made use of bone-marrow derived macrophages obtained from mice globally deficient in TRPC3 (Tano, Smedlund et al. 2011). Macrophages derived from TRPC3 deficient bone marrow ($TRPC3^{-/-}$) exhibited a significant reduction in constitutive cation influx compared to $TRPC3^{+/+}$ cells (Tano, Smedlund et al. 2011). Most importantly, the number of apoptotic macrophages in response to TNFα was significantly higher in $TRPC3^{-/-}$ cultures than in those of $TRPC3^{+/+}$ macrophages, indicating a diminished survival in macrophages lacking TRPC3. Importantly, these observations correlated very well with the activation status of survival signaling: the phosphorylation of IkBα, AKT and BAD was severely reduced in $TRPC3^{-/-}$ macrophages (Tano, Smedlund et al. 2011). Altogether, these findings indicated that TRPC3 has an obligatory role in macrophage survival and that TRPC3 is likely to mediate the constitutive Ca^{2+} influx required for proper operation of survival signaling.

As described above, clearance of apoptotic macrophages by resident phagocytes at the lesion site is fundamental for appropriate inflammation resolution, and is a major factor in determining lesion cellularity. By means of an *in vitro* efferocytosis assay in which $TRPC3^{+/+}$ and $TRPC3^{-/-}$ were used as either phagocytes or apoptotic cells, we observed that the phagocytic function of $TRPC3^{-/-}$ macrophages is drastically impaired when compared to that of $TRPC3^{+/+}$ phagocytes; interestingly, apoptotic $TRPC3^{-/-}$ cells seem to be poor substrates for phagocytosis regardless of the phagocyte's TRPC3 expression status (Tano, Smedlund et al. 2011). Although additional studies are required to clarify TRPC3's role in efferocytosis, these findings suggest a critical requirement for TRPC3 within the signaling associated to phagocytic activity and/or cell-cell recognition processes that underlie efferocytosis.

4. TRPC3 as a prospective target in atherosclerosis: Roadmap of an exciting TRiP

The rapid advance in elucidating signaling mechanisms associated to atherogenesis was enthusiastically perceived as an opportunity to develop anti-inflammatory strategies to manage the disease. However, the multifactorial nature of atherosclerosis makes such therapeutic strategies, often aimed at interfering on single targets, of limited efficacy and it is likely that multiple targeting is necessary to achieve clinically significant outcomes (Yonekawa and Harlan 2005; Preiss and Sattar 2007; Recio-Mayoral, Kaski et al. 2007). This is not surprising if we take in consideration the multifactorial nature of atherosclerosis and the diverse repertoire of signaling molecules and cell types that contribute to its pathogenesis. In that context, identifying new components of signaling events linked to monocyte recruitment and/or modulation of macrophage survival/apoptosis at the lesion site is of fundamental importance to move forward in the search for additional potential targets that could make those alternative therapeutic strategies a reality. Furthering our knowledge on the potential new roles of TRPC3, as well as other TRPC members, in atherogenesis can make a significant contribution to the search for new targets for the disease. Although ubiquitously expressed throughout tissues, TRPC3 on endothelial or macrophage surface could be used as a molecular target of relatively easy access for therapeutic and/or diagnostic purposes or may be exploited as a marker in non-invasive imaging, as it has been applied to other cell surface proteins (Kaufmann, Carr et al.; Saraste, Nekolla et al. 2009). The potential advantages of TRPC3 vs. traditional channel blockers as a prospective target for atherosclerosis has recently been discussed by us (Vazquez 2011). The exploration of TRPC3 as an atherorelevant signaling molecule is at its infancy, and several additional studies will be required to determine the impact of TRPC3 expression/function on atherorelevant events. The generation and characterization of new mouse models of atherosclerosis with genetically manipulated levels of TRPC3 in the atherorelevant cell or tissue of interest (i.e., conditional knockouts or transgenics) will be a unique contribution to that goal.

5. References

Abramowitz, J. and L. Birnbaumer (2009). "Physiology and pathophysiology of canonical transient receptor potential channels." FASEB J. 23(2): 297-328.

Allen, S., S. Khan, et al. (1998). "Expression of adhesion molecules by Lp(a): a potential novel mechanism for its atherogenicity." FASEB J. 12(15): 1765-1776.

Arai, S., J. M. Shelton, et al. (2005). "A role for the apoptosis inhibitory factor AIM/Sp[alpha]/Api6 in atherosclerosis development." Cell metabolism 1(3): 201-213.

Armesilla, A. L., E. Lorenzo, et al. (1999). "Vascular Endothelial Growth Factor Activates Nuclear Factor of Activated T Cells in Human Endothelial Cells: a Role for Tissue Factor Gene Expression." Mol. Cell. Biol. 19(3): 2032-2043.

Babaev, V. R., J. D. Chew, et al. (2008). "Macrophage EP4 Deficiency Increases Apoptosis and Suppresses Early Atherosclerosis." Cell metabolism 8(6): 492-501.

Bai, D., L. Ueno, et al. (2009). "Akt-mediated regulation of NFκB and the essentialness of NFκB for the oncogenicity of PI3K and Akt." International Journal of Cancer 125(12): 2863-2870.

Chen, N. X., K. D. O'Neill, et al. (2002). "Signal transduction of β2m-induced expression of VCAM-1 and COX-2 in synovial fibroblasts." Kidney International 61(2): 414-424.

Chuluyan, E. H., L. Osborn, et al. (1995). "Domains 1 and 4 of vascular cell adhesion molecule-1 (CD106) both support very late activation antigen-4 (CD49d/CD29)-dependent monocyte transendothelial migration." J Immunol 155: 3135-3144.

Cook-Mills, J. (2002). "VCAM-1 signals during lymphocyte migration: role of reactive oxygen species " Mol Immunol 39: 499-508.

Cook-Mills, J., J. Johnson, et al. (2004). "Calcium mobilization and Rac1 activation are required for VCAM-1 (vascular cell adhesion molecule-1) stimulation of NADPH oxidase activity." Biochem J 378: 539-547.

Cybulsky, M. I., K. Iiyama, et al. (2001). "A major role for VCAM-1, but not ICAM-1, in early atherosclerosis." J. Clin. Invest. 107(10): 1255-1262.

Dansky, H. M., C. B. Barlow, et al. (2001). "Adhesion of Monocytes to Arterial Endothelium and Initiation of Atherosclerosis Are Critically Dependent on Vascular Cell Adhesion Molecule-1 Gene Dosage." Arterioscler Thromb Vasc Biol 21(10): 1662-1667.

Datta, S. R., A. Brunet, et al. (1999). "Cellular survival: a play in three Akts." Genes & Development 13(22): 2905-2927.

Deem, T. L., H. Abdala-Valencia, et al. (2007). "VCAM-1 Activation of Endothelial Cell Protein Tyrosine Phosphatase 1B." J Immunol 178(6): 3865-3873.

Galkina, E. and K. Ley (2007). "Vascular Adhesion Molecules in Atherosclerosis." Arterioscler Thromb Vasc Biol: 107.149179.

Hansson, G. K. (2005). "Inflammation, Atherosclerosis, and Coronary Artery Disease." N Engl J Med 352(16): 1685-1695.

Iiyama, K., L. Hajra, et al. (1999). "Patterns of Vascular Cell Adhesion Molecule-1 and Intercellular Adhesion Molecule-1 Expression in Rabbit and Mouse Atherosclerotic Lesions and at Sites Predisposed to Lesion Formation." Circ Res 85(2): 199-207.

Isabelle Ricard, M. D. P. G. D. (1997). "Clustering the adhesion molecules VLA-4 (CD49d/CD29) in Jurkat T cells or VCAM-1 (CD106) in endothelial (ECV 304) cells activates the phosphoinositide pathway and triggers Ca mobilization." European Journal of Immunology 27(6): 1530-1538.

Kaufmann, B. A., C. L. Carr, et al. Molecular Imaging of the Initial Inflammatory Response in Atherosclerosis: Implications for Early Detection of Disease. [Miscellaneous Article], Arteriosclerosis, Thrombosis & Vascular Biology January 2010;30(1):54-59.

Kim, I., S.-O. Moon, et al. (2001). "Vascular Endothelial Growth Factor Expression of Intercellular Adhesion Molecule 1 (ICAM-1), Vascular Cell Adhesion Molecule 1 (VCAM-1), and E-selectin through Nuclear Factor-kappa B Activation in Endothelial Cells." J. Biol. Chem. 276(10): 7614-7620.

Linton, M. F., V. R. Babaev, et al. (1999). "A Direct Role for the Macrophage Low Density Lipoprotein Receptor in Atherosclerotic Lesion Formation." J. Biol. Chem. 274(27): 19204-19210.

Linton, M. F. and S. Fazio (2003). "Macrophages, inflammation, and atherosclerosis." Int J Obes Relat Metab Disord 27(S3): S35-S40.

Liu, J., D. P. Thewke, et al. (2005). "Reduced Macrophage Apoptosis Is Associated With Accelerated Atherosclerosis in Low-Density Lipoprotein Receptor-Null Mice." Arterioscler Thromb Vasc Biol 25(1): 174-179.

Madrid, L. V., C.-Y. Wang, et al. (2000). "Akt Suppresses Apoptosis by Stimulating the Transactivation Potential of the RelA/p65 Subunit of NF-kappa B." Mol. Cell. Biol. 20(5): 1626-1638.

Matheny, H. E., T. L. Deem, et al. (2000). "Lymphocyte Migration Through Monolayers of Endothelial Cell Lines Involves VCAM-1 Signaling Via Endothelial Cell NADPH Oxidase" J Immunol 164(12): 6550-6559.

Preiss, D. J. and N. Sattar (2007). "Vascular cell adhesion molecule-1: a viable therapeutic target for atherosclerosis?" International Journal of Clinical Practice 61(4): 697-701.

Quinlan, K. L., S. M. Naik, et al. (1999). "Substance P Activates Coincident NF-AT- and NF-{kappa}B-Dependent Adhesion Molecule Gene Expression in Microvascular Endothelial Cells Through Intracellular Calcium Mobilization" J Immunol 163(10): 5656-5665.

Recio-Mayoral, A., J. C. Kaski, et al. (2007). "Clinical Trials Update from the European Society of Cardiology Congress in Vienna, 2007: PROSPECT, EVEREST, ARISE, ALOFT, FINESSE, Prague-8, CARESS in MI and ACUITY." Cardiovascular Drugs and Therapy 21(6): 459-465.

Romashkova, J. A. and S. S. Makarov (1999). "NF-[kappa]B is a target of AKT in anti-apoptotic PDGF signalling." Nature 401(6748): 86-90.

Saraste, A., S. G. Nekolla, et al. (2009). "Cardiovascular molecular imaging: an overview." Cardiovasc Res 83(4): 643-652.

Seimon, T. A., Y. Wang, et al. (2009). "Macrophage deficiency of p38Î± MAPK promotes apoptosis and plaque necrosis in advanced atherosclerotic lesions in mice." The Journal of Clinical Investigation 119(4): 886-898.

Seye, C. I., N. Yu, et al. (2003). "The P2Y2 Nucleotide Receptor Mediates UTP-induced Vascular Cell Adhesion Molecule-1 Expression in Coronary Artery Endothelial Cells." J. Biol. Chem. 278(27): 24960-24965.

Smedlund, K., J.-Y. Tano, et al. (2010). "The Constitutive Function of Native TRPC3 Channels Modulates Vascular Cell Adhesion Molecule-1 Expression in Coronary Endothelial Cells Through Nuclear Factor {kappa}B Signaling." Circ Res 106(9): 1479-1488.

Smedlund, K. and G. Vazquez (2008). "Involvement of Native TRPC3 Proteins in ATP-Dependent Expression of VCAM-1 and Monocyte Adherence in Coronary Artery Endothelial Cells." Arterioscler Thromb Vasc Biol 28(11): 2049-2055.

Smyth, J. T., W. I. DeHaven, et al. (2006). "Emerging perspectives in store-operated Ca2+ entry: Roles of Orai, Stim and TRP." Biochimica et Biophysica Acta (BBA) - Molecular Cell Research 1763(11): 1147-1160.

Tabas, I. (2010). "Macrophage death and defective inflammation resolution in atherosclerosis." Nat Rev Immunol 10(1): 36-46.

Tano, J.-Y., K. Smedlund, et al. (2011). "Impairment of survival signaling and efferocytosis in TRPC3-deficient macrophages." Biochemical and Biophysical Research Communications 410(3): 643-647.

Tano, J.-Y. and G. Vazquez (2011). "Requirement for non-regulated, constitutive calcium influx in macrophage survival signaling." Biochemical and Biophysical Research Communications 407(2): 432-437.

Tano, J. Y., K. Smedlund, et al. (2010). "Endothelial TRPC3/6/7 proteins at the edge of cardiovascular disease." Cardiovascular & Hematological Agents in Medicinal Chemistry 8(1): 76-86.

Tergaonkar, V. (2006). "NF[kappa]B pathway: A good signaling paradigm and therapeutic target." The International Journal of Biochemistry & Cell Biology 38(10): 1647-1653.

Trebak, M., G. Vazquez, et al. (2003). "The TRPC3/6/7 subfamily of cation channels." Cell Calcium 33(5-6): 451-61.

van Wetering, S., N. van den Berk, et al. (2003). "VCAM-1-mediated Rac signaling controls endothelial cell-cell contacts and leukocyte transmigration 10.1152/ajpcell.00048.2003." Am J Physiol Cell Physiol 285(2): C343-352.

Vazquez, G. (2011). "TRPC channels as prospective targets in atherosclerosis: terra incognita." Frontiers in Bioscience In press.

Vazquez, G. and J. W. Putney (2006). "Role of Canonical Transient Receptor Potential Channels (TRPC) in Receptor-Dependent Regulation of Vascular Cell Adhesion Molecule-1 In Human Coronary Artery Endothelium." Art. Thr. Vasc. Biol. 26: 93-94.

Vazquez, G., B. J. Wedel, et al. (2004). "The mammalian TRPC cation channels." Biochimica et Biophysica Acta (BBA) - Molecular Cell Research 1742(1-3): 21-36.

Virmani, R., A. P. Burke, et al. (2006). "Pathology of the Vulnerable Plaque." Journal of the American College of Cardiology 47(8, Supplement 1): C13-C18.

Wang, Z., B. Liu, et al. (2008). "Phospholipase C Î²3 deficiency leads to macrophage hypersensitivity to apoptotic induction and reduction of atherosclerosis in mice." The Journal of Clinical Investigation 118(1): 195-204.

Yancey, P. G., J. Blakemore, et al. (2010). "Macrophage LRP-1 Controls Plaque Cellularity by Regulating Efferocytosis and Akt Activation." Arterioscler Thromb Vasc Biol 30(4): 787-795.

Yao, Y.-G. and E. J. Duh (2004). "VEGF selectively induces Down syndrome critical region 1 gene expression in endothelial cells: a mechanism for feedback regulation of angiogenesis?" Biochemical and Biophysical Research Communications 321(3): 648-656.

Yonekawa, K. and J. M. Harlan (2005). "Targeting leukocyte integrins in human diseases." J Leuk Biol 77(129-140).

Zhang, C. (2008). "The role of inflammatory cytokines in endothelial dysfunction." Basic Research in Cardiology 103(5): 398-406.

Zola, H., B. Swart, et al. (2005). "CD molecules 2005: human cell differentiation molecules." Blood 106(9): 3123-3126.

5

Hypoxia-Regulated Pro- and Anti-Angiogenesis in the Heart

Angela Messmer-Blust and Jian Li
CardioVascular Institute
Beth Israel Deaconess Medical Center /Harvard Medical School
USA

1. Introduction

Maintenance of oxygen homeostasis is essential for the survival of all multicellular organisms. Specialized chemoreceptor cells can sense increased (hyperoxia) or decreased (hypoxia) oxygen levels and subsequently regulate cardiovascular and ventilatory rates. Additionally, all nucleated cells sense and respond to reduced O_2 availability acutely, through the activation of proteins, and chronically, through the regulation of gene transcription. Decreased oxygen levels stimulate the oxygen delivery system and provide mechanisms to activate cell death or survival pathways, depending on the context of the hypoxia signal. Several responses are developed by cells and tissues faced with a hypoxic challenge, particularly in the heart: 1) increased ventilation and cardiac output, 2) a switch from aerobic to anaerobic metabolism, 3) promotion of improved vascularization via angiogenesis, and 4) enhanced O_2 carrying capacity of the blood. Hypoxia occurs in physiological situations such as during embryonic development, as well as in pathological conditions such as ischemia, wound healing, and cancer.

Angiogenesis is the process by which blood microvessels are formed from existing ones, which is required for development and occurs in pathological conditions. It is also important for reducing myocardial hypoxia due to coronary and ischemic heart disease. In myocardial infarction or chronic ischemic heart disease, angiogenesis responds to tissue hypoxia by new vessel formation, which diminishes myocardial ischemia. Nevertheless, physiological angiogenesis is usually insufficient to re-establish an adequate blood supply to the myocardium, which decreases its proper functioning. Therapeutic angiogenesis in the heart aims at increasing new vessel formation in ischemic myocardium and thus improving myocardial function by increasing blood flow (oxygen and nutrient supply). This may contribute to preventing heart failure and sudden cardiac death. However, hypoxia also stimulates several angiogenic inhibitors in the heart while pro-angiogenic factors are increased. This spontaneous balance reaction is one of the causes for the failure of angiogenic therapy for ischemia heart diseases. Unfortunately, the area of anti-angiogenesis in the heart has remained unclear. This chapter reviews the effects of both angiogenic and anti-angiogenic reactions in the heart dependent on the endothelial response to hypoxic /ischemic stimulation.

2. Hypoxia-regulated angiogenesis in the myocardium

2.1 HIF1-α-mediated angiogenesis

Hypoxia-stimulated myocardial angiogenesis has well been studied in past decades. When the myocardium is deprived of blood, a process of ischemia, infarction, and myocardial remodeling is initiated. Hypoxia-inducible factor 1 (HIF-1) is a transcriptional activator of vascular endothelial growth factor (VEGF) and is critical for initiating early cellular responses to hypoxia in specimens of human heart tissue (Lee *et al.*, 2000). Upon initiation of the hypoxic signal, HIF1-α translocates to the nucleus, dimerizes with HIF1-β to form the HIF-1 complex and induces the expression of its transcriptional targets via binding to hypoxia-responsive elements (HREs) (Chilov *et al.*, 1999). HREs are present in many angiogenic genes, such as VEGF, angiopoietin-2, VEGF receptors (Flt1 and KDR), and neuropilin-1 (Hickey and Simon, 2006; Simons, 2005). Hypoxia can up-regulate these angiogenic molecules by several mechanisms, including direct transcriptional activation by HIFs or indirect up-regulation by HIF-induced molecules. In addition, previous studies suggested that hypoxia/reoxygenation promotes myocardial angiogenesis via an NF kappa B-dependent mechanism in a rat model of chronic myocardial infarction (Sasaki *et al.*, 2001).

Additional transcription factors induced by hypoxia, such as Related Transcription Enhancer Factor-1 (RTEF-1) and early growth response 1 (EGR-1), can both target VEGF to enhance angiogenesis (Shie *et al.*, 2004; Yan *et al.*, 2000). Additional angiogenic growth factors such as IGF are also induced by hypoxia, but can signal through a HIF-1-independent pathway (Slomiany and Rosenzweig, 2006).

Moreover, hypoxia is associated with virtually all forms of vascular disorders, such as coronary and peripheral arterial diseases, including stroke, myocardial and limb ischemia; lung disorders; and diabetes (Fong, 2008). The post-ischemia neovascular response is largely driven by hypoxia-induced up-regulation and stabilization of VEGF, initiated in part by HIF1. In concert with enhanced expression of VEGF and its receptors, other growth factors and cellular receptors, including placental growth factor (PlGF), basic fibroblast growth factor (bFGF), IL-8 and ETS-1 are also differentially regulated in highly specific spatio-temporal expression patterns, orchestrated to acutely minimize parenchymal damage and to optimize subsequent healing and recovery. Physiological stresses such as hypoxia are regulated by a complex balance of both stimulatory and inhibitory signals that promote or inhibit angiogenesis. Specifically, understanding the role and regulation of genes during angiogenesis is becoming increasingly important in elucidating the compensatory hypoxic response.

2.2 Hypoxia upregulated microRNA-mediated angiogenesis

Recent studies have revealed important roles for microRNAs (miRNAs, miRs) in regulating endothelial cell function, especially in angiogenesis. miRNAs are a class of conserved non-coding small RNAs, with the ability to repress gene expression post-transcriptionally by targeting 3'-untranslated regions (3'UTRs) of mRNAs. Almost 700 miRNAs have been identified in humans, and the estimated number of miRNA genes is as high as 1000 in the human genome (Berezikov *et al.*, 2005). Current evidence demonstrates that miRNAs are important regulators of angiogenesis as well as cardiovascular development and disease.

Pro-angiogenic miRs (angiomiRs) regulate angiogenesis, for example, by targeting negative regulators in angiogenic signaling pathways, while anti-angiomiRs inhibit angiogenesis by targeting positive regulators of angiogenesis. Let7-f, miR-27b, mir-130a, miR-424, miR-296, and miR-210 have been shown to be pro-angiomiRs (Fish *et al.*, 2008; Ghosh *et al.*, 2010; Urbich *et al.*, 2008; Wurdinger *et al.*, 2008).

Let-7f and miR-27b exert pro-angiogenic effects as evidenced by the blockade of *in vitro* angiogenesis with 2'-O-methyl oligonucleotide inhibitors (Kuehbacher *et al.*, 2008), while miR-210 is induced by hypoxia in endothelial cells and overexpression enhanced the formation of capillary-like structures. Additionally, overexpression of miR-210 enhanced VEGF-driven migration of normoxic endothelial cells, whereas inhibition of miR-210 decreased tube formation and migration (Fasanaro *et al.*, 2008).

Endothelial overexpression of miR-424 increased proliferation and migration, as a result of autocrine stimulation by HIF-1α–driven VEGF secretion. In addition to the *in vitro* changes in angiogenesis, miR-424 levels were significantly increased during vascular remodeling *in vivo*. Changes in miR-424 were observed in models of experimental myocardial infarction and PAD. Interestingly, the rodent homologue of miR-424, miR-322, was upregulated in peri-infarct cardiac tissues in rats following LAD ligation. Left ventricular tissues harvested away from the infarcted area also showed significantly higher levels of mu-miR-322. Ischemia seems to activate mu-miR-322 expression in the tissues surrounding the site of hypoxic stress as a survival mechanism to initiate collateral vessel growth (Ghosh *et al.* 2010).

Neoangiogenesis is essential for cardiac repair following myocardial infaction, when collateral vessels form at the site of the infarct and can maintain blood flow to ischemic tissue. The endothelial-specific miR-126 plays a role in neoangiogenesis following myocardial infarction and in the maintenance of vascular integrity. miR-126 potentiates MAP kinase signaling downstream of VEGF and FGF via Spred-1, an intracellular inhibitor of the Ras/MAP kinase pathway. miR-126 over-expression relieves the repressive influence of Spred-1 on the signaling pathways activated by VEGF and FGF, inducing angiogenesis. Elevation of miR-126 expression in the ischemic myocardium could enhance cardiac repair (Wang *et al.*, 2008).

3. Therapeutic angiogenesis in the myocardium

In coronary artery disease (CAD), progressive occlusion of arteries can lead to collateral vessel development to supply the ischemic tissue. In spite of this, angiogenesis via neovascularization is not always sufficient as evidenced by the large number of revascularization procedures performed annually. The lack of a sufficient angiogenic response in part may be related to both the decreased production of angiogenic factors as well as a natural negative feedback by the upregulation of anti-angiogenic molecules. Therapeutic angiogenesis involves improving blood flow to ischemic tissue by the induction of neovascularization by angiogenic agents administered as recombinant protein or by gene transfer. To circumvent insufficient collateral vessel development, administration of recombinant protein or the genes that encode these proteins have been used as techniques of angiogenic therapy in preclinical and clinical trials. Yet, results of these trials have only been slightly beneficial for patients.

4. Anti-angiogenic genes in response to hypoxia

While hypoxia-induced VEGF initiates angiogenesis, it also up-regulates expression of molecules within the endothelium that act as negative feedback regulators to modulate excessive vascular sprouting and endothelial cell proliferation (Messmer-Blust *et al.*, 2009). Additionally, a previous report by An et al. demonstrated that Response Gene to Complement (RGC)-32 is another important VEGF-inducible gene that serves as a negative regulator of hypoxia-induced angiogenesis. RGC-32 expression was significantly increased under hypoxic conditions. Hypoxic induction of RGC-32 was also mediated by HIF-1α □at both the transcriptional and posttranscriptional levels (An *et al.*, 2009). While HIF-1-induced RGS5 was not VEGF-mediated (Jin *et al.*, 2009), RGC-32 expression was significantly increased by VEGF but not by factors including TNF-α, FGF2 and IL-1β (An *et al.*, 2009). Unlike genes such as COX-2 (Wu *et al.*, 2003), RGC-32 did not follow the canonical VEGF-induced angiogenic pathway. Overexpression of RGC-32 destabilized vascular structure formation *in vitro* by down-regulating FGF-2 and cyclin E, which caused negative feedback to VEGF activation. Additionally, when angiogenesis was examined *in vivo* in a mouse model, RGC-32 drastically inhibited VEGF-induced angiogenesis in matrigel, attenuated the recovery rate in hindlimb ischemia and reduced tumor size (An *et al.*, 2009).

VEGF also induces Delta-like ligand 4 (Dll4), a part of the Notch signaling pathway expressed in the vascular endothelium, yet has anti-angiogenic properties (Lobov *et al.*, 2007). Lobov, et al. demonstrated that Dll4 is an antagonistic regulator of angiogenesis by injecting a soluble version of Dll4 (Dll4-Fc) that blocks Dll4/Notch interactions into the vitreous membrane of oxygen-induced ischemic retinopathic (OIR) mice. Blocking Dll4 significantly enhanced angiogenic sprouting while suppressing ectopic pathological neo-vascularization in the retinal vasculature (Lobov *et al.*, 2007). Therefore, Dll4 plays a role as a negative regulator of sprouting angiogenesis in response to the release of hypoxia-induced factors such as VEGF (Lobov *et al.*, 2007).

In addition to VEGF-induced anti-angiogenic genes, the hypoxia-induced VEGF itself is also subjected to negative regulation, such as by transcription factor E2F1 (Qin *et al.*, 2006). Under hypoxic conditions, VEGF is induced by HIF-1; however, E2F1 down-regulates expression of VEGF by associating with p53 and specifically down-regulating VEGF expression but not other hypoxia-inducible genes. Studies of E2F1-/- mice under hypoxic conditions revealed enhanced angiogenesis dependent on de-regulated VEGF, which illustrates a novel negative regulation to VEGF.

5. Anti-angiogenesis in myocardial ischemia

Hypoxia, as a result of impaired blood flow, has a hazardous effect on organ structure and function, especially in the heart, i.e. myocardial ischemia. Acute coronary syndromes resulting from occlusion of one of the coronaries exposes the heart to ischemic conditions. Short periods of ischemia (~20 minutes) are reversible if followed by reperfusion. If coronary occlusion is prolonged, necrosis can propagate from subendocardium to subepicardium. Additionally, reperfusion beyond a few hours does not reduce myocardial infarct size.

Functional recovery of the ischemic tissues and organs is dependent on re-establishing collateral networks that sufficiently supply hyper-oxygenated blood to specialized cell populations. In response to ischemic insults, most tissues in the body have the capacity to compensate for low levels of oxygen by mechanisms of vasodilation, angiogenesis, arteriogenesis, vascular remodeling, and hematopoiesis (Boutin *et al.*, 2008; Makino *et al.*, 2001). Coronary collateral vessels can increase blood flow to regions of the heart supplied by arteries with high-grade stenosis, thus protecting the myocardium from ischemia (Heinle *et al.*, 1974). Collateral formation is highly variable between patients and only partially attributable to differences in the degree of the coronary artery occlusive disease. For therapeutic angiogenesis, it is essential to understand the molecular mechanisms of angiogenesis and arteriogenesis in relation to tissue hypoxia.

Angiopoietin-2 (Ang2) is important in the inhibition of angiogenesis induced by hypoxia; previous reports determined that hypoxia enhances Ang2 expression both *in vivo* and *in vitro* (Oh *et al.*, 1999). The angiopoietin ligands/Tie receptors belong to a class of ligand/receptor families that play a critical role in angiogenesis, cell migration, proliferation, and survival. Ang1 and Ang2 are both ligands with a similar binding affinity for the Tie2 receptor, which is a member of the receptor tyrosine kinases (RTKs) and is predominantly expressed by vascular endothelial cells (Maisonpierre *et al.*, 1997). Ang1 induces angiogenesis via autophosphorylation of Tie2, while Ang2 competitively inhibits this effect (Maisonpierre *et al.*, 1997). Ang2 is an antagonist for the Ang1/Tie2 pathway, as supported by data from over-expressing Ang2 mice that showed a very similar phenotype to the Ang1 and Tie2 single knockouts (Yuan *et al.*, 2009). Interestingly, Ang2 possesses both partial agonistic as well as antagonistic action on Tie2 in the endothelium; alone, Ang2 is a weak activator of Tie2, whereas in the presence of Ang1, Ang2 inhibits Tie2 signaling. When the endothelium is stimulated with Ang1 and Ang2, Ang2 dose-dependently inhibits Ang1-induced Tie2 phosphorylation, Akt activation, as well as EC survival.

Though *in vitro* experimental studies have shown that VEGF, Ang-2, and Tie-2 but not Ang-1 expression is upregulated in ischemic myocardium, (Hashimoto *et al.*, 1994; Matsunaga *et al.*, 2003), clinical studies in patients with acute myocardial infarction have only shown increased peripheral blood VEGF (Kranz *et al.*, 2000). However, a more recent study showed that in addition to increased VEGF and Tie-2 levels, Ang-2 levels were also increased. Additionally, patients with evidence of myocardial damage (ie, AMI) had the highest levels of Ang-2, VEGF, and Tie-2 compared with other groups (Lee *et al.*, 2004).

6. Feedback loops in angiogenic inhibition in response to hypoxia in the heart

As a hypoxia-induced transcription factor, HIF-1 both stimulates and represses a multitude of genes important for adaptation to the low oxygen environment. Regulator of G protein Signaling 5 (RGS5) is a HIF-1-dependent, hypoxia-induced angiogenic inhibitor (Jin *et al.*, 2009) that functions as a negative regulator of G protein-mediated signaling (Adams *et al.*, 2000; Bell *et al.*, 2001). Previous reports showed that hypoxia specifically increased RGS5 expression in endothelial cells; RGS5 mRNA expression was induced by hypoxia while two other family members, RGS2 and RGS4, were not impacted (Jin *et al.*, 2009). In addition to changes in oxygen levels, HIF-1α played a key role in hypoxia-induced RGS5 expression by stimulating RGS5 promoter activity in endothelial cells. RGS5 slowed endothelial cell growth and significantly enhanced the apoptotic protein Bax, which led to increased apoptosis due to the change in the Bcl-2/Bax ratio (Jin *et al.*, 2009; Yang and Korsmeyer,

1996). Furthermore, RGS5 inhibited VEGF-induced angiogenesis through the p38 MAPK-dependent pathway *in vitro* and *in vivo.*

Additionally, a more recent report demonstrated that insulin growth factor binding protein-6 (IGFBP-6) was upregulated in vascular endothelial cells in response to prolonged hypoxia and can inhibit angiogenesis *in vitro* and *in vivo* (Zhang *et al.* 2011). Sequence analysis of the human IGFBP-6 promoter suggested that hypoxia induces the expression of IGFBP-6 in VECs, likely via a HIF-1-mediated mechanism, as there are 8 canonical HREs located in the promoter region of human IGFBP-6 gene. Interestingly, hypoxia has been shown to rapidly induce IGFBP-1 (Kajimura *et al.*, 2005; Tazuke *et al.*, 1998), whereas the up-regulation of the IGFBP-6 gene is not observed until 48 h of hypoxia, implying that IGFBP-6 induction by hypoxia may act as a negative feedback mechanism in hypoxia-induced angiogenesis.

Furthermore, previous studies suggest that HIF1α function is regulated by mitogen activated protein (MAP) kinases (Berra *et al.*, 2000; Minet *et al.*, 2000; Richard *et al.*, 1999). Specifically, the closely related MAP kinase, BMK1/ERK5, is necessary for vasculature remodeling and maintenance. Embryos deficient for the BMK1 MAP kinase die between E10.5 and E11.5 due to angiogenic failure and cardiovascular defects. BMK1 deficiency leads to increased VEGF dysregulation, which impedes angiogenic remodeling and vascular stabilization. Additionally, BMK1 negatively regulates transcription from VEGF during hypoxia. Further research confirmed BMK negative regulation using a conditional BMK1 knockout mouse, which revealed that vascular integrity was compromised and EC apoptosis was increased (Hayashi *et al.*, 2004; Pi *et al.*, 2004; Sohn *et al.*, 2002). Upregulation of BMK1 negatively regulates HIF1α and angiogenesis by increasing HIF1α ubiquitination and degradation in endothelial cells (Pi *et al.*, 2005).

7. Hypoxia-induced apoptosis

During angiogenesis, endothelial cells undergo proliferation, reorganization, and stabilization to establish a mature vascular network. Apoptosis occurring in endothelial cells causes an inhibitory effect on cell proliferation, which has a similar impact to that of anti-angiogenic factors. Hypoxia promotes apoptosis in endothelial cells, as demonstrated by changes in p53 protein levels (Hammond and Giaccia, 2005; Stempien-Otero *et al.*, 1999). Several studies suggest that HIF-1α stabilizes p53 and contributes to hypoxia-induced p53-dependent apoptosis (Xenaki *et al.*, 2008). A recent report proposed that P300/CBP-associated factor (PCAF), an HIF-1α cofactor, regulates the balance between cell cycle arrest and apoptosis in hypoxia by modulating the activity and protein stability of both p53 and HIF-1α (Xenaki *et al.*, 2008). Previous reports demonstrated that p53 can also inhibit angiogenesis by the following mechanisms: elevating thrombospondin-1 levels, repressing both VEGF and FGF-2, and by inducing degradation of HIF-1 (Folkman, 2006).

HIF-1α mediates hypoxia-induced apoptosis through the up-regulation of genes as well as suppression of genes such as Bcl-2 (Carmeliet *et al.*, 1998; Jin *et al.*, 2009). One member of the Bcl-2 family, Bcl-2/E1B interacting protein (BNIP3) is up-regulated under hypoxic conditions (Chen *et al.*, 1997; Kothari *et al.*, 2003). Kothari and colleagues showed that blocking hypoxia-induced BNIP3 expression using siRNA or a mutant BNIP3 inhibits hypoxia-induced cell death. Additionally, hypoxia-mediated BNIP3 expression occurs by direct binding to an HRE in the human BNIP3 promoter, and mutation of this HRE site eliminates the hypoxic responsiveness of the promoter. Furthermore, hypoxia-induced BNIP3 expression was detectable 24 h after initial up-regulation of HIF-1α, indicating that BNIP3 expression occurs much later in the hypoxic response than genes such as VEGF (Kothari *et al.*, 2003).

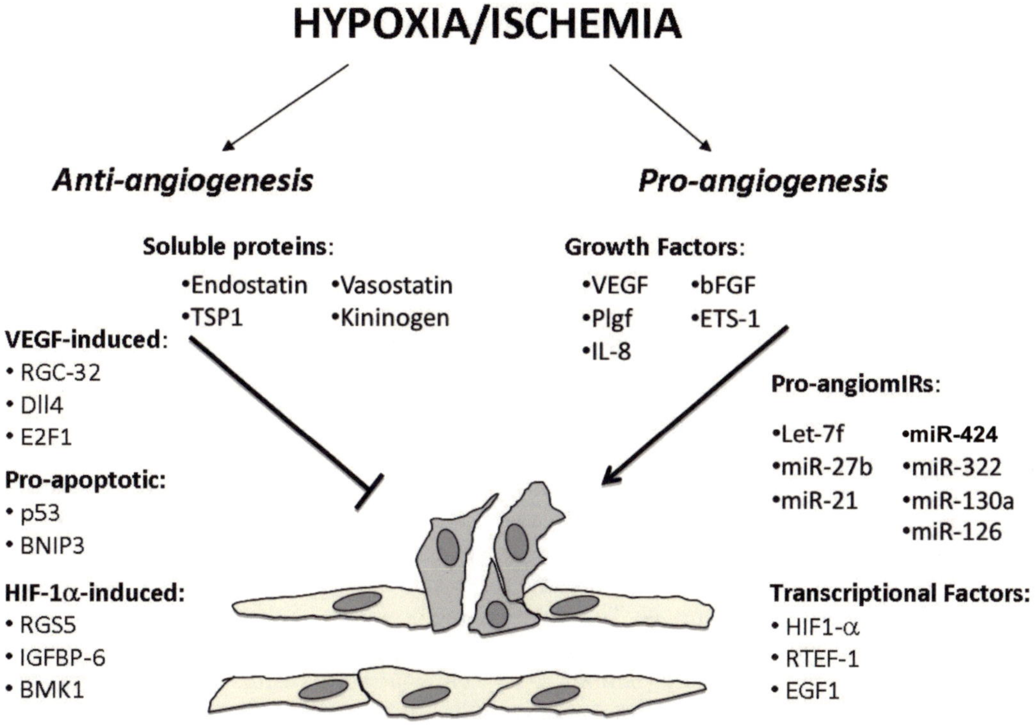

Fig. 1. Schematic illustration of hypoxia/ischemia-induced factors that can balance the decision between pro- and anti-angiogenesis in endothelial cells (EC). It is classified by direct indirect induction through molecules such as HIF-1, VEGF and transcription factors. This delicate equilibrium can easily be influenced by diverse factors, including angiogenic cytokines, local remodeling of the ECM, growth factors, inflammation, and most importantly, exposure to hypoxia.

While HIF-1 mainly targets pro-angiogenic genes, there are feedback molecules to counteract this up-regulation, such as endostatin, which down-regulates HIF-1α (Abdollahi *et al.*, 2004). Hypoxia-induced endostatin inhibits VEGF-induced angiogenesis by preventing proliferation and migration of endothelial cells (Abdollahi *et al.*, 2004; Heljasvaara *et al.*, 2005; Morbidelli *et al.*, 2003) and simultaneously up-regulates anti-angiogenic genes, including thrombospondin (TSP1), vasostatin, and kininogen (Abdollahi *et al.*, 2004). Reduced oxygen supply in FVB mice exposed to a hypobaric hypoxia chamber showed enhanced MMP production leading to a subsequent increase of endostatin generation in the lung and aorta (Paddenberg *et al.*, 2006). These results were confirmed by Suhr et. al, who reported a significant increase in the endostatin and MMP-9 plasma concentration following hypoxic conditions in human cyclists (Suhr *et al.*, 2007). Further studies done on TSP-1 by Morgan-Rowe et. al. showed that it is induced in hypoxia-conditioned media and blocks proliferation of HMEC-1 cells. Increased TSP-1 levels were found following 24 hours of hypoxia in the HMEC-1 media. Additionally, caspase 3 levels were increased followed by inhibition of proliferation and subsequent apoptosis, despite the elevation of VEGF (Morgan-Rowe *et al.*, 2011).

8. Equilibrium between hypoxia-induced angiogenesis and anti-angiogenesis/apoptosis in the heart

Hypoxia promotes pro- and anti-angiogenesis as well as apoptosis in endothelial cells. Apoptosis occurring in endothelial cells causes an inhibitory effect on cell proliferation, which has a similar impact to that of anti-angiogenic factors, as demonstrated by changes in p53 levels in hypoxia. It is important for these three reactions to remain in equilibrium during myocardial ischemia. Additionally, several factors can be both pro- and anti-angiogenic in subsequent studies illustrating the intricacies innate to blood vessel growth.

9. Clinical relevance to coronary artery diseases

Current approaches available for patients with ischemic heart disease include medical therapy or coronary revascularization by percutaneous coronary angioplasty or coronary artery bypass grafting. Problems with these approaches include that many of the patients are not candidates for coronary revascularization procedures or achieve incomplete revascularization with these procedures. It is necessary to discover candidate molecules able to stimulate myocardial angiogenesis for therapeutic application. Preliminary clinical experiences suggest that therapeutic angiogenesis may provide additional blood flow to incompletely revascularized areas. Therapeutic angiogenesis with either HIF-1 or VEGF resulted in a marked increase in blood flow and improved cardiac function in animal studies without apparent toxicity (Simons, 2005). However, the results of clinical trials have been inconsistent and largely disappointing (Simons, 2005), presumably because the negative feedback of angiogenesis during hypoxia may explain the inadequate natural collateral circulation in hypoxic coronary diseases, in which upregulated VEGF inhibits other proangiogenic signaling or triggers angiogenic inhibitor signaling.

10. References

Abdollahi A, Hahnfeldt P, Maercker C, Grone HJ, Debus J, Ansorge W, Folkman J, Hlatky L, Huber PE. 2004. Endostatin's antiangiogenic signaling network. Mol Cell 13:649-663.

Adams LD, Geary RL, McManus B, Schwartz SM. 2000. A comparison of aorta and vena cava medial message expression by cDNA array analysis identifies a set of 68 consistently differentially expressed genes, all in aortic media. Circ Res 87:623-631.

An X, Jin Y, Guo H, Foo SY, Cully BL, Wu J, Zeng H, Rosenzweig A, Li J. 2009. Response gene to complement 32, a novel hypoxia-regulated angiogenic inhibitor. Circulation 120:617-627.

Bell SE, Mavila A, Salazar R, Bayless KJ, Kanagala S, Maxwell SA, Davis GE. 2001. Differential gene expression during capillary morphogenesis in 3D collagen matrices: regulated expression of genes involved in basement membrane matrix assembly, cell cycle progression, cellular differentiation and G-protein signaling. J Cell Sci 114:2755-2773.

Berezikov E, Guryev V, van de Belt J, Wienholds E, Plasterk RH, Cuppen E. 2005. Phylogenetic shadowing and computational identification of human microRNA genes. Cell 120:21-24.

Berra E, Milanini J, Richard DE, Le Gall M, Vinals F, Gothie E, Roux D, Pages G, Pouyssegur J. 2000. Signaling angiogenesis via p42/p44 MAP kinase and hypoxia. Biochem Pharmacol 60:1171-1178.

Boutin AT, Weidemann A, Fu Z, Mesropian L, Gradin K, Jamora C, Wiesener M, Eckardt KU, Koch CJ, Ellies LG, Haddad G, Haase VH, Simon MC, Poellinger L, Powell FL, Johnson RS. 2008. Epidermal sensing of oxygen is essential for systemic hypoxic response. Cell 133:223-234.

Carmeliet P, Dor Y, Herbert JM, Fukumura D, Brusselmans K, Dewerchin M, Neeman M, Bono F, Abramovitch R, Maxwell P, Koch CJ, Ratcliffe P, Moons L, Jain RK, Collen D, Keshert E. 1998. Role of HIF-1alpha in hypoxia-mediated apoptosis, cell proliferation and tumour angiogenesis. Nature 394:485-490.

Chen G, Ray R, Dubik D, Shi L, Cizeau J, Bleackley RC, Saxena S, Gietz RD, Greenberg AH. 1997. The E1B 19K/Bcl-2-binding protein Nip3 is a dimeric mitochondrial protein that activates apoptosis. J Exp Med 186:1975-1983.

Chilov D, Camenisch G, Kvietikova I, Ziegler U, Gassmann M, Wenger RH. 1999. Induction and nuclear translocation of hypoxia-inducible factor-1 (HIF-1): heterodimerization with ARNT is not necessary for nuclear accumulation of HIF-1alpha. J Cell Sci 112 (Pt 8):1203-1212.

Fasanaro P, D'Alessandra Y, Di Stefano V, Melchionna R, Romani S, Pompilio G, Capogrossi MC, Martelli F. 2008. MicroRNA-210 modulates endothelial cell response to hypoxia and inhibits the receptor tyrosine kinase ligand Ephrin-A3. J Biol Chem 283:15878-15883.

Fish JE, Santoro MM, Morton SU, Yu S, Yeh RF, Wythe JD, Ivey KN, Bruneau BG, Stainier DY, Srivastava D. 2008. miR-126 regulates angiogenic signaling and vascular integrity. Dev Cell 15:272-284.

Folkman J. 2006. Angiogenesis. Annu Rev Med 57:1-18.

Fong GH. 2008. Mechanisms of adaptive angiogenesis to tissue hypoxia. Angiogenesis 11:121-140.

Ghosh G, Subramanian IV, Adhikari N, Zhang X, Joshi HP, Basi D, Chandrashekhar YS, Hall JL, Roy S, Zeng Y, Ramakrishnan S. 2010 Hypoxia-induced microRNA-424 expression in human endothelial cells regulates HIF-alpha isoforms and promotes angiogenesis. J Clin Invest 120:4141-4154.

Hammond EM, Giaccia AJ. 2005. The role of p53 in hypoxia-induced apoptosis. Biochem Biophys Res Commun 331:718-725.

Hashimoto E, Ogita T, Nakaoka T, Matsuoka R, Takao A, Kira Y. 1994. Rapid induction of vascular endothelial growth factor expression by transient ischemia in rat heart. Am J Physiol 267:H1948-1954.

Hayashi M, Kim SW, Imanaka-Yoshida K, Yoshida T, Abel ED, Eliceiri B, Yang Y, Ulevitch RJ, Lee JD. 2004. Targeted deletion of BMK1/ERK5 in adult mice perturbs vascular integrity and leads to endothelial failure. J Clin Invest 113:1138-1148.

Heinle RA, Levy RI, Gorlin R. 1974. Effects of factors predisposing to atherosclerosis on formation of coronary collateral vessels. Am J Cardiol 33:12-16.

Heljasvaara R, Nyberg P, Luostarinen J, Parikka M, Heikkila P, Rehn M, Sorsa T, Salo T, Pihlajaniemi T. 2005. Generation of biologically active endostatin fragments from human collagen XVIII by distinct matrix metalloproteases. Exp Cell Res 307:292-304.

Hickey MM, Simon MC. 2006. Regulation of angiogenesis by hypoxia and hypoxia-inducible factors. Curr Top Dev Biol 76:217-257.

Jin Y, An X, Ye Z, Cully B, Wu J, Li J. 2009. RGS5, a hypoxia-inducible apoptotic stimulator in endothelial cells. J Biol Chem 284:23436-23443.

Kajimura S, Aida K, Duan C. 2005. Insulin-like growth factor-binding protein-1 (IGFBP-1) mediates hypoxia-induced embryonic growth and developmental retardation. Proc Natl Acad Sci U S A 102:1240-1245.

Kothari S, Cizeau J, McMillan-Ward E, Israels SJ, Bailes M, Ens K, Kirshenbaum LA, Gibson SB. 2003. BNIP3 plays a role in hypoxic cell death in human epithelial cells that is inhibited by growth factors EGF and IGF. Oncogene 22:4734-4744.

Kranz A, Rau C, Kochs M, Waltenberger J. 2000. Elevation of vascular endothelial growth factor-A serum levels following acute myocardial infarction. Evidence for its origin and functional significance. J Mol Cell Cardiol 32:65-72.

Kuehbacher A, Urbich C, Dimmeler S. 2008. Targeting microRNA expression to regulate angiogenesis. Trends Pharmacol Sci 29:12-15.

Lee KW, Lip GY, Blann AD. 2004. Plasma angiopoietin-1, angiopoietin-2, angiopoietin receptor tie-2, and vascular endothelial growth factor levels in acute coronary syndromes. Circulation 110:2355-2360.

Lee SH, Wolf PL, Escudero R, Deutsch R, Jamieson SW, Thistlethwaite PA. 2000. Early expression of angiogenesis factors in acute myocardial ischemia and infarction. N Engl J Med 342:626-633.

Lobov IB, Renard RA, Papadopoulos N, Gale NW, Thurston G, Yancopoulos GD, Wiegand SJ. 2007. Delta-like ligand 4 (Dll4) is induced by VEGF as a negative regulator of angiogenic sprouting. Proc Natl Acad Sci U S A 104:3219-3224.

Maisonpierre PC, Suri C, Jones PF, Bartunkova S, Wiegand SJ, Radziejewski C, Compton D, McClain J, Aldrich TH, Papadopoulos N, Daly TJ, Davis S, Sato TN, Yancopoulos GD. 1997. Angiopoietin-2, a natural antagonist for Tie2 that disrupts in vivo angiogenesis. Science 277:55-60.

Makino Y, Cao R, Svensson K, Bertilsson G, Asman M, Tanaka H, Cao Y, Berkenstam A, Poellinger L. 2001. Inhibitory PAS domain protein is a negative regulator of hypoxia-inducible gene expression. Nature 414:550-554.

Matsunaga T, Warltier DC, Tessmer J, Weihrauch D, Simons M, Chilian WM. 2003. Expression of VEGF and angiopoietins-1 and -2 during ischemia-induced coronary angiogenesis. Am J Physiol Heart Circ Physiol 285:H352-358.

Messmer-Blust A, An X, Li J. 2009. Hypoxia-regulated angiogenic inhibitors. Trends Cardiovasc Med 19:252-256.

Minet E, Arnould T, Michel G, Roland I, Mottet D, Raes M, Remacle J, Michiels C. 2000. ERK activation upon hypoxia: involvement in HIF-1 activation. FEBS Lett 468:53-58.

Morbidelli L, Donnini S, Chillemi F, Giachetti A, Ziche M. 2003. Angiosuppressive and angiostimulatory effects exerted by synthetic partial sequences of endostatin. Clin Cancer Res 9:5358-5369.

Morgan-Rowe L, Nikitorowicz J, Shiwen X, Leask A, Tsui J, Abraham D, Stratton R. 2011. Thrombospondin 1 in hypoxia-conditioned media blocks the growth of human microvascular endothelial cells and is increased in systemic sclerosis tissues. Fibrogenesis Tissue Repair 4:13.

Oh H, Takagi H, Suzuma K, Otani A, Matsumura M, Honda Y. 1999. Hypoxia and vascular endothelial growth factor selectively up-regulate angiopoietin-2 in bovine microvascular endothelial cells. J Biol Chem 274:15732-15739.

Paddenberg R, Faulhammer P, Goldenberg A, Kummer W. 2006. Hypoxia-induced increase of endostatin in murine aorta and lung. Histochem Cell Biol 125:497-508.

Pi X, Garin G, Xie L, Zheng Q, Wei H, Abe J, Yan C, Berk BC. 2005. BMK1/ERK5 is a novel regulator of angiogenesis by destabilizing hypoxia inducible factor 1alpha. Circ Res 96:1145-1151.

Pi X, Yan C, Berk BC. 2004. Big mitogen-activated protein kinase (BMK1)/ERK5 protects endothelial cells from apoptosis. Circ Res 94:362-369.

Qin G, Kishore R, Dolan CM, Silver M, Wecker A, Luedemann CN, Thorne T, Hanley A, Curry C, Heyd L, Dinesh D, Kearney M, Martelli F, Murayama T, Goukassian DA, Zhu Y, Losordo DW. 2006. Cell cycle regulator E2F1 modulates angiogenesis via p53-dependent transcriptional control of VEGF. Proc Natl Acad Sci U S A 103:11015-11020.

Richard DE, Berra E, Gothie E, Roux D, Pouyssegur J. 1999. p42/p44 mitogen-activated protein kinases phosphorylate hypoxia-inducible factor 1alpha (HIF-1alpha) and enhance the transcriptional activity of HIF-1. J Biol Chem 274:32631-32637.

Sasaki H, Ray PS, Zhu L, Otani H, Asahara T, Maulik N. 2001. Hypoxia/reoxygenation promotes myocardial angiogenesis via an NF kappa B-dependent mechanism in a rat model of chronic myocardial infarction. J Mol Cell Cardiol 33:283-294.

Shie JL, Wu G, Wu J, Liu FF, Laham RJ, Oettgen P, Li J. 2004. RTEF-1, a novel transcriptional stimulator of vascular endothelial growth factor in hypoxic endothelial cells. J Biol Chem 279:25010-25016.

Simons M. 2005. Angiogenesis: where do we stand now? Circulation 111:1556-1566.

Slomiany MG, Rosenzweig SA. 2006. Hypoxia-inducible factor-1-dependent and -independent regulation of insulin-like growth factor-1-stimulated vascular endothelial growth factor secretion. J Pharmacol Exp Ther 318:666-675.

Sohn SJ, Sarvis BK, Cado D, Winoto A. 2002. ERK5 MAPK regulates embryonic angiogenesis and acts as a hypoxia-sensitive repressor of vascular endothelial growth factor expression. J Biol Chem 277:43344-43351.

Stempien-Otero A, Karsan A, Cornejo CJ, Xiang H, Eunson T, Morrison RS, Kay M, Winn R, Harlan J. 1999. Mechanisms of hypoxia-induced endothelial cell death. Role of p53 in apoptosis. J Biol Chem 274:8039-8045.

Suhr F, Brixius K, de Marees M, Bolck B, Kleinoder H, Achtzehn S, Bloch W, Mester J. 2007. Effects of short-term vibration and hypoxia during high-intensity cycling exercise on circulating levels of angiogenic regulators in humans. J Appl Physiol 103:474-483.

Tazuke SI, Mazure NM, Sugawara J, Carland G, Faessen GH, Suen LF, Irwin JC, Powell DR, Giaccia AJ, Giudice LC. 1998. Hypoxia stimulates insulin-like growth factor binding protein 1 (IGFBP-1) gene expression in HepG2 cells: a possible model for IGFBP-1 expression in fetal hypoxia. Proc Natl Acad Sci U S A 95:10188-10193.

Urbich C, Kuehbacher A, Dimmeler S. 2008. Role of microRNAs in vascular diseases, inflammation, and angiogenesis. Cardiovasc Res 79:581-588.

Wang S, Aurora AB, Johnson BA, Qi X, McAnally J, Hill JA, Richardson JA, Bassel-Duby R, Olson EN. 2008. The endothelial-specific microRNA miR-126 governs vascular integrity and angiogenesis. Dev Cell 15:261-271.

Wu G, Mannam AP, Wu J, Kirbis S, Shie JL, Chen C, Laham RJ, Sellke FW, Li J. 2003. Hypoxia induces myocyte-dependent COX-2 regulation in endothelial cells: role of VEGF. Am J Physiol Heart Circ Physiol 285:H2420-2429.

Wurdinger T, Tannous BA, Saydam O, Skog J, Grau S, Soutschek J, Weissleder R, Breakefield XO, Krichevsky AM. 2008. miR-296 regulates growth factor receptor overexpression in angiogenic endothelial cells. Cancer Cell 14:382-393.

Xenaki G, Ontikatze T, Rajendran R, Stratford IJ, Dive C, Krstic-Demonacos M, Demonacos C. 2008. PCAF is an HIF-1alpha cofactor that regulates p53 transcriptional activity in hypoxia. Oncogene 27:5785-5796.

Yan SF, Fujita T, Lu J, Okada K, Shan Zou Y, Mackman N, Pinsky DJ, Stern DM. 2000. Egr-1, a master switch coordinating upregulation of divergent gene families underlying ischemic stress. Nat Med 6:1355-1361.

Yang E, Korsmeyer SJ. 1996. Molecular thanatopsis: a discourse on the BCL2 family and cell death. Blood 88:386-401.

Yuan HT, Khankin EV, Karumanchi SA, Parikh SM. 2009. Angiopoietin 2 is a partial agonist/antagonist of Tie2 signaling in the endothelium. Mol Cell Biol 29:2011-2022.

Zhang C, Lu L, Li Y, Wang X, Zhou J, Liu Y, Fu P, Gallicchio MA, Bach LA, Duan C. 2011 IGF binding protein-6 expression in vascular endothelial cells is induced by hypoxia and plays a negative role in tumor angiogenesis. Int J Cancer.

6

Paraoxonase 1 (PON1) Activity, Polymorphisms and Coronary Artery Disease

Nidhi Gupta, Kiran Dip Gill and Surjit Singh
Post Graduate Institute of Medical Education and Research, Chandigarh, India

1. Introduction

Cardiovascular disorders (CVD) which include coronary artery disease (CAD), heart failure (HF) and stroke are the leading cause of morbidity and mortality both in developed and developing countries and by 2020 CAD is expected to become the number one cause of death worldwide [1-3]. As per WHO, CVD kills nearly 17.5 million persons worldwide each year and is likely to continue to remain number one cause of overall mortality in near future [4, 5].

CAD is the single most important contributor to this increasing burden of CVD. It leads to more deaths than any other disease, including cancer. It can manifest as angina, silent ischemia, unstable angina, myocardial infarction (MI), HF and sudden death. CAD accounts for 52% of 870,000 deaths that occur annually due to CVD in USA i.e. 1 in 5 deaths [6] and nearly accounts for 30 % of all deaths globally. Among American Indians in age group (45-74) the incidence of CVD ranges from 1.5%- 2.8% for men and 0.9- 1.5% for women [7].

Ethnic and regional variations are known to exist in risk factors for developing CVD. The Asian Indians are 3- 4 times more susceptible to develop CAD than Caucasians, 6- times more than Chinese, and 20- times more than Japanese and tend to develop CAD at a younger age [8, 9] as shown by several studies [10-13]. The study SHARE (Study of Health Assessment and Risk in Ethnic groups) has shown a significant higher risk of cardiovascular events among South Asians as compared to Europeans and Chinese [13].

2. Pathophysiology of CAD

The most important underlying pathogenetic mechanism for CVD is atherosclerosis [14, 15]. CAD occurs due to atheromatous narrowing and subsequent occlusion of the coronary arteries. Atheroma [from the Greek athera (porridge) and oma (lump)] starts developing in the first decade of life. A mature plaque has a lipid core which comes from necrotic "foam cells" i.e. monocyte derived macrophages which migrate to intima and ingest lipids (fig. I) [16].

Epidemiological studies have shown an inverse correlation between serum HDL-C levels and risk for developing CAD [17, 18]. The protective effect of HDL-C against the development of CAD appears to be complex. A large part of research in this field is centered on the lipid transport function of HDL-C, particularly in reverse cholesterol transport (RCT). In addition, several studies suggest that HDL-C protects LDL-C from peroxidation, thereby protecting cell membranes from lipid peroxide induced vascular damage. This protection of LDL-C from oxidation by HDL-C possibly potentially impedes the initiation and progression of CAD. Recent studies into the mechanism of the prevention of CAD by HDL-C have revealed that its antioxidant effect is because of its association with an enzyme "paraoxonase".

3. Paraoxonase (PON1; EC 3.1.8.1)

In 1946, Abraham Mazur was the first to report the presence of an enzyme in animal tissues which could hydrolyze organophosphates [19] which ultimately led to the identification of human serum paraoxonase (PON1) enzyme in early 1950's [20]. PON1 is a HDL-C associated serum enzyme whose primary role is to protect LDL-C from oxidative modification [21].

PON1 was first identified in the field of toxicology as it could hydrolyze the organophosphates such as paraoxon, and oxon metabolite of chlorpyriphos, diazinon and nerve gases (e.g., sarin and soman)[22]. Indeed, the enzyme (EC 3.1.8.1) was initially characterized as organophosphate hydrolaze and it still derives its name from its *in vitro* used substrate, paraoxon. Recently, in addition to its role in hydrolyzing organophosphorus compounds, PON1 has been shown to play an important role in lipid metabolism and thus in atherosclerosis and cardiovascular disease.

The PON1 cDNA encodes a protein of 355 amino acids from which only the amino-terminal methionine residue is removed during secretion and maturation[23]. The retained leader sequence is required for the association of PON1 with HDL particle [24]. In human serum, PON1 remains entirely associated with HDL [25].

PON1 lowers the risk of CAD by preventing oxidation of LDL-C which is involved in the initiation and progression of atherosclerosis [26] (Fig. I). Studies have shown that PON1 can prevent accumulation of oxidized LDL-C *in vitro* and *in vivo* [27-29]. In addition, it has also been shown to hydrolyze the oxidized lipids [30]. Serum PON1 activity is reduced in diabetes mellitus and familial hypercholesterolemia[31,32], diseases which are associated with accelerated atherogenesis.

3.1 PON1 structure

The first information about the structure of PON1 was the finding that it retained its signal sequence following secretion from the liver [23]. Sorenson *et al.*, [24] demonstrated that this signal sequence provided a hydrophobic anchor for attachment of PON1 to HDL. Josse *et al.*, [33, 34] identified the following amino acid residues which are essential for PON1's catalytic activity: W280, H114, H154, H242, D53, D168, D182, D268, D278, E52, E194 and the two cysteine residues C41 and C352 that are in disulfide linkage.

A major breakthrough in PON1 structural study came with the engineering of a directed evolution[35] of a form of PON1 that could be crystallized and subjected to X-ray crystallography [36] resulting in determination of crystal structure of the recombinant PON variant, making PON1 the first HDL-associated protein whose three-dimensional structure could be determined [36]. PON has a six-bladed β- propeller with each blade consisting of four β-sheets. In the central tunnel of the enzyme there are two calcium atoms which are needed for the stabilization of the structure and catalytic activity [36]. Three α helices, located at the top of the propeller are involved in its anchoring to the HDL particle [36]

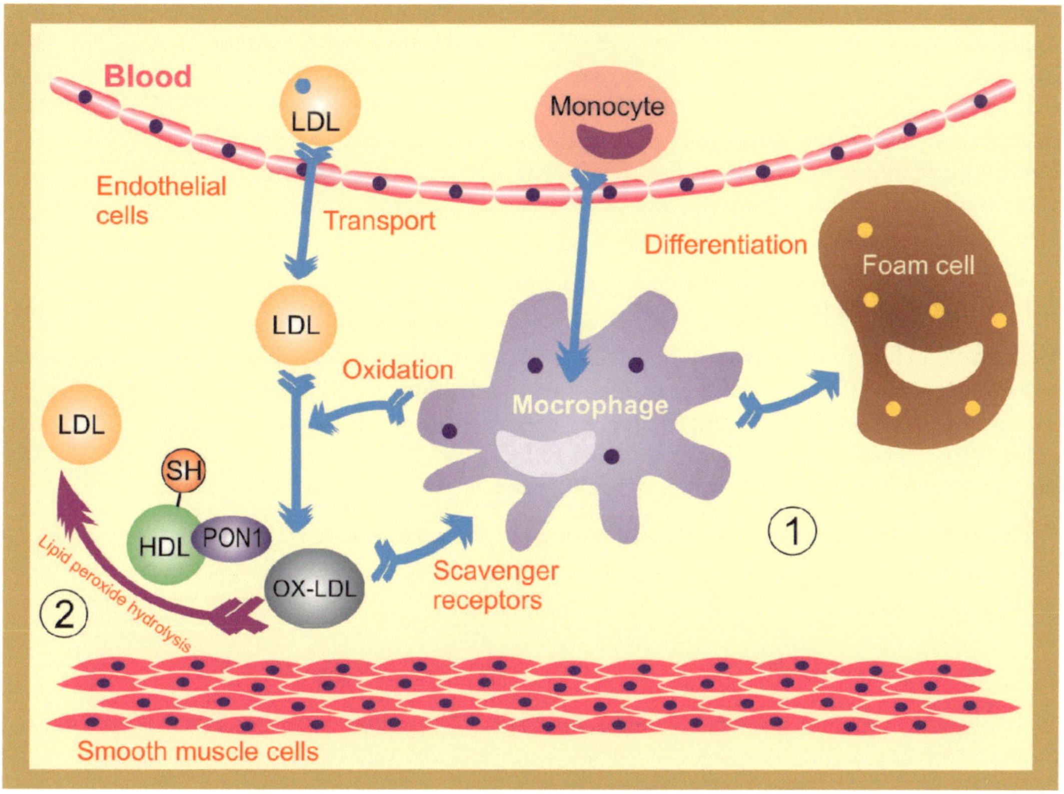

Fig. 1. (1). Normal development of atherosclerosis. (2). Protection from atherosclerosis by PON1.

PON1 contains three Cys residues with one at position 284, having a free sulfhydryl group (Fig. I). PON1 is the only one whose allozymes are found in serum. A unique feature of PON1 in comparison to the other secreted proteins is the retention of its N-terminal hydrophobic signal-leader sequence. Immunological techniques have revealed that PON1 accumulates in the human arterial wall during the development of atherosclerosis [37].

3.2 PON gene cluster

In addition to the known human PON1 gene, two additional PON-like genes, designated as PON2 and PON3 have been identified and all these three genes are located on the long arm of chromosome 7q 21.3–22.1 [38]. These genes share a considerable structural homology and may have arisen from the tandem duplication of a common evolutionary precursor. Within a given mammalian species PON1, PON2 and PON3 share approximately 60% identity at the amino acid level and 70% identity at the nucleotide level. However, between mammalian species each of three genes shares 79-90% identity at the amino acid level and 81-90% identity at nucleotide levels [26].

3.3 Paraoxonase 2 (PON2)

PON2 is a widely expressed intracellular protein with a molecular mass of approximately 44kDa [39]. PON2 mRNA is ubiquitously expressed in nearly every human tissue with highest expression in liver, lung, placenta, testis, and heart. PON2 is able to lower the intracellular oxidative stress of a cell and prevent the cell-mediated oxidation of LDL. Cells over expressing PON2 are less able to oxidize LDL-C and show considerably less intracellular oxidative stress when exposed to either H_2O_2 or oxidized phospholipids. Since PON2 is ubiquitously expressed not just in cells of the artery but in tissues throughout the body, it is likely that PON2 plays a role in reducing local oxidative stress [39] and thereby protects cells from oxidative stress. However, the mechanism by which this effect is produced is not clearly understood.

3.4 Paraoxonase 3 (PON3)

Human PON3 is an approximately 40kDa protein, synthesized primarily in the liver and is associated with HDL in circulation, albeit at much lower level than PON1 [40, 41]. PON3 is interposed between PON1 and PON2 in the PON gene cluster and is the least studied compared to PON1 and PON2. In contrast to PON1, PON3 has very limited arylesterse and no paraoxonase activity but it rapidly hydrolyzes lactones such as statin prodrug.

All the three PON's are thus important players in the maintenance of a low oxidative state in circulating blood, therefore playing role in prevention of atherosclerosis [42]. However, as exact mechanism of action is not clear ,they remain the focus of research in recent years.

4. PONs substrates

PON's native enzyme activity is lactonase [43, 44]. Phylogenetic studies have revealed that PON2 is the oldest member of family from which PON3 and PON1 arose [45]. Draganov *et al.,*, [46] found that PON's have distinct substrate specificity. Dihydrocoumarin (DHC), long chain fatty acid lactones and acyl- homoserine lactones (AHLs) are hydrolyzed by all the three PONs and represent their natural substrates [44]. Additionally, PON1 also hydrolyzes organophosphates and aromatic carboxylic acid esters such as paraoxon and phenylacetate respectively [47] thereby having paraoxonase (PONase) and arylesterase (AREase) activities [48].

4.1 Paraoxonase (PONase) activity

There exists a wide variation in PONase activity in different ethnic groups and within individuals in the same ethnic group [49]. The PONase activity has been shown to be lower after acute myocardial infarction [50]. It is also lower in patients with familial hypercholesterolemia and diabetes mellitus, who are more prone to CAD [31]. This has led to the hypothesis that the lower the PON1 activity, higher is the accumulation of oxidized LDL and risk of CAD.

Nearly 200 single nucleotide polymorphisms (SNPs) of PON1 gene have been identified so far, [51] of which the most studied are -909G/C [rs854572], -162A/G [rs705381], -108C/T [rs 705379] located in the promoter region and Q192R [rs662], L55M [rs 854560] located in the coding region [52]. Serum PONase activity has been found to be influenced by the coding Q192R polymorphism [53]. The PON1 R192 allozyme hydrolyzes paraoxon more rapidly than

PON1 Q192 allozyme whereas PON1 Q192 allozyme hydrolyzes diazoxon, soman and sarin more rapidly than the R192 allozyme [54, 55].

4.2 Arylesterase (AREase) activity

Serum enzyme PON1 activity is not affected towards phenylacetate (AREase) substrate across Q192R polymorphism [56]. Richter *et al.*, [51] have stated that measurement of AREase activity of PON1 or determination of PON1 protein levels by ELISA are the minimum measure that should be carried out in any epidemiological study. Thus it can act as measure of PON levels and this has been used in a number of studies. [48, 51, 56-58].

4.3 Lactonase activity

Lactonase activity is possibly the common enzymatic activity preserved during evolution of the PON proteins. Recent findings suggest that the name PON is infact a misnomer, since PON2 and PON3 lack any significant paraoxonase activity [39-41]. At the molecular level PON1, PON2 and PON3 share an ability to hydrolyze aromatic and long-chain aliphatic lactones, and thus the term lactonase may be more appropriate [44, 45].

Further, the binding of PON1 to HDL particles i.e. the natural carrier of PON1 in blood, has been shown to greatly enhance its lactonase activity. However arylesterase or phosphotriesterase activities are not affected by this. PON1 and PON3 hydrolyze over twenty aromatic and aliphatic lactones with a high degree of overlapping substrate specificity, whereas PON2 lactonase activity is much more restricted.

5. PON1 activity/ levels and CAD

There have been several epidemiological studies to find the relation between PON1 status and CAD. PON1 status can be distinguished into PON1 activity towards paraoxon and PON1 concentration, which is mainly determined in serum by ELISA or can be estimated from phenylacetate hydrolysis activity. The first study on the relation between PON1 activity and CAD was conducted in 1985 [50]. The outcome of this study indicated that lower the PON1 activity, higher was risk of CAD. Subsequently Navab *et al.*, [59] showed that patients with higher HDL-C but low PON1 activity were more susceptible to CAD than patients with low HDL-C but high PON1activity, suggesting that PON1 activity may be more important than HDL protein for protection against CAD. In subsequent, three studies, investigating the relationship of PON1 status and CAD found that low PON1 activity or levels were associated with an increased risk of CAD [60-62] suggesting that PON1 activity predicted coronary events independent of HDL-C.

There is a wide variation (up to 13 –fold) in PON1 serum concentration and activity between individuals even within the same genotype [55, 61]. In addition to genetic polymorphism, PON1 levels can be modified by acquired factors such as diet, lifestyle and disease. It is likely to be the functionality of the enzyme and not simply the genotype that is important in the interaction of PON1 with CAD. A small number of recent studies which include PON1 concentration and/or activity, have found that PON1 levels are reduced in CAD and found this effect is independent of PON1 genotype [61, 63]. In a case-control study of CAD, Jarvik *et al.*,[61] could not find any genotype effect unless PON1 activity was also considered.

A functional genomic analysis as measurement of an individual's PON1 function (serum activity) takes into account all the polymorphisms which might affect its activity. This can be accomplished by use of a high-throughput enzyme assay involving two PON1 substrates usually diazoxon and paraoxon [55]. This, in addition to providing a functional assessment of the serum PON1 192, alloforms also provide the levels of PON1 for each individual, thus encompassing the two factors which affect PON1 levels or activity (position 192 amino acid and serum alloform level). This approach has been referred to as the determination of PON1 'status' of an individual [55]. Measurement of PON1 status, coupled with PCR analysis of codon 192, has been shown to detect genotypes / activity discrepancies that can be explained by the presence of recently discovered mutations in the PON1 gene [63].

Fundamental biochemical principal dictates that it is the catalytic efficiency with which PON1 degrades toxic organophosphates and metabolizes oxidized lipids that determines the degree of protection provided by PON1 against insults from physiological or xenobiotic toxins. In addition, the higher concentration of PON1 provides better protection. Thus, for adequate risk assessment it is important to know PON1 level and activity.

The importance of PON1 status in determining susceptibility or protection from toxicity or disease points to the relevance of factors affecting PON1 activity and its levels of expression. Though genetic determinants such as polymorphisms play a primary role in determining an individual's PON1 status, contribution of other factors in modulating PON1 activity and levels is also important [21, 64].

6. PON1 gene polymorphisms and CAD

6.1 PON1 coding region polymorphisms and CAD

There is 10-40 -fold interindividual variation in serum PON1 activity [53, 65] and this variation in part is determined by 2 common polymorphisms in the coding region of the PON1 gene. The first polymorphism involves glutamine ("A genotype") (Q) → arginine ("B genotype") (R) substitution at position 192, giving rise to 2 allozymes [53, 66]. These allozymes have different activity for different substrates. Some substrates such as paraoxon and fenitroxon are hydrolyzed faster by R allozyme, whereas other substrates such as phenylacetate are hydrolyzed at the same rate by both allozymes [22]. However, others such as diazoxon and nerve gases soman and sarin are hydrolyzed more rapidly by the Q allozyme [22]. The Q192R polymorphism may be playing a role in CAD etiology because this genotype is associated with LDL oxidation and hydrolysis of lipid peroxides. The PON1 192R isoform is less effective at hydrolyzing lipid peroxides than Q isoform [67, 68]. A second polymorphism of the PON1 gene is present at the amino acid position 55, a leucine ("L genotype") (L)→ methionine ("M genotype") (M) substitution, independently influences PON1 activity and has been defined as the molecular basis for this interindividual variability [53, 66]. It is independent of the 192 polymorphism and appears to be the major determinant of the well known biochemical polymorphism in serum PON1 activity towards various organophosphates.

The frequency of PON1 alleles varies greatly across the human population. The distribution of two polymorphisms is significantly different between white and black women. The frequency of the PON1 M55 allele is higher in whites than in blacks, whereas the frequency of the PON1 R192 allele is reverse [69]. The lowest frequency of the PON1 M55 allele has been reported in Chinese. The relatively high frequency of the PON R192 allele in blacks is similar to that reported in Chinese and Japanese varying from 58% to 65% [70, 71]. However, Ferre *et al.*, [72] found no significant differences in genotype and allele frequencies for PON1 polymorphisms at position 55 and 192 between control subjects and patients with myocardial infarction in a Spanish population. The frequencies were similar to those described for other Caucasian populations. These two polymorphisms have significant linkage disequilibrium. Several case-control studies conducted in Caucasians and in Japanese have shown that the Q192R is associated with increased risk of CAD [73-77], although others have failed to replicate this association [71, 78-82]. Other studies have indicated that Q192R polymorphism is associated with altered PON1 enzyme activity for paraoxon as a substrate [53, 66]. On the other hand, Garin *et al.*, [83] reported that in a French population L55M polymorphism may be a major genetic determinant of PON1 enzyme activity and of increased risk for CAD whereas discordant results were obtained in Singapore in Asian Indians and Chinese [84] and in Japanese [73]. In North- West Indian Punjabi's, Q192R was independently associated with CAD (QR (OR: 2.73 (1.57-4.72)) and RR (OR, 16.24 (6.41-41.14) [58]. These results suggest that PON1 R might be an independent risk factor for CAD only in certain populations. Thus, the association between the PON1 polymorphism and CAD is not clear and continues to remain controversial.

The dramatic alteration in enzyme activity caused by this single amino acid change is explained by the structure of the enzyme. Amino acid 192R is an important active site residue [36]. The Q192R polymorphism alters the enzyme's ability to protect LDL-C from oxidation in vivo with the Q form being the most protective [67].

The PON1 L55M polymorphism does not affect the interaction of PON1 with its substrates, but is associated with lower serum PON1 activity and concentration of the enzyme [83]. Leviev *et al.*, [85] found lower PON1 mRNA levels in individuals carrying the M alleles. Subsequent analysis showed a strong linkage disequilibrium with the C (-108)T polymorphisms in the promoter region of the gene. Clinical reports have demonstrated that PON1 activity is reduced in patients with acute myocardial infarction [60], fish eye disease [86] and tangier disease [87]. Lower paraoxonase activity has been observed in Type 2 diabetes mellitus patients with peripheral neuropathy[32] and retinopathy [88-90].

Watson *et al.*, [29] have shown that purified PON1 can prevent the pro-inflammatory effects of oxidized LDL when incubated in a vascular cell co-culture system, probably due to the mechanism of oxidized-arachidonic acid derivatives in the Sn-2position of LDL-phospholipids. Of the PON1 192 allozymes the R allozyme proved to be more efficient at protecting LDL-C from oxidation. Numerous case-control studies have therefore been conducted to determine whether the PON1 192R polymrphism is more closely associated with CAD than the Q polymorphism. Some studies have shown association whereas others have not [21]. However, a recent meta-analysis has revealed a statistically significant increased likelihood of CAD with the PON1 192R allele. Some studies suggest that the PON1 R allele may increase susceptibility to other established CAD risk factors, such as diabetes mellitus [88], cigarette-smoking [91] and age [92]. The PON1 55L allozyme is also more effective in vivo in protecting LDL-C against oxidation than M allozyme. Few case-control studies of the 55 polymorphism have been done. Some have shown an association between the PON1 55L allele and atherosclerosis [83, 93], but others have not [84, 94]. However, no prospective studies of CAD and PON1 polymorphisms are available. Moreover the association between CAD and

PON1 genotype although largely confirmatory is not the only test for hypothesis that PON1 protects against CAD. This may be due to acquired factors acting either on the composition of the lipid environment of HDL, in which PON1 operates, or on the promoter region of the PON1 gene or in some manner as yet to be identified. When PON1 activity is measured directly in patients with CAD, it is about half that of the disease-free controls [50, 60]. Ayub *et al.*, [60] have observed low PON1 activity within few hours of the onset of myocardial infarction, suggesting a low serum PON1 activity to precede the event. Low serum PON1 activity independent of genotype has been reported in several other disorders, which are known to be associated with CAD. These include experimental and clinical diabetes mellitus [31, 32, 88, 95, 96], hypercholesterolemia [31] and renal failure [97].

Interestingly, in addition to preventing LDL-C oxidation, PON1 may also stimulate cellular cholesterol efflux, the first step in reverse cholesterol transport. Thus, PON1 might affect the efficiency of lipid transfer between HDL-C and LDL-C [26]. Also, Rodrigo *et al.*, [98] demonstrated that PON1 may play a role in protecting against bacterial endotoxins and may have a stabilizing property for cellular membranes that undergo either acute or chronic exposure to oxidative agents and free radicals.

6.2 PON1 promoter region polymorphisms and CAD

Sequencing of the promoter PON1 gene led to the discovery of at least five polymorphisms with varying degree of influence over gene expression. These polymorphisms are located at -909(G/C), -832 (A/G), -162 (A/G), -126(C/G) and -108 (C/T) [99-101] of PON1 gene. Promoter containing polymorphisms GAAC, as opposed to CGGT, at positions -909,-832, -162 and -108 respectively, are up to two times more active [99-101]. These variations in promoter activity have been shown to be physiologically relevant as they correlate with significant differences in serum PON1 concentration and activity [99-101].

Identification of clinically significant polymorphisms has been hampered by the fact that there is significant linkage disequilibrium between all the promoter polymorphisms. Haplotype analysis of two populations showed that the C(-108)T polymorphism was the main contributor to the serum PON1 variation, accounting for 23-24% of the total variation [100]. Brophy *et al.*, [100] also reported a slight contribution (1.1% total variation) from the A (-162) G site. The sites at -909 and -832 made little or no difference to serum PON1 levels [100, 102].

Reporter gene assays using promoter regions of varying length have shown that approximately 200 base pair region covering the -108 and -162 polymorphism is sufficient for transcription of the PON1 gene [102-104]. Deleting this region completely abolishes promoter activity, indicating that it is an essential regulatory region of the promoter [102] site of PON1 gene.

As the -108 site appears to be the most significant contributor to the PON1 serum variation, it has been the subject of further investigation. The polymorphism is located in the center of a consensus binding site for the ubiquitous transcription factor sp1 and sp3. This consensus site is abolished by the presence of the -108T variant [99, 100].

Binding of the sp1 to the -108 site is weaker in the presence of T than C, suggesting an effect of the polymorphism on sp1 binding [102]. There are multiple Sp1 sites in this region of the

PON1 promoter, so the effect of the polymorphism is likely to be positional. The -162 polymorphism lies over a potential NF-1 (nuclear factor-1) binding site, with the high activity A variant forming the site and the low-activity G variant disrupting it [103]. This may explain the effect of the change at -162 on gene expression. Other polymorphisms in the promoter region (-162A/G, and -909G/C) may have less significant effect on PON1 expression. They are in strong disequilibrium with C-108T [105].

The increasing role attributed to PON1 in assuring protective mechanisms associated with HDL-C underlines the need to clarify fully the factors which control gene expression and thus modulate the serum PON1 concentration.

6.3 PON1 haplotypes and CAD

Determination of haplotypes is gaining attention because multiple linked SNP's have the potential to provide significantly more power to genetic analysis than individual SNP's [106]. Information is lacking regarding PON1 haplotypes and CAD risk. In North-West Indian Punjabi's L-T-G-Q-C (carrying 4 variant and 1 wild type allele) and L-T-G-R-G (carrying 4 variant and 1 wild type allele) haplotypes are associated with 3.2 and 2.8 fold increase in the risk of CAD whereas haplotypes M-C-A-Q-G (carrying all wild type allele), L-T-A-Q-G (carrying 2 variant and 3 wild type allele) and L-C-A-Q-G (carrying 1 variant and 4 wild type allele) which are more prevalent in controls could be protective of CAD[58].

7. PON1 polymorphisms and lipoproteins

Many studies have suggested that variation in serum PON1 activity is associated with variation in serum lipoprotein concentration including the serum apoA1, LDL-C and HDL-C. Several studies have been conducted to determine the relationship between PON1 gene polymorphisms and serum lipoproteins in Hutterite North American population genetically isolated by religious belief. Further analysis of this population using several candidate genes led [107] to reveal that PON1 was one of nine genes which was responsible for between 3.2 and 7.8% of the total variation in plasma lipoproteins in them. The PON1 genotypes were significantly associated with variation in the plasma concentration of HDL-C, LDL-C, TG and apo B [107]. Homozygotes for the low activity variant of PON1 had significantly lower levels of plasma triglycerides, LDL and apo-B than heterozygotes and homozygotes for the high activity variant. Furthermore, homozygotes for the low-activity variant had significantly lower ratios of total cholesterol/HDL-C, LDL -C/HDL- C and apo B/apo A1 indicating that homozygotes for the low activity allele had a less atherogenic lipoprotein profile than heterozygotes and homozygotes for the high activity allele.

More recently, Leus *et al.,* [108] found that a significant difference in mean TC and LDL-C levels between subjects with the PON1 LL55 and MM55 genotype, and PON1 MM55 had a better plasma lipoprotein profile.

Watson *et al.,* [29] (the Fogelman group) have reported that PON1 in HDL may block inflammatory response by preventing the oxidation of LDL. The same group has also shown that during an acute-phase response, there was a significant loss of the PON1 activity, thus accounting for the failure of HDL to protect LDL from oxidation during it [109]. More recently the same group [59] have reported a failure of HDL to protect LDL from oxidation in patients with CAD, which they propose is due to low serum PON1 activity in them.

8. Modulation of PON1 by exogenous compounds

8.1 Environmental chemicals

PON1 activity is completely dependent upon Ca++ and EDTA, irreversibly abolishes its activity. Other cations, also, have been shown to have an inhibitory effect on PON1 activity. The barium, lithium, copper, zinc and mercurials have been found to inhibit PON1 activity in rat and human liver [110]. In case of mercurials and copper, studies suggest that a free thiol group on the Cys 285 residue may be the molecular target [110, 111]. More recent experiments have revealed that cadmium, iron, zinc and mercurials are highly potent in vitro inhibitors of PON1 192R activity and can inhibit upto 80% of activity. However, in vivo the PON Q192 appears to be less sensitive to inhibition by metals, with the exception of lead [112]. In vivo exposures of mice to cadmium, methylmercury or dietary iron leading to metal serum concentration of higher than 1μM has failed to alter PON1 activity in plasma and liver [112]. This is probably due to binding of metal to proteins in plasma leading to protection of PON1.

8.2 Classical inducers

A few studies have investigated whether PON1 is an inducible enzyme. Phenobarbital, a classical enzyme inducer which is particularly effective toward certain isozymes of cytochrome P450 (e.g. CYP2B), caused a modest (20-150%) increase in hepatic PON1 activity [113], with a concomitant increase in liver RNA levels [114]. However, serum PON1 activity has been found to be decreased in patients on (40-50%) phenobarbital treatment [113-116].

9. Modulation of PON1 by life-style factors

Enzyme inducers, environmental chemicals, physiological and pathological states, and dietary and lifestyle factors have shown their effects on PON1 activity.

9.1 Age

In humans, PON1 serum arylesterase activity increases from birth to 15-25 months of age, when it seems to reach a plateau whose level is determined by the 5′ regulatory-region polymorphisms and the genetic background of the individual [114]. In an adult, PON1 levels remain stable as no significant changes have been observed with age [117, 118].

9.2 Enzme inducers and environmental chemicals

3-Methylcholantherene has been found to increase both serum and liver PON1 level in rats [98] but not in mice [114]. Administration of lipopolysaccharide, which mimics gram-negative infection, causes a transient decrease in serum and liver PON1 activity and in hepatic mRNA levels [114, 119]. The phytoalexin resveratrol is considered to be a major biologically active component contributing to the beneficial effect of wine [120] and is known to modulate gene expression.

PON1 activity can vary depending on physiological conditions or pathological states. Serum PON1 activity is significantly decreased during pregnancy [121].

9.3 Smoking

Cigarette smoke extract is known to inhibit PON1 activity in vitro [122], suggesting that smoking may be detrimental to enzyme activity in vivo. James *et al.*,[91] showed that PON1 serum concentration and activity were reduced in smokers compared with non-smokers. Ex-smokers had activities and concentrations comparable with those of non-smokers, suggesting a reversible influence of smoking on PON1. In vitro experiments found that inhibition of PON1 activity by a cigarette-smoke extract was antagonized by reduced glutathione (GSH), N-acetylcysteine, and 2-mercaptoethanol, suggesting that free thiols are central to the inhibitory effects [122].

9.4 Alcohol

Moderate wine consumption appears to have potential beneficial effects related to the prevention of CAD [123]. Wine consumption increases serum PON1 activity [124, 125]. Ethanol and other aliphatic alcohols have been shown to inhibit serum PON1 activity [126]; however, in middle aged men daily moderate alcohol consumption increased serum PON1 activity, with no differences between wine, beer, and spirits [127]. This increase may be due to the consumption of alcohol itself or to that of antioxidants, as similar results were obtained after consumption of red wine [128] or pomegranate juice [129, 130].

9.5 Diet

In both rabbit and transgenic mouse model, a proatherogenic diet caused a significant fall in PON1 activity, which correlated with a reduction in HDL-cholesterol [89, 131-133]. Diets with a high trans-unsaturated fat content can reduce PON1 activity [134]. In contrast, oleic acid from olive oil is associated with increased activity [135, 136]. Meals rich in used cooking fat which contains a high content of oxidized lipids, is followed by a significant fall in PON1 activity when fed to healthy men [137].

PON1 is highly susceptible to inactivation by oxidation. In vitro, PON1 activity is protected by the anti-oxidant polyphenols quercetin and glabridin [138], suggesting that dietary antioxidants may play a similar role in vivo. Some studies have shown that consumption of pomegranate juice which is rich in polyphenols and other antioxidants, can raise PON1 activity up to 20% in both humans and apoE knockout mice [130].

10. Conclusions and future prospects

Human epidemiological studies and experimental work carried out so far provides convincing evidence that PON(s) play an important role in protection against atherosclerosis. Studies are required to elucidate the role of the PON genetic polymorphisms in this potentially important function of PON(s) and role in CAD and other related diseases. Since nutritional and environmental factors explain some of the individual variations in serum PON 1 activity, the enzyme is considered as a promising target for pharmaceutical intervention. Therefore, pharmacological modulation of PON1 activity or PON 1 gene expression could constitute a useful approach for the prevention of CAD.

11. Acknowledgement

Council of Scientific and Industrial Research- University Grants Commission (CSIR-UGC), New- Delhi, India provided research fellowship to Nidhi Gupta.

12. References

[1] Murray, C. J. and Lopez, A. D., Alternative projections of mortality and disability by cause 1990-2020: Global Burden of Disease Study, Lancet, 1997, 349: 1498-1504.

[2] Kullo, I. J. and Ding, K., Mechanisms of disease: The genetic basis of coronary heart disease, Nat Clin Pract Cardiovasc Med, 2007, 4: 558-569.

[3] Tunstall-Pedoe, H., Vanuzzo, D., Hobbs, M., Mahonen, M., Cepaitis, Z., Kuulasmaa, K. and Keil, U., Estimation of contribution of changes in coronary care to improving survival, event rates, and coronary heart disease mortality across the WHO MONICA Project populations, Lancet, 2000, 355: 688-700.

[4] Libby, P., Ridker, P. M. and Maseri, A., Inflammation and atherosclerosis, Circulation, 2002, 105: 1135-1143.

[5] Wang, Q., Advances in the genetic basis of coronary artery disease, Curr Atheroscler Rep, 2005, 7: 235-241.

[6] Rosamond, W., Flegal, K., Friday, G., Furie, K., Go, A., Greenlund, K., Haase, N., Ho, M., Howard, V., Kissela, B., Kittner, S., Lloyd-Jones, D., McDermott, M., Meigs, J., Moy, C., Nichol, G., O'Donnell, C. J., Roger, V., Rumsfeld, J., Sorlie, P., Steinberger, J., Thom, T., Wasserthiel-Smoller, S. and Hong, Y., Heart disease and stroke statistics--2007 update: a report from the American Heart Association Statistics Committee and Stroke Statistics Subcommittee, Circulation, 2007, 115: e69-171.

[7] Thomas K. Welty, E. T. L., Jeunliang Yeh, Linda D. Cowan, Oscar Go, Richard R., Fabsitz, NgoC-Anh Le, Arvo J. oopik, David C. Robbins and Barbara V. Howard., Cardiovasculat Disease Risk Factors among American Indians: The Strong Heart Study., Am J Epidemiol, 1995, 142: 269-287.

[8] McKeigue, P. M., Ferrie, J. E., Pierpoint, T. and Marmot, M. G., Association of early-onset coronary heart disease in South Asian men with glucose intolerance and hyperinsulinemia, Circulation, 1993, 87: 152-161.

[9] Janus, E. D., Postiglione, A., Singh, R. B. and Lewis, B., The modernization of Asia. Implications for coronary heart disease. Council on Arteriosclerosis of the International Society and Federation of Cardiology, Circulation, 1996, 94: 2671-2673.

[10] Enas, E. A., Garg, A., Davidson, M. A., Nair, V. M., Huet, B. A. and Yusuf, S., Coronary heart disease and its risk factors in first-generation immigrant Asian Indians to the United States of America, Indian Heart J, 1996, 48: 343-353.

[11] Hughes, K., Yeo, P. P., Lun, K. C., Sothy, S. P., Thai, A. C., Wang, K. W. and Cheah, J. S., Ischaemic heart disease and its risk factors in Singapore in comparison with other countries, Ann Acad Med Singapore, 1989, 18: 245-249.

[12] Balarajan, R., Ethnic differences in mortality from ischaemic heart disease and cerebrovascular disease in England and Wales, BMJ, 1991, 302: 560-564.

[13] Anand, S. S., Yusuf, S., Vuksan, V., Devanesen, S., Teo, K. K., Montague, P. A., Kelemen, L., Yi, C., Lonn, E., Gerstein, H., Hegele, R. A. and McQueen, M., Differences in risk factors, atherosclerosis, and cardiovascular disease between ethnic groups in Canada: the Study of Health Assessment and Risk in Ethnic groups (SHARE), Lancet, 2000, 356: 279-284.

[14] Dawber, T. R., Meadors, G. F. and Moore, F. E., Jr., Epidemiological approaches to heart disease: the Framingham Study, Am J Public Health Nations Health, 1951, 41: 279-281.

[15] Ross, R., The pathogenesis of atherosclerosis--an update, N Engl J Med, 1986, 314: 488-500.

[16] Grech, E. D., ABC of interventional cardiology: percutaneous coronary intervention. I: history and development, BMJ, 2003, 326: 1080-1082.

[17] Tanne, D., Yaari, S. and Goldbourt, U., High-density lipoprotein cholesterol and risk of ischemic stroke mortality. A 21-year follow-up of 8586 men from the Israeli Ischemic Heart Disease Study, Stroke, 1997, 28: 83-87.

[18] Assmann, G., Schulte, H., von Eckardstein, A. and Huang, Y., High-density lipoprotein cholesterol as a predictor of coronary heart disease risk. The PROCAM experience and pathophysiological implications for reverse cholesterol transport, Atherosclerosis, 1996, 124 Suppl: S11-20.

[19] Mazur, A., An enzyme in animal tissue capable of hydrolyzing the phosphorus-fluorine bond of alkyl fluorophosphates., J. Biol. Chem., 1946, 164: 271-289.

[20] Aldridge, W. N., Serum esterases. I. Two types of esterase (A and B) hydrolysing p-nitrophenyl acetate, propionate and butyrate, and a method for their determination, Biochem J, 1953, 53: 110-117.

[21] Durrington, P. N., Mackness, B. and Mackness, M. I., Paraoxonase and atherosclerosis, Arterioscler Thromb Vasc Biol, 2001, 21: 473-480.

[22] Davies, H. G., Richter, R. J., Keifer, M., Broomfield, C. A., Sowalla, J. and Furlong, C. E., The effect of the human serum paraoxonase polymorphism is reversed with diazoxon, soman and sarin, Nat Genet, 1996, 14: 334-336.

[23] Hassett, C., Richter, R. J., Humbert, R., Chapline, C., Crabb, J. W., Omiecinski, C. J. and Furlong, C. E., Characterization of cDNA clones encoding rabbit and human serum paraoxonase: the mature protein retains its signal sequence, Biochemistry, 1991, 30: 10141-10149.

[24] Sorenson, R. C., Bisgaier, C. L., Aviram, M., Hsu, C., Billecke, S. and La Du, B. N., Human serum Paraoxonase/Arylesterase's retained hydrophobic N-terminal leader sequence associates with HDLs by binding phospholipids : apolipoprotein A-I stabilizes activity, Arterioscler Thromb Vasc Biol, 1999, 19: 2214-2225.

[25] Blatter, M. C., James, R. W., Messmer, S., Barja, F. and Pometta, D., Identification of a distinct human high-density lipoprotein subspecies defined by a lipoprotein-associated protein, K-45. Identity of K-45 with paraoxonase, Eur J Biochem, 1993, 211: 871-879.

[26] Mackness, B., Durrington, P. N. and Mackness, M. I., The paraoxonase gene family and coronary heart disease, Curr Opin Lipidol, 2002, 13: 357-362.

[27] Mackness, M. I., Arrol, S. and Durrington, P. N., Paraoxonase prevents accumulation of lipoperoxides in low-density lipoprotein, FEBS Lett, 1991, 286: 152-154.

[28] Mackness, M. I., Arrol, S., Abbott, C. and Durrington, P. N., Protection of low-density lipoprotein against oxidative modification by high-density lipoprotein associated paraoxonase, Atherosclerosis, 1993, 104: 129-135.
[29] Watson, A. D., Berliner, J. A., Hama, S. Y., La Du, B. N., Faull, K. F., Fogelman, A. M. and Navab, M., Protective effect of high density lipoprotein associated paraoxonase. Inhibition of the biological activity of minimally oxidized low density lipoprotein, J Clin Invest, 1995, 96: 2882-2891.
[30] Aviram, M., Rosenblat, M., Bisgaier, C. L., Newton, R. S., Primo-Parmo, S. L. and La Du, B. N., Paraoxonase inhibits high-density lipoprotein oxidation and preserves its functions. A possible peroxidative role for paraoxonase, J Clin Invest, 1998, 101: 1581-1590.
[31] Mackness, M. I., Harty, D., Bhatnagar, D., Winocour, P. H., Arrol, S., Ishola, M. and Durrington, P. N., Serum paraoxonase activity in familial hypercholesterolaemia and insulin-dependent diabetes mellitus, Atherosclerosis, 1991, 86: 193-199.
[32] Abbott, C. A., Mackness, M. I., Kumar, S., Boulton, A. J. and Durrington, P. N., Serum paraoxonase activity, concentration, and phenotype distribution in diabetes mellitus and its relationship to serum lipids and lipoproteins, Arterioscler Thromb Vasc Biol, 1995, 15: 1812-1818.
[33] Josse, D., Xie, W., Renault, F., Rochu, D., Schopfer, L. M., Masson, P. and Lockridge, O., Identification of residues essential for human paraoxonase (PON1) arylesterase/organophosphatase activities, Biochemistry, 1999, 38: 2816-2825.
[34] Josse, D., Lockridge, O., Xie, W., Bartels, C. F., Schopfer, L. M. and Masson, P., The active site of human paraoxonase (PON1), J Appl Toxicol, 2001, 21 Suppl 1: S7-11.
[35] Aharoni, A., Gaidukov, L., Yagur, S., Toker, L., Silman, I. and Tawfik, D. S., Directed evolution of mammalian paraoxonases PON1 and PON3 for bacterial expression and catalytic specialization, Proc Natl Acad Sci U S A, 2004, 101: 482-487.
[36] Harel, M., Aharoni, A., Gaidukov, L., Brumshtein, B., Khersonsky, O., Meged, R., Dvir, H., Ravelli, R. B., McCarthy, A., Toker, L., Silman, I., Sussman, J. L. and Tawfik, D. S., Structure and evolution of the serum paraoxonase family of detoxifying and anti-atherosclerotic enzymes, Nat Struct Mol Biol, 2004, 11: 412-419.
[37] Mackness, B., Hunt, R., Durrington, P. N. and Mackness, M. I., Increased immunolocalization of paraoxonase, clusterin, and apolipoprotein A-I in the human artery wall with the progression of atherosclerosis, Arterioscler Thromb Vasc Biol, 1997, 17: 1233-1238.
[38] Rowles, J., Scherer, S. W., Xi, T., Majer, M., Nickle, D. C., Rommens, J. M., Popov, K. M., Harris, R. A., Riebow, N. L., Xia, J., Tsui, L. C., Bogardus, C. and Prochazka, M., Cloning and characterization of PDK4 on 7q21.3 encoding a fourth pyruvate dehydrogenase kinase isoenzyme in human, J Biol Chem, 1996, 271: 22376-22382.
[39] Ng, C. J., Wadleigh, D. J., Gangopadhyay, A., Hama, S., Grijalva, V. R., Navab, M., Fogelman, A. M. and Reddy, S. T., Paraoxonase-2 is a ubiquitously expressed protein with antioxidant properties and is capable of preventing cell-mediated oxidative modification of low density lipoprotein, J Biol Chem, 2001, 276: 44444-44449.

[40] Draganov, D. I., Stetson, P. L., Watson, C. E., Billecke, S. S. and La Du, B. N., Rabbit serum paraoxonase 3 (PON3) is a high density lipoprotein-associated lactonase and protects low density lipoprotein against oxidation, J Biol Chem, 2000, 275: 33435-33442.

[41] Reddy, S. T., Wadleigh, D. J., Grijalva, V., Ng, C., Hama, S., Gangopadhyay, A., Shih, D. M., Lusis, A. J., Navab, M. and Fogelman, A. M., Human paraoxonase-3 is an HDL-associated enzyme with biological activity similar to paraoxonase-1 protein but is not regulated by oxidized lipids, Arterioscler Thromb Vasc Biol, 2001, 21: 542-547.

[42] Precourt, L. P., Amre, D., Denis, M. C., Lavoie, J. C., Delvin, E., Seidman, E. and Levy, E., The three-gene paraoxonase family: physiologic roles, actions and regulation, Atherosclerosis, 214: 20-36.

[43] Khersonsky, O. and Tawfik, D. S., Structure-reactivity studies of serum paraoxonase PON1 suggest that its native activity is lactonase, Biochemistry, 2005, 44: 6371-6382.

[44] Draganov, D. I., Teiber, J. F., Speelman, A., Osawa, Y., Sunahara, R. and La Du, B. N., Human paraoxonases (PON1, PON2, and PON3) are lactonases with overlapping and distinct substrate specificities, J Lipid Res, 2005, 46: 1239-1247.

[45] Draganov, D. I. and La Du, B. N., Pharmacogenetics of paraoxonases: a brief review, Naunyn Schmiedebergs Arch Pharmacol, 2004, 369: 78-88.

[46] Draganov, D. I., Lactonases with organophosphatase activity: structural and evolutionary perspectives, Chem Biol Interact, 2010, 187: 370-372.

[47] La Du, B. N., Human Serum paraoxonase/arylesterase. In, Pharmacogenetics of Drug metabolism (W. Kalow.ed.) Pergamon Press, New York USA pp51-91, 1992.

[48] Richter, R. J., Jarvik, G. P. and Furlong, C. E., Determination of paraoxonase 1 status without the use of toxic organophosphate substrates, Circ Cardiovasc Genet, 2008, 1: 147-152.

[49] MacKness, B., Mackness, M. I., Durrington, P. N., Arrol, S., Evans, A. E., McMaster, D., Ferrieres, J., Ruidavets, J. B., Williams, N. R. and Howard, A. N., Paraoxonase activity in two healthy populations with differing rates of coronary heart disease, Eur J Clin Invest, 2000, 30: 4-10.

[50] McElveen, J., Mackness, M. I., Colley, C. M., Peard, T., Warner, S. and Walker, C. H., Distribution of paraoxon hydrolytic activity in the serum of patients after myocardial infarction, Clin Chem, 1986, 32: 671-673.

[51] Richter, R. J., Jarvik, G. P. and Furlong, C. E., Paraoxonase 1 status as a risk factor for disease or exposure, Adv Exp Med Biol, 2010, 660: 29-35.

[52] Costa, L. G., Cole, T. B., Jarvik, G. P. and Furlong, C. E., Functional genomic of the paraoxonase (PON1) polymorphisms: effects on pesticide sensitivity, cardiovascular disease, and drug metabolism, Annu Rev Med, 2003, 54: 371-392.

[53] Humbert, R., Adler, D. A., Disteche, C. M., Hassett, C., Omiecinski, C. J. and Furlong, C. E., The molecular basis of the human serum paraoxonase activity polymorphism, Nat Genet, 1993, 3: 73-76.

[54] Aviram, M., Hardak, E., Vaya, J., Mahmood, S., Milo, S., Hoffman, A., Billicke, S., Draganov, D. and Rosenblat, M., Human serum paraoxonases (PON1) Q and R selectively decrease lipid peroxides in human coronary and carotid atherosclerotic lesions: PON1 esterase and peroxidase-like activities, Circulation, 2000, 101: 2510-2517.

[55] Richter, R. J. and Furlong, C. E., Determination of paraoxonase (PON1) status requires more than genotyping, Pharmacogenetics, 1999, 9: 745-753.

[56] Furlong, C. E., Holland, N., Richter, R. J., Bradman, A., Ho, A. and Eskenazi, B., PON1 status of farmworker mothers and children as a predictor of organophosphate sensitivity, Pharmacogenet Genomics, 2006, 16: 183-190.

[57] Berkowitz, G. S., Wetmur, J. G., Birman-Deych, E., Obel, J., Lapinski, R. H., Godbold, J. H., Holzman, I. R. and Wolff, M. S., In utero pesticide exposure, maternal paraoxonase activity, and head circumference, Environ Health Perspect, 2004, 112: 388-391.

[58] Gupta, N., Singh, S., Maturu, V. N., Sharma, Y. P. and Gill, K. D., Paraoxonase 1 (PON1) Polymorphisms, Haplotypes and Activity in Predicting CAD Risk in North-West Indian Punjabis, PLoS ONE, 2011, 6: e17805.

[59] Navab, M., Hama-Levy, S., Van Lenten, B. J., Fonarow, G. C., Cardinez, C. J., Castellani, L. W., Brennan, M. L., Lusis, A. J., Fogelman, A. M. and La Du, B. N., Mildly oxidized LDL induces an increased apolipoprotein J/paraoxonase ratio, J Clin Invest, 1997, 99: 2005-2019.

[60] Ayub, A., Mackness, M. I., Arrol, S., Mackness, B., Patel, J. and Durrington, P. N., Serum paraoxonase after myocardial infarction, Arterioscler Thromb Vasc Biol, 1999, 19: 330-335.

[61] Jarvik, G. P., Rozek, L. S., Brophy, V. H., Hatsukami, T. S., Richter, R. J., Schellenberg, G. D. and Furlong, C. E., Paraoxonase (PON1) phenotype is a better predictor of vascular disease than is PON1(192) or PON1(55) genotype, Arterioscler Thromb Vasc Biol, 2000, 20: 2441-2447.

[62] Mackness, B., Davies, G. K., Turkie, W., Lee, E., Roberts, D. H., Hill, E., Roberts, C., Durrington, P. N. and Mackness, M. I., Paraoxonase status in coronary heart disease: are activity and concentration more important than genotype?, Arterioscler Thromb Vasc Biol, 2001, 21: 1451-1457.

[63] Jarvik, G. P., Hatsukami, T. S., Carlson, C., Richter, R. J., Jampsa, R., Brophy, V. H., Margolin, S., Rieder, M., Nickerson, D., Schellenberg, G. D., Heagerty, P. J. and Furlong, C. E., Paraoxonase activity, but not haplotype utilizing the linkage disequilibrium structure, predicts vascular disease, Arterioscler Thromb Vasc Biol, 2003, 23: 1465-1471.

[64] Ferre, N., Camps, J., Fernandez-Ballart, J., Arija, V., Murphy, M. M., Ceruelo, S., Biarnes, E., Vilella, E., Tous, M. and Joven, J., Regulation of serum paraoxonase activity by genetic, nutritional, and lifestyle factors in the general population, Clin Chem, 2003, 49: 1491-1497.

[65] Mackness, M. I., Mackness, B., Durrington, P. N., Connelly, P. W. and Hegele, R. A., Paraoxonase: biochemistry, genetics and relationship to plasma lipoproteins, Curr Opin Lipidol, 1996, 7: 69-76.

[66] Adkins, S., Gan, K. N., Mody, M. and La Du, B. N., Molecular basis for the polymorphic forms of human serum paraoxonase/arylesterase: glutamine or arginine at position 191, for the respective A or B allozymes, Am J Hum Genet, 1993, 52: 598-608.

[67] Aviram, M., Billecke, S., Sorenson, R., Bisgaier, C., Newton, R., Rosenblat, M., Erogul, J., Hsu, C., Dunlop, C. and La Du, B., Paraoxonase active site required for protection against LDL oxidation involves its free sulfhydryl group and is different from that required for its arylesterase/paraoxonase activities: selective action of human paraoxonase allozymes Q and R, Arterioscler Thromb Vasc Biol, 1998, 18: 1617-1624.

[68] Mackness, B., Durrington, P. N. and Mackness, M. I., Polymorphisms of paraoxonase genes and low-density lipoprotein lipid peroxidation, Lancet, 1999, 353: 468-469.
[69] Ahmed, Z., Ravandi, A., Maguire, G. F., Emili, A., Draganov, D., La Du, B. N., Kuksis, A. and Connelly, P. W., Apolipoprotein A-I promotes the formation of phosphatidylcholine core aldehydes that are hydrolyzed by paraoxonase (PON-1) during high density lipoprotein oxidation with a peroxynitrite donor, J Biol Chem, 2001, 276: 24473-24481.
[70] Imai, Y., Morita, H., Kurihara, H., Sugiyama, T., Kato, N., Ebihara, A., Hamada, C., Kurihara, Y., Shindo, T., Oh-hashi, Y. and Yazaki, Y., Evidence for association between paraoxonase gene polymorphisms and atherosclerotic diseases, Atherosclerosis, 2000, 149: 435-442.
[71] Ko, Y. L., Ko, Y. S., Wang, S. M., Hsu, L. A., Chang, C. J., Chu, P. H., Cheng, N. J., Chen, W. J., Chiang, C. W. and Lee, Y. S., The Gln-Arg 191 polymorphism of the human paraoxonase gene is not associated with the risk of coronary artery disease among Chinese in Taiwan, Atherosclerosis, 1998, 141: 259-264.
[72] Ferre, N., Tous, M., Paul, A., Zamora, A., Vendrell, J. J., Bardaji, A., Camps, J., Richart, C. and Joven, J., Paraoxonase Gln-Arg(192) and Leu-Met(55) gene polymorphisms and enzyme activity in a population with a low rate of coronary heart disease, Clin Biochem, 2002, 35: 197-203.
[73] Zama, T., Murata, M., Matsubara, Y., Kawano, K., Aoki, N., Yoshino, H., Watanabe, G., Ishikawa, K. and Ikeda, Y., A 192Arg variant of the human paraoxonase (HUMPONA) gene polymorphism is associated with an increased risk for coronary artery disease in the Japanese, Arterioscler Thromb Vasc Biol, 1997, 17: 3565-3569.
[74] Odawara, M., Tachi, Y. and Yamashita, K., Paraoxonase polymorphism (Gln192-Arg) is associated with coronary heart disease in Japanese noninsulin-dependent diabetes mellitus, J Clin Endocrinol Metab, 1997, 82: 2257-2260.
[75] Sanghera, D. K., Saha, N., Aston, C. E. and Kamboh, M. I., Genetic polymorphism of paraoxonase and the risk of coronary heart disease, Arterioscler Thromb Vasc Biol, 1997, 17: 1067-1073.
[76] Serrato, M. and Marian, A. J., A variant of human paraoxonase/arylesterase (HUMPONA) gene is a risk factor for coronary artery disease, J Clin Invest, 1995, 96: 3005-3008.
[77] Ruiz, J., Blanche, H., James, R. W., Garin, M. C., Vaisse, C., Charpentier, G., Cohen, N., Morabia, A., Passa, P. and Froguel, P., Gln-Arg192 polymorphism of paraoxonase and coronary heart disease in type 2 diabetes, Lancet, 1995, 346: 869-872.
[78] Suehiro, T., Nakauchi, Y., Yamamoto, M., Arii, K., Itoh, H., Hamashige, N. and Hashimoto, K., Paraoxonase gene polymorphism in Japanese subjects with coronary heart disease, Int J Cardiol, 1996, 57: 69-73.
[79] Herrmann, S. M., Blanc, H., Poirier, O., Arveiler, D., Luc, G., Evans, A., Marques-Vidal, P., Bard, J. M. and Cambien, F., The Gln/Arg polymorphism of human paraoxonase (PON 192) is not related to myocardial infarction in the ECTIM Study, Atherosclerosis, 1996, 126: 299-303.

[80] Antikainen, M., Murtomaki, S., Syvanne, M., Pahlman, R., Tahvanainen, E., Jauhiainen, M., Frick, M. H. and Ehnholm, C., The Gln-Arg191 polymorphism of the human paraoxonase gene (HUMPONA) is not associated with the risk of coronary artery disease in Finns, J Clin Invest, 1996, 98: 883-885.

[81] Rice, G. I., Ossei-Gerning, N., Stickland, M. H. and Grant, P. J., The paraoxonase Gln-Arg 192 polymorphism in subjects with ischaemic heart disease, Coron Artery Dis, 1997, 8: 677-682.

[82] Ombres, D., Pannitteri, G., Montali, A., Candeloro, A., Seccareccia, F., Campagna, F., Cantini, R., Campa, P. P., Ricci, G. and Arca, M., The gln-Arg192 polymorphism of human paraoxonase gene is not associated with coronary artery disease in italian patients, Arterioscler Thromb Vasc Biol, 1998, 18: 1611-1616.

[83] Garin, M. C., James, R. W., Dussoix, P., Blanche, H., Passa, P., Froguel, P. and Ruiz, J., Paraoxonase polymorphism Met-Leu54 is associated with modified serum concentrations of the enzyme. A possible link between the paraoxonase gene and increased risk of cardiovascular disease in diabetes, J Clin Invest, 1997, 99: 62-66.

[84] Sanghera, D. K., Saha, N. and Kamboh, M. I., The codon 55 polymorphism in the paraoxonase 1 gene is not associated with the risk of coronary heart disease in Asian Indians and Chinese, Atherosclerosis, 1998, 136: 217-223.

[85] Leviev, I., Negro, F. and James, R. W., Two alleles of the human paraoxonase gene produce different amounts of mRNA. An explanation for differences in serum concentrations of paraoxonase associated with the (Leu-Met54) polymorphism, Arterioscler Thromb Vasc Biol, 1997, 17: 2935-2939.

[86] Mackness, M. I., Walker, C. H. and Carlson, L. A., Low A-esterase activity in serum of patients with fish-eye disease, Clin Chem, 1987, 33: 587-588.

[87] Mackness, M. I., Peuchant, E., Dumon, M. F., Walker, C. H. and Clerc, M., Absence of "A"-esterase activity in the serum of a patient with Tangier disease, Clin Biochem, 1989, 22: 475-478.

[88] Ikeda, Y., Suehiro, T., Inoue, M., Nakauchi, Y., Morita, T., Arii, K., Ito, H., Kumon, Y. and Hashimoto, K., Serum paraoxonase activity and its relationship to diabetic complications in patients with non-insulin-dependent diabetes mellitus, Metabolism, 1998, 47: 598-602.

[89] Mackness, B., Durrington, P. N., Abuashia, B., Boulton, A. J. and Mackness, M. I., Low paraoxonase activity in type II diabetes mellitus complicated by retinopathy, Clin Sci (Lond), 2000, 98: 355-363.

[90] Mackness, M. I., Durrington, P. N., Ayub, A. and Mackness, B., Low serum paraoxonase: a risk factor for atherosclerotic disease?, Chem Biol Interact, 1999, 119-120: 389-397.

[91] James, R. W., Leviev, I. and Righetti, A., Smoking is associated with reduced serum paraoxonase activity and concentration in patients with coronary artery disease, Circulation, 2000, 101: 2252-2257.

[92] Senti, M., Tomas, M., Vila, J., Marrugat, J., Elosua, R., Sala, J. and Masia, R., Relationship of age-related myocardial infarction risk and Gln/Arg 192 variants of the human paraoxonase1 gene: the REGICOR study, Atherosclerosis, 2001, 156: 443-449.

[93] Salonen, J. T., Malin, R., Tuomainen, T. P., Nyyssonen, K., Lakka, T. A. and Lehtimaki, T., Polymorphism in high density lipoprotein paraoxonase gene and risk of acute myocardial infarction in men: prospective nested case-control study, BMJ, 1999, 319: 487-489; discussion 490.

[94] Arca, M., Ombres, D., Montali, A., Campagna, F., Mangieri, E., Tanzilli, G., Campa, P. P., Ricci, G., Verna, R. and Pannitteri, G., PON1 L55M polymorphism is not a predictor of coronary atherosclerosis either alone or in combination with Q192R polymorphism in an Italian population, Eur J Clin Invest, 2002, 32: 9-15.

[95] Mackness, B., Mackness, M. I., Arrol, S., Turkie, W., Julier, K., Abuasha, B., Miller, J. E., Boulton, A. J. and Durrington, P. N., Serum paraoxonase (PON1) 55 and 192 polymorphism and paraoxonase activity and concentration in non-insulin dependent diabetes mellitus, Atherosclerosis, 1998, 139: 341-349.

[96] Patel, B. N., Mackness, M. I., Harty, D. W., Arrol, S., Boot-Handford, R. P. and Durrington, P. N., Serum esterase activities and hyperlipidaemia in the streptozotocin-diabetic rat, Biochim Biophys Acta, 1990, 1035: 113-116.

[97] Mackness, B., Durrington, P. N. and Mackness, M. I., Human serum paraoxonase, Gen Pharmacol, 1998, 31: 329-336.

[98] Rodrigo, L., Hernandez, A. F., Lopez-Caballero, J. J., Gil, F. and Pla, A., Immunohistochemical evidence for the expression and induction of paraoxonase in rat liver, kidney, lung and brain tissue. Implications for its physiological role, Chem Biol Interact, 2001, 137: 123-137.

[99] Leviev, I. and James, R. W., Promoter polymorphisms of human paraoxonase PON1 gene and serum paraoxonase activities and concentrations, Arterioscler Thromb Vasc Biol, 2000, 20: 516-521.

[100] Brophy, V. H., Hastings, M. D., Clendenning, J. B., Richter, R. J., Jarvik, G. P. and Furlong, C. E., Polymorphisms in the human paraoxonase (PON1) promoter, Pharmacogenetics, 2001, 11: 77-84.

[101] Suehiro, T., Nakamura, T., Inoue, M., Shiinoki, T., Ikeda, Y., Kumon, Y., Shindo, M., Tanaka, H. and Hashimoto, K., A polymorphism upstream from the human paraoxonase (PON1) gene and its association with PON1 expression, Atherosclerosis, 2000, 150: 295-298.

[102] Deakin, S., Leviev, I., Brulhart-Meynet, M. C. and James, R. W., Paraoxonase-1 promoter haplotypes and serum paraoxonase: a predominant role for polymorphic position - 107, implicating the Sp1 transcription factor, Biochem J, 2003, 372: 643-649.

[103] Brophy, V. H., Jampsa, R. L., Clendenning, J. B., McKinstry, L. A., Jarvik, G. P. and Furlong, C. E., Effects of 5' regulatory-region polymorphisms on paraoxonase-gene (PON1) expression, Am J Hum Genet, 2001, 68: 1428-1436.

[104] Gouedard, C., Koum-Besson, N., Barouki, R. and Morel, Y., Opposite regulation of the human paraoxonase-1 gene PON-1 by fenofibrate and statins, Mol Pharmacol, 2003, 63: 945-956.

[105] James, R. W., Leviev, I., Ruiz, J., Passa, P., Froguel, P. and Garin, M. C., Promoter polymorphism T(-107)C of the paraoxonase PON1 gene is a risk factor for coronary heart disease in type 2 diabetic patients, Diabetes, 2000, 49: 1390-1393.

[106] Cambien, F., Genes in population. In: Malcolm,S.Goodship, J. (eds), Genotype to Phenotype. Academic Press, Guildford, UK, pp 31-53, 2001.

[107] Hegele, R. A., Brunt, J. H. and Connelly, P. W., A polymorphism of the paraoxonase gene associated with variation in plasma lipoproteins in a genetic isolate, Arterioscler Thromb Vasc Biol, 1995, 15: 89-95.

[108] Leus, F. R., Zwart, M., Kastelein, J. J. and Voorbij, H. A., PON2 gene variants are associated with clinical manifestations of cardiovascular disease in familial hypercholesterolemia patients, Atherosclerosis, 2001, 154: 641-649.

[109] Van Lenten, B. J., Hama, S. Y., de Beer, F. C., Stafforini, D. M., McIntyre, T. M., Prescott, S. M., La Du, B. N., Fogelman, A. M. and Navab, M., Anti-inflammatory HDL becomes pro-inflammatory during the acute phase response. Loss of protective effect of HDL against LDL oxidation in aortic wall cell cocultures, J Clin Invest, 1995, 96: 2758-2767.

[110] Gonzalvo, M. C., Gil, F., Hernandez, A. F., Villanueva, E. and Pla, A., Inhibition of paraoxonase activity in human liver microsomes by exposure to EDTA, metals and mercurials, Chem Biol Interact, 1997, 105: 169-179.

[111] Debord, J., Bollinger, J. C., Merle, L. and Dantoine, T., Inhibition of human serum arylesterase by metal chlorides, J Inorg Biochem, 2003, 94: 1-4.

[112] Furlong, C. E., Cole, T. B., Jarvik, G. P. and Costa, L. G., Pharmacogenomic considerations of the paraoxonase polymorphisms, Pharmacogenomics, 2002, 3: 341-348.

[113] Kaliste-Korhonen, E., Torronen, R., Ylitalo, P. and Hanninen, O., Inhibition of cholinesterases by DRP and induction of organophosphate-detoxicating enzymes in rats, Gen Pharmacol, 1990, 21: 527-533.

[114] Costa, L. G. and Furlong, C. E., Paraoxonase (PON1) in Health and Disease: Basic and Clinical Aspects. Kluwer Academic Publishers, Boston, USA., 2002.

[115] Kaliste-Korhonen, E., Tuovinen, K. and Hanninen, O., Effect of phenobarbital and beta-naphthoflavone on activities of different rat esterases after paraoxon exposure, Gen Pharmacol, 1998, 31: 307-312.

[116] Vitarius, J. A., O'Shaughnessy, J. A. and Sultatos, L. G., The effects of phenobarbital pretreatment on the metabolism and toxicity of paraoxon in the mouse, Pharmacol Toxicol, 1995, 77: 16-22.

[117] Playfer, J. R., Powell, C. and Evans, D. A., Plasma paroxonase activity in old age, Age Ageing, 1977, 6: 89-95.

[118] Zech, R. and Zurcher, K., Organophosphate splitting serum enzymes in different mammals, Comp Biochem Physiol B, 1974, 48: 427-433.

[119] Feingold, K. R., Memon, R. A., Moser, A. H. and Grunfeld, C., Paraoxonase activity in the serum and hepatic mRNA levels decrease during the acute phase response, Atherosclerosis, 1998, 139: 307-315.

[120] Pervaiz, S., Resveratrol: from grapevines to mammalian biology, FASEB J, 2003, 17: 1975-1985.

[121] Weitman, S. D., Vodicnik, M. J. and Lech, J. J., Influence of pregnancy on parathion toxicity and disposition, Toxicol Appl Pharmacol, 1983, 71: 215-224.

[122] Nishio, E. and Watanabe, Y., Cigarette smoke extract inhibits plasma paraoxonase activity by modification of the enzyme's free thiols, Biochem Biophys Res Commun, 1997, 236: 289-293.

[123] Aviram, M. and Fuhrman, B., Wine flavonoids protect against LDL oxidation and atherosclerosis, Ann N Y Acad Sci, 2002, 957: 146-161.

[124] Durrington, P. N., Mackness, B. and Mackness, M. I., The hunt for nutritional and pharmacological modulators of paraoxonase, Arterioscler Thromb Vasc Biol, 2002, 22: 1248-1250.

[125] Fuhrman, B. and Aviram, M., Preservation of paraoxonase activity by wine flavonoids: possible role in protection of LDL from lipid peroxidation, Ann N Y Acad Sci, 2002, 957: 321-324.

[126] Debord, J., Dantoine, T., Bollinger, J. C., Abraham, M. H., Verneuil, B. and Merle, L., Inhibition of arylesterase by aliphatic alcohols, Chem Biol Interact, 1998, 113: 105-115.

[127] van der Gaag, M. S., van Tol, A., Scheek, L. M., James, R. W., Urgert, R., Schaafsma, G. and Hendriks, H. F., Daily moderate alcohol consumption increases serum paraoxonase activity; a diet-controlled, randomised intervention study in middle-aged men, Atherosclerosis, 1999, 147: 405-410.

[128] Hayek, T., Fuhrman, B., Vaya, J., Rosenblat, M., Belinky, P., Coleman, R., Elis, A. and Aviram, M., Reduced progression of atherosclerosis in apolipoprotein E-deficient mice following consumption of red wine, or its polyphenols quercetin or catechin, is associated with reduced susceptibility of LDL to oxidation and aggregation, Arterioscler Thromb Vasc Biol, 1997, 17: 2744-2752.

[129] Aviram, M., Dornfeld, L., Rosenblat, M., Volkova, N., Kaplan, M., Coleman, R., Hayek, T., Presser, D. and Fuhrman, B., Pomegranate juice consumption reduces oxidative stress, atherogenic modifications to LDL, and platelet aggregation: studies in humans and in atherosclerotic apolipoprotein E-deficient mice, Am J Clin Nutr, 2000, 71: 1062-1076.

[130] Kaplan, M., Hayek, T., Raz, A., Coleman, R., Dornfeld, L., Vaya, J. and Aviram, M., Pomegranate juice supplementation to atherosclerotic mice reduces macrophage lipid peroxidation, cellular cholesterol accumulation and development of atherosclerosis, J Nutr, 2001, 131: 2082-2089.

[131] Forte, T. M., Subbanagounder, G., Berliner, J. A., Blanche, P. J., Clermont, A. O., Jia, Z., Oda, M. N., Krauss, R. M. and Bielicki, J. K., Altered activities of anti-atherogenic enzymes LCAT, paraoxonase, and platelet-activating factor acetylhydrolase in atherosclerosis-susceptible mice, J Lipid Res, 2002, 43: 477-485.

[132] Hedrick, C. C., Hassan, K., Hough, G. P., Yoo, J. H., Simzar, S., Quinto, C. R., Kim, S. M., Dooley, A., Langi, S., Hama, S. Y., Navab, M., Witztum, J. L. and Fogelman, A. M., Short-term feeding of atherogenic diet to mice results in reduction of HDL and paraoxonase that may be mediated by an immune mechanism, Arterioscler Thromb Vasc Biol, 2000, 20: 1946-1952.

[133] Shih, D. M., Gu, L., Hama, S., Xia, Y. R., Navab, M., Fogelman, A. M. and Lusis, A. J., Genetic-dietary regulation of serum paraoxonase expression and its role in atherogenesis in a mouse model, J Clin Invest, 1996, 97: 1630-1639.

[134] de Roos, N. M., Schouten, E. G., Scheek, L. M., van Tol, A. and Katan, M. B., Replacement of dietary saturated fat with trans fat reduces serum paraoxonase activity in healthy men and women, Metabolism, 2002, 51: 1534-1537.

[135] Wallace, A. J., Sutherland, W. H., Mann, J. I. and Williams, S. M., The effect of meals rich in thermally stressed olive and safflower oils on postprandial serum paraoxonase activity in patients with diabetes, Eur J Clin Nutr, 2001, 55: 951-958.

[136] Tomas, M., Senti, M., Elosua, R., Vila, J., Sala, J., Masia, R. and Marrugat, J., Interaction between the Gln-Arg 192 variants of the paraoxonase gene and oleic acid intake as a determinant of high-density lipoprotein cholesterol and paraoxonase activity, Eur J Pharmacol, 2001, 432: 121-128.

[137] Sutherland, W. H., Walker, R. J., de Jong, S. A., van Rij, A. M., Phillips, V. and Walker, H. L., Reduced postprandial serum paraoxonase activity after a meal rich in used cooking fat, Arterioscler Thromb Vasc Biol, 1999, 19: 1340-1347.

[138] Aviram, M., Rosenblat, M., Billecke, S., Erogul, J., Sorenson, R., Bisgaier, C. L., Newton, R. S. and La Du, B., Human serum paraoxonase (PON 1) is inactivated by oxidized low density lipoprotein and preserved by antioxidants, Free Radic Biol Med, 1999, 26: 892-904.

Part 2

Acute Coronary Syndrome

7

Acute Coronary Syndrome: Pathological Findings by Means of Electron Microscopy, Advance Imaging in Cardiology

Mohaddeseh Behjati[1] and Iman Moradi[2]
[1]Isfahan University of Medical Sciences,
[2]NCDC Center,
[1]Iran
[2]Italy

1. Introduction

Acute coronary syndrome (ACS) caused by a blockage in coronary arteries as a result of atherosclerosis or thrombosis, is one of the leading causes of death worldwide [Rajapakse et al., 2010]. Due to the altered trends of ischemic heart disease and emergence of some new cardiovascular risk factors in depth understanding of the underlying pathophysiological mechanisms is needed. In this way, inspection of the anatomical structures responsible for the development of acute coronary events is highly deemed and electron microscope is the right instrument for this purpose.

For a long while, electron microscopy has been used as one of the best instruments for pathologic diagnostics. These scientific instruments use a beam of highly energetic electrons to examine objects on very fine scales. Limitations of light microscopes due to the physics of light with limited 500X or 1000X magnification and a resolution of 200 nanometer let scientist to search for development of Electron Microscopes. Basic steps involved in all EMs, regardless of type, include a stream of electrons made by electron source which is accelerated toward the specimen using a positive electrical potential. This stream is restricted and focused into a thin beam using metal apertures and magnetic lenses. Electron beams are affected by interactions occurred inside the irradiated sample. These interactions are transformed to the final image [www.upesh.edu.pk].

Transmission Electron Microscope (TEM) was the first type of Electron Microscope developed by Max Knoll and Ernst Ruska in Germany in 1931. It was patterned exactly on the Light Transmission Microscope except application of a focused beam of electrons instead of light in order to "see through" the specimen. TEM functions with a high voltage electron beam in order to create images [McMullan, 1993]. Emitted electrons by electron gun fitted with a tungsten alloy filament cathode as electron source. An anode typically at 100 KeV accelerates electron beams with respect to the cathodes, are focused by electrostatic and electromagnetic lenses and transmitted through the specimens. Thus, scattered electron beams carries information about the structure of specimen which is magnified by objective lens system of microscope. The final image will be appeared on a screen coated by fluorescent material. This specific screen is necessary as the regular images of electrons are not visible for our eyes. Images detected by CCD (charge-coupled devices) camera might be displayed on a monitor or computer [Wikipedia]. The resolution of TEM is partly limited by spherical aberrations but using aberration correctors, achievement of higher resolutions became possible. This correction using hardware made it possible to achieve images with resolution values below 0.5 angstrom and magnifications above 50 million times by for high-resolution TEM (HRTEM) [Erni et al., 2009, Wikipedia].

Freeze-fracturing also known as freeze-etch or freeze-and-break is another preparation method valuable for evaluation of lipid membranes and their incorporated proteins in "face on" view [Severs, 2007, Sekiya et al., 1979]. It reveals proteins embedded in lipid bi-layer [Sekiya et al., 1979]. Fresh tissue or cell suspension is frozen promptly (cryofixed), then fractured by simple breaking or using a microtome at liquid nitrogen temperature [Osumi et al., 2006, Dempsey & Bullivant, 1976]. Cold fractured surface is consequently "etched" by increasing the temperature to about -95°C for a few minutes, in order to reveal microscopic details by subliming surface ice. One rotary-shadowed with evaporated platinum at low angle (typically about 6°) in a high vacuum evaporator is required for TEM as an extra- step that is not needed for SEM. To improve the stability of replica coating, a second carbon coating is generally performed. Thereafter, chemical digestion with acids, hypochlorite solution or SDS detergent is used to release the extremely fragile "shadowed" metal replica of the fracture surface. Washed floating replica is picked up on EM grid and used for TEM evaluation after complete drying [Wikipedia]. Freeze-etched preparation of vessels can be investigated using this method to demonstrate altered intimal cushions in cases with and without ACS. Immune localization study of deep-etch replicas of frozen vessels will enhance our knowledge regarding pathologic changes during the process of ACS development. This method is highly suitable for depiction of fat deposits in vessel walls (Guyton & Klemp, 1992). Actually, the hypothesis of fused lipoproteins in the extracellular space to form larger lipid deposits has been first proposed by Frank and Fogelman using this technique [Guyton & Klemp, 1992].

Scanning Electron Microscope (SEM), first debuted around 1965, works exactly as their optical counterparts except using a focused beam of electrons rather than light to image specimens and gain informatics details about their composition and structure. It images samples by scanning it with high-energy electron beams in a raster scan pattern. Signals made by interaction of electron beams with samples' atoms bring information about the sample's surface topography, composition, and other properties as electrical conductivity. The final image resolution of SEM is poorer than that achieved by TEM. Since SEM images rely on surface processes rather than transmission, bulk imaging of samples up to many centimeters in size with great depth of field is possible. Thus, images with good representation of three-dimensional shape of samples can be achieved [Wikipedia]. SEMs equipped with cold stage for cryo-microscopy can be used for cryofixation as low temperature SEM [Read & Jeffree, 1991]. Cryo-fixed specimens can also be cryo-fractured under vacuum to reveal internal structures [Faulkner et al., 2008]. Sputter coated cryo-fractured specimens are transferred onto cryo-staged SEM in frozen state [Faulkner et al., 2008]. Low-temperature SEM can be used effectively for imaging temperature-sensitive materials as fats, thus fatty athermanous plaques might be good subjects for this kind of imaging [Hindmarsh et al., 2007].

One of the fundamental progresses in the field of SEM has been related to the development of environmental scanning electron microscope (ESEM). Since conventional SEM needs high vacuum for proper imaging, samples that produce significant amounts of vapor like wet or oily biological samples need to be either dried or cryogenically frozen. ESEM developed in late 1980s, allowed samples to be observed in high relative humidity and low-pressure gaseous environments [Mohankumar, 2010]. This capability has been attributed to the presence of secondary-electron detectors operating in the presence of water vapor and pressure-limiting apertures supplemented with differential pumping in the path of electron beams in order to separate vacuum region from the sample chamber [Mohankumar, 2010]. Bypassing the need for coating with carbon or gold, ESEM became a useful instrument for investigation of non-metallic and biological materials [Ishidi et al., 2011]. Irreversibility of coating process with concealing effects on sample surface might reduce value of obtained results and the advantage of ESEM is bypassing this step [Ishidi et al., 2011]. In contrary with SEM, ESEM allows X-ray microanalysis on uncoated non-conductive specimens [Wikipedia]. In this case, polymer or surface damage induced after intravascular deployment of drug eluting stent has been visualized using ESEM [Wiemer et al, 2010]. Indeed, evaluation of qualitative surface morphology and elemental analysis of intravascular stents designed for the treatment of ACS is possible through ESEM [Sojitra et al, 2009]. Despite of these advancements, there is still plenty room for further applications of ESEM in revealing the underlying pathophysiological mechanisms of ACS.

Meanwhile, SEM plays a main role in characterization of athermanous lesions containing oily and volatile materials through a new approach called wet SEM technique. It is ideal for examination of fully-hydrated or liquid-containing samples - as biological cells, tissues, and fluid suspensions [Bergmans et al., 2005]. Wet SEM technique provides researchers by an accurate and detailed structural evaluation of pathological processes involved in development and progression of atherosclerosis [KAMARI et al., 2008]. In wet SEM, wet samples are protected from high vacuum conditions applied in conventional EMs [Bergmans et al., 2005]. Conventional EMs, need samples to be evaluated at high vacuum conditions, wet specimens are not suitable for evaluation using this today's primary tool for high-resolution imaging. This is one major drawback for application of EM in biomedical research. Previously, wet specimens were evaluating using freezing or drying. This time-consuming, costly and artifact-prone procedure was associated with changing specimen's nature and consequently. Wet SEM has reduced the preparation needs required for high-resolution of such wet specimens which consequently made easier and faster imaging possible. Less occurred artifacts are also note worthy. This technique is cheap and widely applicable for various samples [Bogner et al., 2007].

Other developed EM variations are also useful for investigation of ACS, which are included here. EM-immunohistochemistry serves in distinct subcellular localization of proteins in heart as at the level of sarcomer, A-, I-, H- bands and Z-, M-line. It needs labeling of ultrathin sections with purified polyclonal antibodies. This helps in understanding the cell function in normal and pathologic conditions. Immune gold EM is based on the application of antibodies against the desired element and densities of immune labeling reflected by number of gold particles per unit area of respective structural component. It has been applied for determination of proteins in myofibrils associated with actin, myosin filaments and with sarcomers (Z-lines), in sarcoplasmic reticulum and in mitochondria [Maco et al., 2001].

EM-TUNEL serves a fundamental role in definite distinguishing apoptotic cells and their remnants from necrosis. Indeed, it can detect apoptotic cell death without nuclear condensation or DNA fragmentation. Immune gold particles in normal cells are slightly accumulated on nuclear heterochromatin, contrary with apoptotic cells in which gold particles are significantly accumulated on condensed chromatin. Due to high electron density of apoptotic nucleolus, fainter prints with attenuated contrast of background are recommended. Evaluation of myocytes and smooth muscle cells (SMCs) isolated from primary coronary lesions using EM-TUNEL showed rich glycogen granules in cytoplasm, condensated chromatin clumped to the nuclear envelope with clearing of central nuclear region, fragmentation of internucleosomal DNA, cell fragmentation into small membrane-bound vesicles in the presence of undamaged mitochondria and without rupture of cell membrane at early stages [Ohno et al., 1998]. Matrix vesicles also known as apoptotic detritus vary in size and shape but are often speckled appearance reflect final phase of apoptosis [Bauriedel et al., 1999]. Cell shrinkage, subsequent formation of membrane bound apoptotic bodies and phagocytosis are observed in final stages [Ohno et al., 1998].

For biological specimens, sample preparation is necessary. Inside the electron microscope is under high vacuum suitable for travelling of electron beams in a straight line which makes sample processing a prerequisite step. Applied processing procedure highly depends on the specimen, mentioned analyses and type of applied microscope. The quality of final electron micrograph is a function of the quality of preparation. EM is an expensive technique due to the complexity of process and the cost of applied materials, but it is still profitable because of its power for diagnostics purposes. Biological specimens should be dried completely for evaluation under high vacuum condition of SEM. Living cells, tissues and soft-bodied organisms often need chemical fixation prior to preservation and stabilization of their structure. For evaluation of pathologic and reparative alterations during ACS, samples taken from infarcted regions, periinfarct site regions bordering the infarction, are at risk, the center of non-risk area, subendocardial, subepicardial or transmural portions and healthy tissue in the left ventricular myocardium or anterior superior intraventricular septum as positioning control samples are valuable. Samples could be taken using paunch biopsy or by cutting the region of interest under direct visualization, based on the characteristics of the sample source. Transmural biopsies could be taken during coronary intervention, percutaneous atherectomy or bypass graft surgery. Obviously, direct tissue sampling from heart can be achieved through post-mortem analysis of research animal models or expired humans suffered from ACS. Samples should be taken immediately after killing animals. In addition to myocytes, coronary arteries can also be evaluated after AMI by subdividing them into infarct related artery (IRA) and non –IRA. Stenotic segments can be cutted and decalcified if necessary. Animal models of acute ischemia and ischemia-reperfusion injury (wild type or knocked-out and transgenic) facilitated these kinds of investigation, especially in the case of evaluation of temporal changes after ACS. Models of temporarily ischemia, reversibly vs. irreversible injury, gentle vs. abrupt reperfusion and other intended study models can be generated in vivo. Animal hearts can be fixed with vascular perfusion of fixative agents through abdominal aorta. Perfusion fixation allows usage of vascular system of a deeply anesthetized animal to deliver fixative agents to tissues of interest. Since tissues are fixed before autolysis begins, this technique is considered as the optimal method of tissue preservation. Perfused tissues are less vulnerable to artifact injuries caused by handling. Fixation techniques vary depending on the organ, tissue and the desired processing. Appropriate literature review should be done to determine the ideal technique for the organ of concern. With perfusion fixation in contrast to direct immersion fixation, no cell rupture during mincing prior to fixation will occur.

Immediately fixed cardiac endothelium presents an invariable surface throughout the interior of the heart. Smooth predominant nuclear bulges and attenuated peripheral plasmalemma with occasional marginal ruffles, scattered microvilli and small blebs can also be seen. Various stages of systole and diastole lead to some physiological local variations in SEM of endocardium. Great liability of endocardial surface is seen in response to classic "holding solution" often used in preparatory technique. Thus, caution must be paid in preparing soft tissues for SEM in the case of applied "holding solution" [Peine & Low, 1975]. Some tissues need pretreatment before fixation step, as SMCs which should be collected after trypsinization [Tran et al., 2004].

Harvested samples should be immediately transferred to cold fixative agent. Samples can also be freezed rapidly, typically to liquid nitrogen temperatures or below, that water forms ice (cryofixation) [Mitsuoka, 2011]. This preserves the specimen with the minimal of artifacts. With cryo-electron microscopy, it is possible to observe any biological specimen close to its native state. Anyway, preserved samples are then dissected into small cubes when lying in the fixative and fixed. Fixation is a general term used to describe the process of preserving a sample at a moment in time and to prevent further deterioration so that it appears as close as possible to what it would be like in the living state, although it is now dead. Fixation is performed by incubation of samples in a solution of a buffered chemical aldehyde-based fixative, such as glutaraldehyde, paraformaldehyde, or formaldehyde or combinations of these [Read & Jeffree, 1991, Karnovsky, 1965, Kiernan, 2000]. For primary fixation, glutaraldehyde buffered (pH 7.4) in sodium cacodylate, Sucrose or phosphate buffers (PBS, HEPES, and PIPES), are used. Glutaraldehyde and osmium tetroxide are often used to crosslink protein molecules and to preserve lipids, respectively. This step is followed by post-fixation with osmium tetroxide (OsO4) [Read & Jeffree, 1991]. A buffer containing sodium cacodylate, Sucrose and 2-Mercaptoethanol is recommended if precipitation is visible in final sections. Secondary fixation with OsO4 can be performed either in aqueous or in the same buffer as used in the primary fixative. Osmium-based procedures should be performed under a fume hood with worn gloves due to the toxicity and fixation capability of the Osmium fumes. Aqueous Uranyl acetate can be used for tertiary fixation or en-bloc staining. This can enhance membranes preservation by serving both as a fixative and stain. Fixed tissues are then dehydrated in graded series of ethanol or through using an acetone gradient or propylene oxide. It is a stepping stone towards total drying infiltration with resin for subsequent embedding for SEM or TEM analysis, respectively. Samples are treated with propylene oxide in a mixture of EM grade resin and Succinic anhydride as the transition solvent before embedding. Samples are then embedded in an adhesive such as epoxy resin, EPON medium, Spurr's Resin, LR White and so on.

Since air-drying causes sample collapse and shrinkage, critical point drying (CPD) is used commonly for dehydration step. CPD replaces intracellular water with organic solvents as acetone. These solvents replace in turn with a transitional fluid as liquid carbon dioxide at high pressure. By removing of carbon dioxide in a supercritical state, no gas-liquid interface will be present within the sample during drying [ProSciTech]. After heat polymerization, ultrathin sections, typically under 90 nm, which are semitransparent to electrons, are preferred. Using ultramicrotomes or diamond knives, these sections are prepared from selected blocks. Glass knives and are much cheaper than diamond and can be easily made in laboratory, but they blunt frequently and need replacing. Optimal timing of serial sectioning after AMI should be kept in mind. After 24 hrs the edges of infarct becomes very narrow and easily missed on biopsy specimens [Hoffstein et al., 1975]. In contrast, biopsy specimens from marginal zones are easily taken in early hours after AMI [Hoffstein et al., 1975]. For SEM, sample size must be considered due to limitations of microscope chamber size and specimen exchange. Sections are then collected on metallic grids. Grids are mesh-like metallic discs for holding the ultrathin sections. The number of meshes varies from one for calibration of instrument to 1000 for studying the viruses. Therefore, the number of meshes depends on the size of specimen and accuracy of the study. For tissues like athermanous plaques and heart we recommend 200-mesh grids which may be made of gold, Nickel, silver, copper or other conductive metals. In SEM, dry specimens are usually mounted on stubs using electrically-conductive double-sided adhesive tape. Tissues are stained with the salt of Uranyl acetate and followed by lead citrate in double staining. Experimentally, Uranyl acetate provides better membrane perseveration and contrast but it leaves empty spaces in cells due to glycogen extraction [Vye & Fischman, 1970]. Indeed, the acidic pH of the stain leads in calcium extraction which subsequently results in un-visualization of mitochondrial granular dense bodies using en blocks stained it aqueous Uranyl acetate [Kloner et al., 1974].

Since biological samples are nearly transparent to electron beams, heavy metals give contrast between different structures by scattering imaging electrons. By staining using heavy metals, added electron density results in better contrast by providing more interaction between primary beam and those of sample. Then, samples are sputter coated using electrically-conducting materials, deposited on the surface of samples by low vacuum coating, in order to prevent specimen charging during imaging process due to accumulation of static electric fields by irradiated electrons. In this way, the amount of detectable secondary electrons from the surface of samples and consequently signal to noise ratio are increased [Mancuso et al., 1988]. Generally, gold or gold alloys, silver and iridium are used for this purpose [Suzuki, 2002]. Gold with high atomic number provide a coating with high topographic contrast and resolution [Wikipedia]. However, this coating with a few nanometer thicknesses can obscure the underlying through details of samples at very high magnification. Imaging without coating has been possible using low-vacuum SEMs with differential pumping apertures [Schatten & Pawley, 2007]. Thus, coating induced loss of contrast is obviated but the obtained resolution will be less than SEM with conventional sample coating [Schatten et al., 2008]. Ultimately, processed samples undergo observation and photography using a perspective electron microscope. Attention should be paid regarding possible loss of agents from tissues during fixation and embedding.

Due to the complexity of sample preparation, a technique so-called cryoultramicrotomy facilitates this process. Cryofixation, cryoultramicrotomy, and appropriate transfer of cryosections into the electron microscope are vial for proper ultrastructure and measurement of subcellular elemental distributions [Hagler et al., 1986]. All of these stages seem fundamental for experimental analysis of ultrastructural modification of heart prior, within and after acute ischemic insult. In cryo-ultramicrotomy or cryo-sectioning samples are sectioned at temperatures below 273K in order to avoid damaging effects of temperatures above this threshold on ultrastructure by lipid melting [Hagler et al., 1986]. Rapid section freezing leads to occurrence of minimal or no ice damage during the cryofixation step. Hagler et al., 1986]. This technique facilitates the process to cut objects, hardened by cooling, without the need for deleterious fixation, dehydration, and embedding. In this way, a favorable basis for x-ray microanalysis of electrolytes and soluble cell constituents and histochemical and immunocytochemical localization of molecules is gained from frozen sections. But this technique is not confined to frozen sections and non-aqueous components embedded in a water matrix can also be used. Preparation of plastics, polymers, and elastomers either liquid or highly flexible at ambient temperatures is allowed by technique. Mechanical strength of object has been increased by applied low temperature which is associated with attenuated viscosity and plastic flow. It will convert essentially liquid materials to solids, if enough low temperature is reached [Adelide University, 2011]. An important issue which should be cared while handing with cryoultramicrotomy and cryo-sectioning, is proper cryotransfer stage for transfer of sectioned pieces from cryoultramicrotome to the electron microscope [Hagler et al., 1986]. By application of this stage, potential problems with rehydration damage to freeze-dried sections are avoided [Hagler et al., 1986]. Indeed, possible lipid melting in sections is also prohibited [Hagler et al., 1986]. In this way, tissue morphology and *in situ* elemental distribution are well preserved within tissues [Hagler et al., 1986].

Since tissue antigenecity is preserved using cryo-ultramicrotomy, this technique is suitable for in-depth investigation of mechanisms involved in the pathogenesis of ACS [Russell. et al., 1998]. This technique has been previously used for structural analysis of cardiac muscle [Luther, 2007]. Cryoultramicrotomy of myocardium using a cryosystem interfaced with an ultramicrotome was performed by BUJA et al to investigate microanalysis of the elemental composition of rabbit myocytes in hypoxic conditions. In this study, a knife temperature as low as $-100^{0}C$ was applied [Buja et al., 1983]. Substructure of inner mitochondrial membranes of myocardial cells has also been depicted using cryo-ultramicrotomy [Sætersdal et al., 1978]. This technique can provide good facilities for depiction of ultrastructural modifications during the process of development and progression of ACS.

Depiction of some sub-cellular elements needs more manipulation. Mitochondrial pellet preparation is partly a complex process. Heart pieces after mincing with scissors are immersed and homogenized in isolation buffer containing sucrose, mannitol, EDTA in Tris/HCL pH 7.4. For optimal homogenization, tissue grinder can be used. Supernatant of centrifugated homogenate is poured through cheesecloth, re-centrifugated and re-suspended in above buffer. Mitochondria are washed in that buffer and centrifugated. Isolated mitochondria are stored on ice prior investigation [Bopassa et al., 2006]. For depiction of ribosomes, residual glycogen storage should be extracted [Vye & Fischman, 1970]. Evaluation of glycogen content is performed using PAS-staining [Sherman et al., 2000]. Masson tri-chrome staining can be used for collagen staining [Toumpoulis et al., 2009].

Acute coronary syndrome is mainly evolved from insidious development of atherosclerotic nidus. Each plaque is composed mainly from a fatty core, a fibrous cap with partly calcified shell. It is the proportion of fatty core to the fibrous cap that determines the plaque stability. Using SEM, cholesterol crystals (CCs) with intima perforation and tearing have been demonstrated within plaques prepared with ethanol or vacuum dehydration [Abela et al.,

2009]. Cholesterol crystals vary in shape and size, perforating the intima of coronary arteries and are strongly associated with acute coronary syndrome and cardiac death as well as with thrombus at rupture and/or erosion sites [Schmid et al, 1980, [Ewence et al., 2008]. This suggests that cholesterol crystallization is critical to plaque rupture and/or erosion and is associated with thrombosis and clinical events [Abela et al., 2006]. Cholesterol materials expand with crystallization tearing and perforating fibrous tissues [Abela et al., 2009]. Acute coronary syndromes are mainly attributed to plaque rupture or erosion [Sun et al., 2011]. Thus, plaque morphology determines plaque phenotype. These events are commonly known as plaque disruption (PD) [Abela et al., 2006]. The role of CCs in triggering and development of PD is yet unknown. Recently, it has been observed that large plate-like calcified areas are correlated with stable plaque phenotype [Ewence et al., 2008]. In contrary, speckled or spotty calcified deposits are commonly observed in ruptured atherosclerotic plaques [Virmani et al., 2003, Ehara et al., 2004, Vengrenyuk et al., 2006]. It has been suggested that microcalcifications exert local stress in atherosclerotic fibrous caps [Virmani et al., 2003, Ehara et al., 2004, Vengrenyuk et al., 2006]. Calcium phosphate micro- and nanoparticles and hydroxyapatite-containing "atherosclerotic gruel" lead to apoptosis of plaque vascular SMC (VSMCs) which is linked with weakening of the fibrous cap and plaque rupture and instability [Ewence et al., 2008]. Multiplication of SMC nuclei have been observed in atherosclerotic plaques, but SMCs "hurry on to their own destruction" as Virchow has stated, which brings plaque instability [Virchow, 1860]. SEM evaluation of calcified extracts from ruptured plaques demonstrated that small non-aggregated particles are more cytotoxic to VSMCs than larger deposits [Ewence et al., 2008]. Indeed, small crystals are more potent than large ones in activating inflammatory cascades driven by macrophages [Nadra et al., 2008]. Calcium phosphate crystals lead in rapid rise in intracellular calcium ion concentration [Ewence et al., 2008]. Un-sequestrated calcium leads to loss of function of membrane pumps and consequently cell death [Ewence et al., 2008]. VSMC death potentiates calcification by providing a nidus for further nucleation and activation of various downstream inflammatory pathways as release of cytokines [Proudfoot et al., 2000, Park et al., 2006, Zhou et al., 2008, Porto et al., 2006]. In addition to size, crystal composition is also of paramount importance. Similar effects in reducing VSMC viability was seen by synthetic carbonated or noncarbonated forms of hydroxyapatite [Ewence et al., 2008]. Hydroxyapatite crystals are found to be less damaging than more soluble forms of calcium phosphate [Ewence et al., 2008]. In this regard, analytic EM played a great role. Analytical EM clarifies the correlation of structure and elemental content in thin sections of normal and diseased tissues [Buja et al., 1976]. Through detection of specific elemental traces, it helps in localization of histological reactions [Buja et al., 1976]. Subtle changes of electrolyte homeostasis can be identified through this technique [Buja et al., 1976]. Indeed, cryo-ultramicrotomy techniques for preparation of unfixed, unstained thin section allow elucidation of very early stages in formation of calcium-containing inclusion bodies [Buja et al., 1976].

Other factors as surface crystal properties and containing factors like anti-apoptotic and calcification-regulatory proteins as fetuin might attenuate their detrimental effects [Ewence et al., 2008]. In design of research on the mechanisms of plaque calcification and identification of treatments to ameliorate plaque calcification, it should be kept in mind that tissues should be prepared without ethanol solvents that dissolve CCs, are highly recommended [Abela et al., 2009]. Accumulated calcium in tissues leads to mitochondrial damage and prevention of cell recovery [Duchen, 2004]. SEM analysis of fixed mitochondrial suspension demonstrated opening of mitochondrial transition pores in response to calcium-induced permeability [Hüser et al., 1998]. This mitochondrial damage is associated with formation of two types of mitochondrial inclusion bodies as necrotic cell type inclusion and viable cell type inclusions. The former which occupies enlarged matrix spaces, masks crista membrane profiles and often invaded intracristal spaces of disrupted mitochondria has been observed in aneurysmal ventricular wall. The second type of inclusion materials occurred in the presence of various focal ultrastructural changes has been observed in hearts with old myocardial infarctions or unstable angina [Kawamura et al., 1978].

Typical phenotypic characteristics of normal fixed cardiomyocytes revealed by SEM and TEM include ovoid nucleus with irregular shallow indentation and evenly distributed nuclear chromatins with small amounts of heterochromatin clustered near inner nuclear envelope, regularly ordered myofibrils with intact sarcolemma, contracted sarcomers, prominent I bands, intact intercalated discs with narrow interspaces and regularly patterned honeycombs of sarcoplasmic reticulum over the periphery of myofibrils are observed [Sherman et al., 2000, Sage & Jennings, 1988]. In addition, lysosomes with variable amounts of lipid and dense materials, dense granules of glycogen particles distributed through the cell mainly in perinuclear regions, abundant mitochondria elongated between myofibrils, rounded in perinuclear areas with intact double membrane, numerous tightly packed orderly cristae, small condensed homogenous matrix space and tiny dense randomly scattered intra-mitochondrial matrix granules are also visible [Sherman et al., 2000, Li et al., 2001, Sage & Jennings, 1988]. Patent and empty capillaries with few collagen fibers in a relatively clear matrix are other findings in normal myocytes [Sage & Jennings, 1988].

In myocytes suffered from ischemic or reperfusion injury SEM and TEM analyses marked intracellular and extracellular edema, parenchymal cell swelling, hemorrhage, endothelial cell swelling, intraluminal bleb formation, disappeared Lysosomal enzymes from lateral sacs of vesiculated sarcoplasmic reticulum, disintegrated sarcolemma membrane, appearance of electron dense materials in capillary lumen, membrane-bound vesicles disintegrated plasma membrane, partial or complete depletion of glycogen granules, nuclear chromatin indentation are identified [Sherman et al., 2000, Sage & Jennings, 1988, Hoffstein et al, 1975]. In swollen cells contraction bands with few thick filaments in the A band and disarrayed sarcomers with preferential loss of myosin thick filaments, relaxed I bands, some hypercontractile areas in adjoining "unaffected" myocytes, abnormally contracted myofibrils, disrupted myofibrils with interfilamental edema and large intracellular vacuoles are apparent [Sage & Jennings, 1988, Sherman et al., 2000]. Empty electron lucent spaces seen between myofibrils around mitochondria and free cell margin are attributed to the appearance of wide clear interstitial spaces separating myocytes [Sage & Jennings, 1988]. Large subsarcolemmal bleb-like fluid spaces, possibly derived from dilated sarcoplasmic reticulum, appear tom compress adjacent capillaries [Sherman et al., 2000, Sage & Jennings, 1988]. In ischemic tissue, collapsed vessels with reduced capillary lumen are visible [Sage & Jennings, 1988].

Presence of normal or slightly damaged mitochondria in cells with severely injured cytoplasm implies the occurrence of mitochondrial damage subsequent to cytoplasmic damage [Hoffstein et al., 1975]. Spectrum of inspected mitochondrial changes seen using

SEM, TEM and STEM during AMI include denudation of mitochondrial structure as well as reorganized and processed mitochondria with mitochondrial swelling, loss of matrix density, formation of large annular, granular and amorphous intramitochondrial dense bodies, mitochondrial calcification, complete loss of tubular cristae (cristolysis), extensive swelling and appearance of mitochondria containing mitochondria remnants [Kloner et al., 1974, Buja et al., 1976]. No trace element was detected in moderately electron-dense amorphous inclusion bodies in mitochondria isolated from centers as well as the peripheries of myocardial infarcts [Buja et al., 1976]. Appearance of flocculent granules or "amorphous matrix" within mitochondrial cristae reflects server irreversible mitochondrial injury as a result of precipitation of denatured proteins [Buja et al., 1976].

In spite of plaque composition, EM evaluation could be applied to display other players in evolution from stable plaque to ACS. Inflammation is a tightly bound element to the progression of stable towards unstable plaques. Leukocyte margiantion and migration into nascent atherosclerotic plaques are correlated with severity of atherosclerosis and extent of endothelial cell turnover [Jerome et al., 1983]. The sites of rapid endothelial cell turnover with enhanced leukocyte adherence were depicted using stereological analysis of conventional SEM preparations [Jerome et al., 1983]. Although accumulation of leukocytes and inflammatory cells occurs in area susceptible to atherosclerosis, critical congestion of these cells is particularly evident at the growing edge of lesions [Jerome et al., 1983].

Another participant factor in the scenario of ACS is activation of thrombotic cascades. Thrombus formation occludes capillary lumen at the site of plaque rupture due to the exposure of sub-intima collagen with circulating and recruited platelets [Tselepis et al., 2011]. Clots extracted from occluded vessels have been evaluated in terms of fiber diameter and thickness. Clot samples were incubated for 1 hr in room temperature in a mixture of HBS, CaCl2, fibrinogen and thrombin [Dugan et al., 2006]. These observations might gain therapeutic insights. SEM allows visualization of full three-dimensional image the severely altered collagen structures of heart in temporal intervals after AMI. Ultrastructure of Infarct scar tissue and collagen fibers can be investigated in various time intervals after AMI. SEM can also used for demonstration of the pathogens suggested to be associated with progression of atherosclerosis. Presence of C. pneumonia (CP) in the cytoplasm of cardiomyocytes, with large abnormal reticular bodies surrounded by abundant mitochondria and numerous electron dense sites reflecting nucleoid condensation near the CP cell wall, are displayed using TEM [Spagnoli et al., 2007]. EM evaluation can also be applied for ultrastructural analysis of cell-to-cell contacts, basement membranes, membrane channels, receptor proteins, lipid rafts, cholesterol-rich plasma domains and plasma invaginations within acute ischemic event. Volume fraction (vV) of different tissue components and cell organelles could be quantified using stereological analysis of TEM [Lindal et al., 1990]. SEM provided with a rectilinear grid can calculate volume densities of intact and disrupted myofibrils [Sherman et al., 2000].

TEM with a standardized in vitro method can be used to evaluate the degree of blood platelet reactivity. Through this technique the number of circulating platelets/mm^3 is also determined. Three distinct types of platelets are observed when platelets are classified at the magnification level of TEM. The round type is compact, has a smooth contour, uniformly electron-dense and corresponded to the disc-shaped circulating platelet. Dendritic type is characterized by a compact, electron-dense central area from which pseudopodia extruded.

The spread type shows varying degrees of cytoplasmic spreading between adjacent pseudopodia accompanies by relocation of internal organelles. Platelet differential count includes the percent of round, dendritic and spread type platelets. Also the number of platelet aggregates counted during classification of the 100 single platelets can be recorded through this technique [Riddle et al., 1983]. TEM can also be used for acute ischemic events related to cardiotoxic compounds. TEM has potential to be used for molecular characterization of disease mechanisms involved in the development and progression of ACS. Indeed, myocardial autophagy variation and drug effects on mitochondrial function, apoptosis and in one word cytoprotection can also be seen using SEM [Zhang et al., 2009]. An example is beneficial effects of Carvedilol on mitochondrial function [Zhang et al., 2009]. EM analysis provided structural insights to the beneficial effects of Glucose-Insulin-Potassium infusion on myocardium with reduced mitochondrial flocculent granules and diminished infarct size [Sybers et al., 1973]. Effects of applied angiogenic factors, growth factors and engrafted regenerating stem cells for the treatment of ACS could be investigated using EM. TEM analysis displayed progression of cardiac progenitor cells displayed elongated uninucleated beating cells with myosin filaments radiating outward from dense bodies into an organizing sarcomer and copious mitochondria [Winitsky et al., 2005]. EM analysis provides valuable information from co-cultured stem cells with cardiomyocytes which can gain insights into the in depth understanding of regenerative medicine and its therapeutic opportunities. Characterization of cardiomyocyte progenitors and their niches is possible through application of SEM. These cells show ultrastructurally thin filaments organized by desmine-like structures, thick filaments, Z-line dense structures and confluent intracytoplasmic vesicles recognized as primordial T tubules [Popescu et al., 2009].

TEM analysis made progress in evaluation of protective effects of ischemic preconditioning (IPC) on ACS outcomes. Mitochondria isolated directly from IPC rabbit hearts showed a delayed mitochondrial pore opening by exposure to Calcium-overload [Argaud et al., 2004]. Thus less mitochondria sweltering, cristolysis and lost membrane integrity was occurred [Argaud et al., 2004]. Subsequently, improved myocardial salvage with less apoptosis and necrosis was occurred [Argaud et al., 2004]. Using EM analysis, it is possible to evaluate complications of ACS as rupture of papillary muscles, intraventricular septum and free wall by samples taken from these segments post-mortem or during reparative interventions. It is possible to observe changes made in vessels and organs remote from heart during acute coronary attacks using EM. EM can also be used for evaluation of adaptive and non-adaptive responses to acute ischemia. Myocardial hibernation is a condition that heart tries to restore an approximately normal oxygen supply/demand ratio in order to preserve myocardial viability [McFalls et al., 2007]. This is achieved by down-regulation of cardiac contractile function in response to diminished blood supply [Heusch & Schulz, 2009]. Observed ultrastructural changes in nonreperfused hibernated myocytes are altered nucleoplasm with homogenously dispersed heterochromatin and heterochromatin clumping which are consistent with adoption of dedifferentiated state resembling fetal cardiomyocytes [Borgers, 2002, Sherman et al., 2000]. Other changes include reappearance of strands of rough endoplasmic reticulum, reappearance and accretion of glycogen masses, transformed mitochondrial structure into numerous small dark and elongated mitochondria with condensed matrix, presence of large areas with non-specific cytoplasm, vacuoles, lipid droplets, lost myofibrils from perinuclear area, depletion of myocytes (myolysis) and slightly enlarged endothelial cell space [Elsässer et al., 1997, Dispersyn et al., 2001, Sherman et al., 2000]. Loss of sarcoplasmic reticulum and T-tubules, disrupted and disassembled myofibrillar structures with apparent irregularly oriented thick filaments aggregates in perinuclear and between myofibrils, reduced sarcoplasmic A-band length without obvious scar tissue are in favor of hibernation [Borgers, 2002, Sherman et al., 2000]. The end-diastolic lengthening of subendocardial segments during flow reduction and mechanical loads determine the frequency of myofibrillar disruption [Sherman et al., 2000].

Apoptotic cell death has been shown in portions of the myocardium remote from the infarct site which is attributed to remodeling [Schwarz et al., 2006]. EM showed abundant macrophages in vulnerable lesions accompanied by lower proportion of viable SMCs [Bauriedel et al., 1999]. In these cases, macrophage apoptosis was also observed in intimal cell pool [Bauriedel et al., 1999]. Higher proportion of apoptotic SMCs in intimal cell pool is parallel with increased frequency of apoptotic remnants in ruptured and eroded plaques [Bauriedel et al., 1999]. Based on the concept of cross-talk between apoptosis and inflammatory necrosis, depletion of SMC and collagen with high density of inflammatory cells reflects incorporation of both apoptosis and necrosis pathways [Bauriedel et al., 1999]. Presence of multi-lammelated basal laminae encircling apoptotic SMCs implies loss of SMC/matrix adhesion [Bauriedel et al., 1999]. This cell detaching from surrounding extracellular matrix is so-called anoikis [Bauriedel et al., 1999]. Engulfed apoptotic bodies were observed using TEM in SMCs and macrophages [Bauriedel et al., 1999]. Paucity of cell debris on normal extracellular matrix indicates an effective sealing of apoptotic structures [Bauriedel et al., 1999]. Typical finding of cellular necrosis showed by EM include shrunken cells with marginated and clumped nuclear chromatin, disrupted cytoplasmic membranes, dispersed cytoplasmic organelles, degraded pericellular matrix, stretched fibers with wide I bands and contraction bands [Bauriedel et al., 1999, Trump et al., 1997, Ohno et al., 1998]. In these cells large round spaces with residual central structures presumably due to residual protein or lipid components of decalcified granular dense bodies have been shown in mitochondria [Kloner et al., 1974].

Generally, cell injury progresses from an initially reversible phase (pre-lethal phase) to early stage of an irreversible phase (point of return) and ultimately into end stage irreversible phase (postmortem phase) [Trump et al., 1997]. All of these three death phases have been figured out using EM, but ultrastructural features seen in reperused myocytes implicates a cell death pattern compatible with oncosis [Sayk & Bartels, 2004]. It progresses from reversible oncosis without DNA fragmentation to irreversible oncosis with or without DNA fragmentation [Makowski, 2005]. It is in contrast with early stages of apoptotic cell death which no DNA fragmentation is visible [Hwang et al., 2011]. Other ultrastructural features of ischemic-reperfusion injury include increased total volume fraction of capillaries accompanied with decreased capillary fraction of endothelial cells [Lindal et al., 1990].

2. References

Adelide University. 2011. Cryo-ultramicrotomy or Cryo-sectioning, Microscopy department of Adelide university, https://www.adelaide.edu.au/microscopy/techniques/cryoultramicrotomy.html

Abela. G., Aziz. K. & DeJong. J. (2006). Cholesterol Crystals Cause Acute Coronary Events by Perforating the Arterial Intima. Circulation. 114:II_22.

Abela GS., Aziz. K., Vedre. A., Pathak. DR., Talbott. JD. & Dejong. J. (2009). Effect of cholesterol crystals on plaques and intima in arteries of patients with acute coronary and cerebrovascular syndromes. Am J Cardiol 103:959-68.

Argaud. L., Gateau-Roesch. O., Chalabreysse. L., Gomez. L., Loufouat. J., Thivolet-Béjui. F., Robert. D. & Ovize. M. (2004). Preconditioning delays Ca2+-induced mitochondrial permeability transition. Cardiovasc Res 61:115-22.

Bauriedel. G., Hutter. R., Welsch. U., Bach. R., Sievert. H. & Lüderitz. B. (1999). Role of smooth muscle cell death in advanced coronary primary lesions: implications for plaque instability. Cardiovasc Res 41:480-8.

Bergmans. L., Moisiadis. P., Van Meerbeek. B., Quirynen. M. & Lambrechts. P. (2005). Microscopic observation of bacteria: review highlighting the use of environmental SEM. Int Endod J 38:775-88.

Bogner. A., Jouneau. PH., Thollet. G., Basset. D. & Gauthier. C. (2007). A history of scanning electron microscopy developments: towards "wet-STEM" imaging. Micron 38:390-401.

Bopassa. JC., Vandroux. D., Ovize. M. & Ferrera. R. (2006). Controlled reperfusion after hypothermic heart preservation inhibits mitochondrial permeability transition-pore opening and enhances functional recovery. Am J Physiol Heart Circ Physiol 291:H2265-71.

Buja. LM., Dees. JH., Harling. DF. & Willerson. JT. (1976). Analytical electron microscopic study of mitochondrial inclusions in canine myocardial infarcts. J Histochem Cytochem. 24:508-16.

Buja. LM., Burton KP, Hagler HK & Willerson JT. (1983). Quantitative x-ray microanalysis of the elemental composition of individual myocytes in hypoxic rabbit myocardium. Circulation 68, No. 4, 872-88.

Borgers. LM. (2002). Hibernating myocardium: Programmed cell survival or programmed cell death? Exp Clin Cardiol 7:69-72.

Luther. PK. (2007). Structural analysis of cardiac muscle by modern electron microscopy. British Society for Cardiovascular Research Bulletin, 20:4-10.

Faulkner. C., Akman. OE., Bell. K., Jeffree. C. & Oparka. K. (2008). "Peeking into Pit Fields: A Multiple Twinning Model of Secondary Plasmodesmata Formation in Tobacco". Plant Cell 20: 1504.

Dempsey. GP. & Bullivant. S. (1976). A copper block method for freezing non-cryoprotected tissue to produce ice-crystal-free regions for electron microscopy. II. Evaluation using freeze fracturing with a cryo-ultramicrotome. J Microsc 106:261-71.

Dispersyn. GD., Geuens. E., Ver Donck. L., Ramaekers. FC. & Borgers. M. (2001). Adult rabbit cardiomyocytes undergo hibernation-like dedifferentiation when co-cultured with cardiac fibroblasts. Cardiovasc Res 51(2):230-40.

Duchen. MR. (2004). Roles of mitochondria in health and disease. Diabetes 53 Suppl 1:S96-102.

Dugan. TA, Yang. VW., McQuillan. DJ. & Höök. M. (2006). Decorin modulates fibrin assembly and structure. J Biol Chem 281:38208-16.

Ehara. S., Kobayashi. Y., Yoshiyama. M., Shimada. K., Shimada. Y., Fukuda. D., Nakamura. Y., Yamashita. H., Yamagishi. H., Takeuchi. K., Naruko. T., Haze. K., Becker. AE., Yoshikawa. J. & Ueda. M. (2004). Spotty calcification typifies the culprit plaque in patients with acute myocardial infarction: an intravascular ultrasound study. Circulation 110: 3424–3429.

Elsässer. A., Schlepper. M., Klövekorn. WP., Cai. WJ., Zimmermann. R., Müller. KD., Strasser. R., Kostin. S., Gagel. C., Münkel. B., Schaper. W. & Schaper. J. (1997). Hibernating myocardium: an incomplete adaptation to ischemia. Circulation. 96:2920-31.

Erni. R., Rossell. MD., Kisielowski. C. & Dahmen. U. (2009). Atomic-resolution imaging with a sub-50-pm electron probe. Phys Rev Lett 102:096101.

Ewence. AE., Bootman. M., Roderick. HL., Skepper. JN., McCarthy. G., Epple. M., Neumann. M., Shanahan. CM. & Proudfoot. D. (2008). Calcium phosphate crystals induce cell death in human vascular smooth muscle cells: a potential mechanism in atherosclerotic plaque destabilization. Circ Res 103:e28-34.

Guyton.JR. & Klemp. KF. (1992). Early extracellular and cellular lipid deposits in aorta of cholesterol-fed rabbits. Am J Pathol 141:925-36.

Hagler. HK & Buja. LM. (1986). Effect of specimen preparation and section transfer techniques on the preservation of ultrastructure, lipids and elements in cryosections. Journal of Microscopy 141: 311–317,

Hwang. B., Hwang. JS., Lee. J., Kim. JK., Kim. SR., Kim. Y. & Lee. DG. (2011). Induction of yeast apoptosis by an antimicrobial peptide, Papiliocin. Biochem Biophys Res Commun 408:89-93.

Heusch G & Schulz R. (2009) Hibernation or repetitive stunning - does it matter? The basic perspective Heart Metab 42:32–33

Hindmarsh. JP., Russell. AB. & Chen XD. (2007). "Fundamentals of the spray freezing of foods—microstructure of frozen droplets". Journal of Food Engineering 78: 136–150.

Hüser. J., Rechenmacher. CE. & Blatter. LA. (1998). Imaging the permeability pore transition in single mitochondria. Biophys J 74:2129-37.

Hoffstein. S., Gennaro. DE., Weissmann. G., Hirsch. J., Streuli. F. & Fox. AC. (1975). Cytochemical localization of lysosomal enzyme activity in normal and ischemic dog myocardium. Am J Pathol 79:193-206.

Ishidi E, Adamu I, Kolawale E, Sunmonu K & Yakubu M. (2011). Morphology and Thermal Properties of Alkaline Treated Palm Kernel Nut Shell - HDPE Composites. Journal of Emerging Trends in Engineering and Applied Sciences (JETEAS) 2 (2): 346-350

Jerome. WG., Lewis. JC., Taylor. RG. & White. MS. (1983). Concurrent endothelial cell turnover and leukocyte margination in early atherosclerosis. Scan Electron Microsc Pt 3:1453-9.

KAMARI. Y., Cohen. H., Shaish. A., Bitzur. R., Afek. A., Shen. S., Vainshtein. A. & Harats. D. (2008). Characterisation of atherosclerotic lesions with scanning electron microscopy (SEM) of wet tissue. Diab Vasc Dis Res 5:44-7.

Karnovsky. MJ. (1965). "A formaldehyde-glutaraldehyde fixative of high osmolality for use in electron microscopy". Journal of Cell Biology 27: 137A.

Kawamura. K., Cowley. MJ., Karp. RB., Mantle. JA., Logic. JR., Rogers. WJ., Russel RO., Rackley. CE. & Tames. TN. (1978). Intramitochondrial inclusions in the myocardial cells of human hearts and coronary disease. J Mol Cell Cardiol 10:797-811.

Kiernan. JA. (2000). "Formaldehyde, formalin, paraformaldehyde and glutaraldehyde: What they are and what they do". Microscopy Today: 8–12.

Kloner. RA., Ganote. CE., Whalen D, Jennings. RB. (1974). Effect of a transient period of ischemia on myocardial cells. II. Fine Structture During the First Few Minutes of Reflow. Am J Pathol. 1974 Mar;74(3):399-422.

Li YY, Chen D, Watkins SC & Feldman AM (2001). Mitochondrial abnormalities in tumor necrosis factor-alpha-induced heart failure are associated with impaired DNA repair activity. Circulation 104:2492-7.

Lindal. S., Gunnes. S., Ytrehus. K., Straume BK., Jørgensen. L. & Sørlie. D. (1990). Amelioration of reperfusion injury following hypothermic, ischemic cardioplegia in isolated, infarcted rat hearts. Eur J Cardiothorac Surg 4:33-9.

Maco. B., Mandinova. A., Dürrenberger. MB., Schäfer. BW., Uhrík. B. & Heizmann. CW. (2001). Ultrastructural distribution of the S100A1 Ca2+-binding protein in the human heart. Physiol Res 50:567-74.

Makowski. G. (2005). Advances in Clinical Chemistry, 40, p45, Academic Press, ISBN: 0120103400

Mancuso. J., Maxwell. W. & Danilatos. G. (1988). Secondary Electron Detector for Use in a Gaseous Atmosphere", US patent 4785182 11:15McFalls. EO., Kelly. RF., Hu. Q., Mansoor. A., Lee. J., Kuskowski. M., Sikora. J., Ward. HB. & Zhang. J. (2007). The energetic state within hibernating myocardium is normal during dobutamine despite inhibition of ATP-dependent potassium channel opening with glibenclamide. Am J Physiol Heart Circ Physiol 293:H2945-51.

McMullan. D. (1993). "Scanning Electron Microscopy, 1928–1965". 51st Annual Meeting of the Microscopy Society of America. Cincinnati, OH.

Mohankumar D.2010. Environmental Scanning Electron Microscope –ESEM: *wordpress.*

Nadra. I., Boccaccini. AR., Philippidis. P., Whelan. LC., McCarthy. GM., Haskard. DO. & Landis. RC. (2008). Effect of particle size on hydroxyapatite crystal-induced tumor necrosis factor alpha secretion by macrophages. Atherosclerosis. 196: 98–105.

Ohno. M., Takemura. G., Ohno. A., Misao. J., Hayakawa. Y., Minatoguchi. S., Fujiwara. T. & Fujiwara. H. (1998). "Apoptotic" myocytes in infarct area in rabbit hearts may be oncotic myocytes with DNA fragmentation: analysis by immunogold electron microscopy combined with In situ nick end-labeling. Circulation 98:1422-30.

Osumi. M., Konomi. M., Sugawara. T., Takagi. T. & Baba. M. (2006). High-pressure freezing is a powerful tool for visualization of Schizosaccharomyces pombe cells: ultra-low temperature and low-voltage scanning electron microscopy and immunoelectron microscopy. J Electron Microsc (Tokyo) 55:75-88.

Park. JS., Gamboni-Robertson. F., He. Q., Svetkauskaite. D., Kim. JY., Strassheim. D., Sohn. JW., Yamada. S., Maruyama. I., Banerjee. A., Ishizaka. A. & Abraham. E. (2006). High mobility group box 1 protein interacts with multiple Toll-like receptors. Am J Physiol Cell Physiol 290: C917–924.

Peine. CJ.& Low. FN. (1975) Scanning electron microscopy of cardiac endothelium of the dog. Am J Anat 142:137-57.

Popescu. LM., Gherghiceanu. M., Manole. CG. & Faussone-Pellegrini. MS. (2009). Cardiac renewing: interstitial Cajal-like cells nurse cardiomyocyte progenitors in epicardial stem cell niches. J Cell Mol Med 13:866-86.

ProSciTech: Critical point dryers, freeze dryers". http://www.proscitech.com/cataloguex/online.asp

Porto. A., Palumbo. R., Pieroni. M., Aprigliano. G., Chiesa. R., Sanvito. F., Maseri. A. & Bianchi. ME. (2006). Smooth muscle cells in human atherosclerotic plaques secrete and proliferate in response to high mobility group box 1 protein. Faseb J 20: 2565–2566.

Proudfoot. D., Skepper. JN., Hegyi. L., Bennett. MR., Shanahan. CM. & Weissberg. (2000). PL. Apoptosis regulates human vascular calcification in vitro: evidence for initiation of vascular calcification by apoptotic bodies. Circ Res. 87: 1055–1062.

Rajapakse. S., Rodrigo. PC. & Selvachandran. J. (2010). Management of acute coronary syndrome in a tertiary care general medical unit in Sri Lanka: how closely do we follow the guidelines? J Clin Pharm Ther 35:421-7.

Rame. JE., Barouch. LA., Sack. MN., Lynn. EG., Abu-Asab. M., Tsokos. M., Kern. SJ., Barb. JJ., Munson. PJ., Halushka. MK., Miller. KL., Fox-Talbot. K., Zhang. J., Hare. JM., Solomon. MA. & Danner. RL. (2011). Caloric restriction in leptin deficiency does not correct myocardial steatosis: failure to normalize PPAR{alpha}/PGC1{alpha} and thermogenic glycerolipid/fatty acid cycling. Physiol Genomics 43:726-38.

Read. ND. & Jeffree. CE. (1991). Low-temperature scanning electron microscopy in biology. J Microsc 161:59-72.

Riddle. JM., Stein. PD., Magilligan. DJ. & McElroy. HH. (1983). Evaluation of platelet reactivity in patients with valvular heart disease. J Am Coll Cardiol. 1983 Jun;1(6):1381-4.

Russell. FD., Skepper. JN. & Davenport. AP. (1998). Evidence Using Immunoelectron Microscopy for Regulated and Constitutive Pathways in the Transport and Release of Endothelin. Journal of Cardiovascular Pharmacology: 31: 424-430

Sætersdal. TS., Myklebust. R., Engedal. H. & Ødegaarden. S. (1978). Substructure of inner mitochondrial membranes of myocardial cells as shown by cryo-ultramicrotomy. Cell and Tissue Research 186:13-24

Sage MD & Jennings RB (1988). Cytoskeletal injury and subsarcolemmal bleb formation in dog heart during in vitro total ischemia. Am J Pathol 133:327-37.

Sayk. F. & Bartels. C. (2004). Oncosis rather than apoptosis? Ann Thorac Surg 77:382; author reply 382-3.

Schatten H. & Pawley J. (2007). Biological Low-Voltage Scanning Electron Microscopy. Springer 61–63.

Schwarz. K., Simonis. G., Yu. X., Wiedemann. S. & Strasser. RH. (2006). Apoptosis at a distance: remote activation of caspase-3 occurs early after myocardial infarction. Mol Cell Biochem 281:45-54.

Sekiya. T., Kitajima. Y. & Nozawa. Y. (1979). Effects of lipid-phase separation on the filipin action on membranes of ergosterol-replaced Tetrahymena cells, as studied by freeze-fracture electron microscopy. Biochim Biophys Acta 550:269-78.

Severs. N. (2007). Freeze-fracture electron microscopy, Nature Protocols 2, -547 - 576 (2007)

Mitsuoka. K. (2011). Obtaining high-resolution images of biological macromolecules by using a cryo-electron microscope with a liquid-helium cooled stage. Micron 42:100-6.

Sherman. AJ., Klocke. FJ., Decker. RS., Decker. ML., Kozlowski. KA., Harris. KR., Hedjbeli. S., Yaroshenko. Y., Nakamura. S., Parker. MA., Checchia. PA. & Evans. DB. (2000). Myofibrillar disruption in hypocontractile myocardium showing perfusion-contraction matches and mismatches. Am J Physiol Heart Circ Physiol 278:H1320-34.

Schmid. K., McSharry. WO., Pameijer. CH. & Binette. JP. (1980). Chemical and physicochemical studies on the mineral deposits of the human atherosclerotic aorta. Atherosclerosis 37: 199–210

Sojitra P, Engineer Ch, Raval A, Kothwala D, Jariwala A, Kotadia H, Adeshara S & Mehta G. (2009). Surface Enhancement and Characterization of L-605 Cobalt Alloy Cardiovascular Stent by Novel Electrochemical Treatment. Trends Biomater. Artif. Organ 23:55-64.

Spagnoli. LG., Pucci. S., Bonanno. E., Cassone. A., Sesti. F., Ciervo. A. & Mauriello. A. (2007). Persistent Chlamydia pneumoniae infection of cardiomyocytes is correlated with fatal myocardial infarction. Am J Pathol 170:33-42.

Sun. W., Zheng. L. & Huang. L. (2011). Role of unusual CD4 (+) CD28 (-) T cells in acute coronary syndrome. Mol Biol Rep 22.

Suzuki. E. (2002). "High-resolution scanning electron microscopy of immunogold-labelled cells by the use of thin plasma coating of osmium". Journal of Microscopy 208: 153–157.

Sybers. HD., Maroko. PR., Ashraf. M., Libby. P. & Braunwald. E. (1973). The effect of glucose-insulin-potassium on cardiac ultrastructure following acute experimental coronary occlusion. Am J Pathol 70:401-20.

Toumpoulis. IK., Oxford. JT., Cowan. DB., Anagnostopoulos. CE., Rokkas. CK., Chamogeorgakis. TP., Angouras. DC., Shemin. RJ., Navab. M., Ericsson. M., Federman. M., Levitsky. S. & McCully. JD. (2009). Differential expression of collagen type V and XI alpha-1 in human ascending thoracic aortic aneurysms. Ann Thorac Surg 88:506-13.

Tran. PK., Tran-Lundmark. K., Soininen. R., Tryggvason. K., Thyberg. J. & Hedin. U. (2004). Increased intimal hyperplasia and smooth muscle cell proliferation in transgenic mice with heparan sulfate-deficient perlecan. Circ Res 94:550-8.

Trump. BF., Berezesky. IK., Chang. SH. & Phelps. PC. (1997). The pathways of cell death: oncosis, apoptosis, and necrosis. Toxicol Pathol 25:82-8.

Tselepis. AD., Gerotziafas. G., Andrikopoulos. G., Anninos. H. & Vardas. P. (2011). Mechanisms of platelet activation and modification of response to antiplatelet agents. Hellenic J Cardiol 52:128-40.

Ueno. M., Suzuki. J., Zenimaru. Y., Takahashi. S., Koizumi. T., Noriki. S., Yamaguchi. O., Otsu. K., Shen. WJ., Kraemer. FB. & Miyamori. I. (2008). Cardiac overexpression of hormone-sensitive lipase inhibits myocardial steatosis and fibrosis in streptozotocin diabetic mice. Am J Physiol Endocrinol Metab 294:E1109-18.

Vengrenyuk. Y., Carlier. S., Xanthos. S., Cardoso. L., Ganatos. P., Virmani. R., Einav. S., Gilchrist. L. & Weinbaum. S. (2006). A hypothesis for vulnerable plaque rupture due to stress-induced debonding around cellular microcalcifications in thin fibrous caps. Proc Natl Acad Sci U S A 103: 14678–14683.

Virchow. R. (1860). A more precise account of fatty metamorphosis. In: Chance F, ed. Cellular Pathology. London, Gryphonham 342–366

Virmani. R, Burke. AP., Kolodgie. FD. & Farb. A. (2003). Pathology of the thin-cap fibroatheroma: a type of vulnerable plaque. J Interv Cardiol 16: 267–272.

Vye MV & Fischman DA (1970). The morphological alteration of particulate glycogen by en bloc staining with uranyl acetate. J Ultrastruct Res 33:278-91.

Wiemer M, Butz T, Schmidt W, Schmitz KP, Horstkotte D, Langer C. Scanning electron microscopic analysis of different drug eluting stents after failed implantation: from nearly undamaged to major damaged polymers. Catheter Cardiovasc Interv. 2010 May 1;75(6):905-11.

Winitsky. SO., Gopal. TV., Hassanzadeh. S., Takahashi. H., Gryder. D., Rogawski. MA., Takeda. K., Yu. ZX., Xu. YH. & Epstein. ND. (2005). Adult murine skeletal muscle contains cells that can differentiate into beating cardiomyocytes in vitro. PLoS Biol 3:e87.

www.upesh.edu.pk/academics/researchcenter

Zhang. JL., Lu. JK., Chen. D., Cai. Q., Li. TX., Wu. LS. & Wu. XS. (2009). Myocardial autophagy variation during acute myocardial infarction in rats: the effects of carvedilol. Chin Med J (Engl) 122:2372-9.

Zhou. Z., Han. JY., Xi. CX., Xie. JX., Feng. X., Wang. CY., Mei. L. & Xiong. WC. (2008). HMGB1 regulates RANKL-induced osteoclastogenesis in a manner dependent on RAGE. J Bone Miner Res 23: 1084–1096.

8

Shortened Activated Partial Thromboplastin Time (APTT): A Simple but Important Marker of Hypercoagulable State During Acute Coronary Event

Wan Zaidah Abdullah
Universiti Sains Malaysia, Malaysia

1. Introduction

Haemostatic system has several important functions: to keep blood in a fluid state, to arrest bleeding at the site of vascular injury by formation of a haemostatic plug and to destroy the plug slowly when healing takes place. Normal physiology constitutes a delicate balance between procoagulant and anticoagulant properties of this system, and a deficiency or exaggeration of any one may lead to either haemorrhage or vascular thrombosis respectively. Haemostatic factors have an important role in prothrombotic state and in the pathogenesis of cardiovascular diseases. Vascular, platelet and coagulation factors contribute to the development of coronary artery disease.

The main focus here is on the general implication of acute coronary event on coagulation factors, and its effect to the haemostatic system by inducing a hypercoagulable state. This state (or also described as prothrombotic state) is defined as a tendency or propensity to develop vascular thrombosis due to an abnormality in the coagulation system. Thrombophilia is another terminology describing the same condition. Although hypercoagulable state is commonly referred to venous thrombosis when coagulation system is involved, it is not an exclusive feature to this blood vessel. Its existence will lead to a harmful effect either as recurrent thrombo-embolic (TE) event or tissue damage due to ischaemic complications.

APTT is a simple and widely available test commonly used to screen for hypocoagulable state in bleeding disorders. Whether APTT is suitable as a routine screening test for hypercoagulable state is currently unknown. It is important to understand the pathophysiology of arterial thrombosis triggered by haemostatic factors and how this affect the APTT results particularly during acute coronary event. In addition, clinical consequences of hypercoagulable state in coronary artery disease are well recognized and controlling this condition has been applied successfully to the patient management protocol. Other concern includes potential errors that can falsely lead to shortened APTT results which should be highlighted to improve the clinical and laboratory practices.

2. Haemostasis and laboratory investigations

Formation of haemostatic plug is under a regulated physiological process. Haemostatic plug or blood clot or also known as thrombus is the end product of serial activations of the haemostatic system, starting from an injury or any insult usually to the blood vessel wall or endothelium. The basic physiology of haemostatic system includes the blood vessel, platelets, von Willebrand factor (vWF) and coagulation system. The coagulation system is controlled by inhibitors especially the natural anticoagulant proteins, namely the protein C, protein S, antithrombin and others. Fibrinolytic activity is essential in maintaining the patency of blood vessel lumen by removing the haemostatic plug during its course of recovery. Each of the components in the haemostatic system plays their role at the right time and at the right place that will ensure the haemostatic plug is formed when appropriate. Knowledge on the components and serial activations of the haemostatic system is important in order to understand the pathophysiology of either thrombotic (hypercoagulable) or haemorrhagic (hypocoagulable) disorders.

There are two main types of measurements related to haemostatic disturbances in the investigations of the prothrombotic state in cardiovascular disease: measurement of levels of haemostatic factors and measurement of activation products of haemostasis. In the former type of measurements, the most promising factors identified have been fibrinogen, factor VIII (FVIII), factor VII (FVII), vWF and the fibrinolytic variables i.e tissue-type plasminogen activator (t-PA) and plasminogen activator inhibitor-1 (PAI-1) (Fareed et al., 1998).

Common laboratory findings indicating the presence of hypercoagulable state from the haemostatic point of view include elevated coagulation factors (FVIII and others), vWF, fibrinogen, positive activated protein C resistance (APC-R) assay, shortened APTT (mainly as a result of high factor VIII and other coagulation factors) and etc. The function of protein C system in the anticoagulation pathway can be detected by APC-R assay. In this test, the function of protein C to inactivate factor VIIIa and factor Va is assessed by special coagulation test. In brief, the presence of high FVIII (or other factors) which is usually part of acute phase protein will lead to ineffective inhibition to this factor by protein C and hence the detection of this condition as a positive APC-R assay. There are many other factors that may give rise to a positive APC-R assay but in the context of coronary artery disease, it is partly explained by high factor VIII (see below).

The prothrombotic or hypercoagulable state is not easily detected by routine laboratory tests unlike the hypocoagulable state. So far, no coagulation screening test is available to detect a hypercoagulable state, whether it is due to congenital or acquired thrombotic disorders, with the exception of lupus anticoagulant (LA). In hypocoagulable state, APTT is a useful screening test in the investigation of bleeding disorders. Prolonged APTT and corrected result after mixing test is most likely to be associated with hypocoagulable disorder due to coagulation factor/s deficiency. Previous finding on the association of shortened APTT and venous thrombosis has opened some lights to the possibility of using this routine coagulation test as a screening method for the risk of TE disorder. Unfortunately there is still no consensus to use APTT as a routine screening test in clinical practice for the investigation of hypercoagulable state.

Shortened APTT could be a screening tool to be considered for hypercoagulable state during acute thrombotic episodes. However shortened APTT was also detected during venous TE event free interval (Legnani et al., 2002; Tripodi 2004) among patients who had past history of vascular thrombosis. There was a report that showed the presence of shortened APTT at any time was related to a 10-fold increased incidence of TE events (McKenna et al., 1977). Further investigation including immunological and specialized coagulation tests may be required to find the aetiology of thrombosis in patients presenting with TE disorders.

Shortened APTT was described in acute conditions of both venous and arterial thrombosis. The role of APTT as a screening tool in asymptomatic individuals or during episodes of TE free event is probably justified, though it may not be highly sensitive. Similar application goes to the screening ability of this test in hypocoagulable conditions due to its limitation in detecting mild coagulation factor deficiency. However, using APTT as a screening test in patients with positive LA (antiphospholipid syndrome) is clearly useful and had been established for a long time. In the presence of LA, a paradoxical finding of prolonged APTT is the hallmark of this condition and its presence is strongly associated with hypercoagulable state.

In acute arterial thrombosis such as coronary artery thrombosis, similar finding of shortened APTT was also described as seen in venous thrombosis (Abdullah WZ. et al., 2010). There was a significant negative correlation between APTT and FVIII, which was described in the similar study. APTT is a robust and simple test that is available in most laboratories in all hospitals. However the natural limitation of APTT is the major reason preventing it as a powerful screening tool for both hypo and hypercoagulable states.

Abnormally shortened APTT was reported to be associated with elevated plasma level of FVIII (Ten Boekal & Bartels, 2002). Elevated FVIII levels and probably other coagulation factors play a pathogenic role in the mechanism of abnormally shortened APTT during acute coronary event or related to venous thrombosis (Abdullah WZ et al., 2010; Tripodi et al., 2004)). Hence in arterial thrombosis, presence of high coagulation factors (particularly FVIII) and positive APC-R assay were found similar to the reported findings in venous thrombosis. Majority of the patients with positive APC-R assay also could have high coagulation factors, particularly FVIII.

2.1 APTT test in clinical practice

APTT is a routine screening test for the investigation of bleeding tendency, in both acquired and congenital disorders. It is also indicated pre-operatively to detect a hypocoagulable state that can lead to excessive bleeding during or after surgery. There are many APTT reagents in the market and it is the responsibility of the laboratory personnel to ensure the results produced from this test are accurate and precise.

APTT test was originally performed to screen the function of coagulation system, mainly for the intrinsic pathway factors: factor XII, XI, IX and VIII. Various APTT reagents for different purposes are now available, including for screening of factor deficiencies and lupus anticoagulant. The normal reference ranges are expected to be different from one laboratory to another depending on the types of reagents and coagulometers. There are two major principles of clot detection for APTT test. The mechanical and optical methods, both measure the time to form a fibrin clot after adding the reagents to the test plasma. The time is commonly expressed in second (s). Plasma containing normal levels of clotting factors will clot within the time in normal ranges which should be established according to the reagent and equipment used in the local laboratory. The reference normal range is determined by establishing the values using normal healthy volunteers of the local population. It is important for the clinical personnel to know the normal range of their local laboratory when interpreting the patients' APTT results. The same principle also applies to other coagulation tests like prothrombin time, thrombin time, fibrinogen and etc.

There are limitations with APTT test, for example possible pre-analytical errors that could occur during venepuncture procedure or during sample collection. Inappropriate blood taking procedure may lead to coagulation factors activation and falsely giving a shortened APTT results. Other problem with APTT is the consistency in reporting the results. The coagulation laboratory should practice an appropriate quality procedure, including accuracy and precision testing, participation in internal and external quality assurance programme, establishment of a normal reference ranges and other related requirements.

Validation process should be done regularly whenever changes occur in the reagents (including lot number), equipments and etc. Laboratories running APTT and other haemostatic tests should follow the standard guideline for coagulation study to avoid errors (pre-analytical, analytical and post analytical) by practicing a regular auditing, considering the use of uncertainty of measurement in the results reporting (or when consulted) and verifying the correct normal reference ranges for local use. By doing this, the finding of shortened APTT can be recognized consistently in cases with high coagulation factors or due to other reasons that can contribute to this effect. Ability to detect the evidence of hypercoagulable state through this test is strictly dependent on the laboratory performance in their practice.

2.2 Haemostatic investigations related to hypercoagulable state

TE event involving venous thrombosis is the outcome of a hypercoagulable state and usually related to increased haemostatic factors or decreased natural anticoagulant proteins. Direct and indirect involvements of haemostatic system in arterial thrombosis have been also well recognized and hence hypercoagulable state is a pathological condition present in both arterial and venous thromboses (Virchow's triad). Anti-phospholipid syndrome, APC-R assay, deficiencies of protein C, protein S and antithrombin are the most common causes being investigated when patients present with venous TE disorders.

The group of tests performed in the investigation of hypercoagulable state is also known as thrombophilia study. Congenital protein C, protein S, antithrombin deficiencies, factor V Leiden and prothrombin gene mutations are among the genetic factors associated with venous thrombosis included in the thrombophila study. Among specialised haemostatic tests in the investigation of TE disorders are protein C, protein S, antithrombin activity/antigen assays, APC-R assay and LA tests to detect underlying thrombophilic disorders. Thrombosis is the outcome of multiple contributing factors and hence the above mentioned factors might be compounded with other conditions such as medical diseases, hyperhomocysteinaemia, high levels of coagulation factors (for example secondary to oral contraceptive pills) and etc.

Arterial thrombosis is associated with medical conditions such as smoking, diabetes mellitus, obesity, hypertension and etc. The laboratory investigation for arterial thrombosis is mainly related to the traditional risk factors mentioned above, for example lipid profile, glucose levels, biochemical tests and etc. Some local guidelines include thrombophilia investigation similar to venous thrombosis for young patients presenting with 'premature" arterial thrombosis (for example less than 40 years old) or recurrent arterial events. Currently only homocysteine measurement and antiphospholipid antibodies detection are clearly indicated in the investigation of arterial thrombosis (hypercoagulable risk factors) especially in young patients without other known risk factors. In arterial thrombosis, the association with other conditions (including heritable thrombophilia) is unproven and not sufficient to change therapy for primary or secondary prevention of the disease.

APC-R state can be due to acquired or inherited disorders. APC-R assay is a form of specialised coagulation test which is done mainly for the screening of APC-R state due to factor V Leiden (FVL) mutation. This condition is associated with hypercoagulable state and has been reported to be high among Caucasians. FVL mutation is associated with venous thrombosis and the risk is higher in homozygous state than the heterozygous state. The mutated factor V molecule in FVL results in failure or ineffective inactivation by the protein C (protein S functions as cofactor).

The coagulation assay to detect this FVL mutation is sensitive and was also reported to be specific. However similar to other coagulation studies, there are certain limitations with APC-R assay in which the positive results could be due to other variables (high FVIII & other coagulation factors or protein S deficiency). Confirmation with molecular test is therefore the standard method to diagnose FVL mutation. However in coronary artery thrombosis, its association with FVL mutation was debatable (Cushman et al., 1998). There is probably a weak association of this mutation with coronary artery disease particularly in young smoking females. The presence of high coagulation factors may lead to a positive APC-R assay but not due to the FVL mutation. Hence positive APC-R assay is an evidence of hypercoagulable state, whether it is due to FVL or related to haemostatic factors.

Thromboelastography (TEG) is a haemostatic analyser which has been introduced in clinical practice many years ago, serving as a form of point of care testing. However it is not widely available routinely. TEG parameters reflect the function of the haemostatic components and able to detect both hypo and hypercoagulable states. Previous studies have shown that certain parameters of TEG are useful indicators for the presence of prothrombotic state such as, maximum amplitude (MA). One study showed that this parameter of TEG predicted post operative thrombotic complications including myocardial infarction (McCrath et al., 2005).

So far, basic coagulation tests to detect the presence of hypercoagulable state are still under-utilised but shortened APTT and positive APC-R assay could be applied for this purpose although with some limitations, as described above. Unlike APTT, APC-R assay is usually done in a specialised coagulation laboratory and not easily available in most hospitals. Ideally this investigation should be interpreted by an experienced scientist or haematologist rendering its usefulness as a screening test for hypercoagulable state is limited.

3. Haemostasis and coronary artery disease

Acute coronary syndrome (ACS) is a condition described for coronary artery atherothrombosis which compromised the blood supply to the myocardium and followed by clinical and/or laboratory evidences of ischaemia. ACS comprises of unstable angina, non-ST segment elevation myocardial infarction and ST segment elevation infarction. Association of haemostatic factors with ACS has been widely investigated and thoroughly discussed in the literatures (Cooper *et al.*, 2000; Fuster et al., 2005). The insult on the coronary vessel is mainly from atherosclerotic process and its complication (example plaque rupture) leading to an acute thrombotic event from the haemostatic activation. The formation of blood clot (fibrin) from this activity gives a sudden blockage of the vessel lumen and produced the signs and symptoms of ACS mainly chest pain, electrocardiographic and biochemical changes. The schematic drawing of coagulation cascade activation and fibrinolytic activity is shown in figure 1.

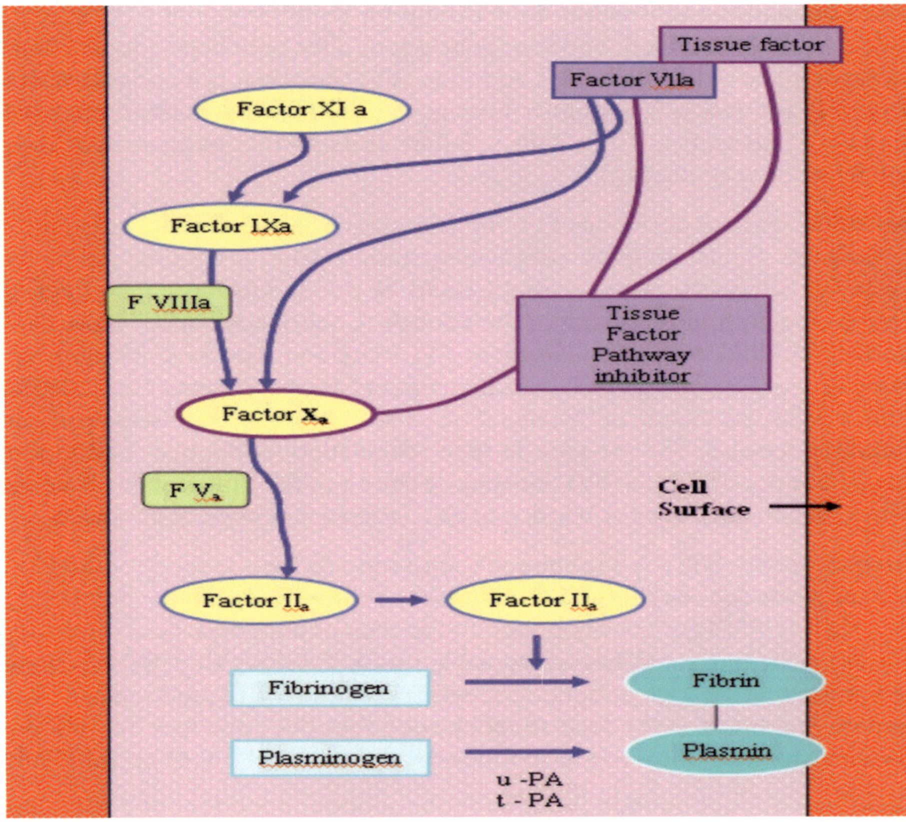

Fig. 1. Coagulation activation, fibrinolysis and tissue factor pathway inhibitor. (u-PA, urokinase plasminogen activator; t-PA, tissue plasminogen activator)

The mechanism of thrombosis according to Virchow's triad explained the hypercoagulable process. Most of the risk factors for venous thrombosis are caused by stasis or changes in overall total blood coagulabality, while vessel wall damage is the main cause of thrombogenicity in arterial thrombosis. Vascular endothelium is involved in a wide range of homoestatic functions including maintaining the balance of anticoagulant and procoagulant forces. On the anticoagulant side, the endothelium releases heparin sulfate and prostacyclin, expresses thrombomodulin, t-PA, tissue factor pathway inhibitor and endothelial nitric oxide synthase which provide a non-thrombogenic cell-surface membrane. On the prothrombotic side, endothelial cells release von Willebrand factor and plasminogen activator inhibitor type-1, expose critical binding sites for coagulation factor complexes and some other functions. The endothelium is capable of integrating multiple feedbacks and capable of shifting the haemostatic balance from time to time that allows the haemostatic system with tremendous flexibility (Rosenberg and Aird, 1999). However the endothelium is also vulnerable to focal dysfunction resulting in many ways including narrowing of the lumen and increased risk of sudden obstruction as seen in the various phases of atherothrombosis.

Although Protein C, protein S and antithrombin do not confer an increased risk of arterial thrombosis, other anticoagulant mechanisms must be responsible for maintaining the patent of vascular lumen, particularly in coronary vessels. Fibrinolytic enzymes play a critical role to keep the lumen patent by preventing fibrin deposition within the vascular bed of the heart. These enzymes are t-PA and urokinase-type plasminogen activator. Binding of t-PA to fibrin enhances the conversion of thrombus-bound plasminogen into plasmin. Plasmin is capable to digest the fibrinogen, fibrin and factor VIII. The anticoagulant property of tissue factor pathway inhibitor helps to control the procoagulant activity of the extrinsic coagulation factors (FVIIa and tissue factor). Similarly APC stimulates fibrinolysis by destroying plasma inhibitors of t-PA. Haemostatic balance within the coronary vessels is controlled by a vascular bed-specific circuit or feedback system. Hence there is a strong possibility that thrombosis in coronary artery arises through the interplay of plaque rupture and an alteration of local haemostatic circuit (Rosenberg and Aird, 1999).

In addition to the consequences of atherosclerotic plaque rupture where the thrombus formed in the coronary artery, the systemic effect of this acute event is seen almost immediately. In one study, shortened APTT was significantly different in ACS patients compared to stable coronary artery disease patients (SCAD) when they presented early to the hospital (Abdullah WZ., et al 2010). High FVIII levels were also found to be significant in ACS patients compared to the SCAD group. None of the SCAD patients had shortened APTT result in their study although some of them were having elevated FVIII levels (which did not affect the APTT results). Significantly high vWF and fibrinogen were seen among ACS patients compared to the SCAD patients and most patients with APCR state also had high FVIII levels. (Abdullah WZ., et al 2011). Interestingly, inversed relationship between FVIII and APTT was shown among coronary heart disease patients indicating that shortened APTT is partly explained by increased FVIII levels (Figure 2 and table 1).

Haemostatic system involves in the initiation of ACS through haemostatic activation (platelet and coagulation system activation) and hypercoagulable state is a finding following this event, as evidenced by high vWF, fibrinogen and FVIII levels. The net outcome of the effect of these hypercoagulable factors is detected as shortened APTT as shown by the above study.

Patients with arterial thrombosis also have a form of hypercoagulable state, manifested by higher baseline concentrations of fibrinogen and elevated factor VII activity. Increased fibrinogen concentration is a strong and independent predictor of cardiovascular risk in apparently healthy person as well as in person manifested as coronary heart disease (Thomas and Roberts, 1997). Clinical studies have shown that subjects with higher plasma levels of procoagulant proteins (including vWF and coagulation factors) had an increased risk of myocardial infarction (Rosenberg and Aird, 1999).

The role of platelet and vWF in arterial thrombosis is not elaborated in details here. Obviously there is an integrated process from various haemostatic components that eventually promote a hypercoagulable state throughout the entire process. Furthermore shortened APTT does not account for the platelet reactivity in atherothrombosis. The contribution of haemostatic system in the development of atherothrombosis has been greatly discussed in literatures. It is also interesting that this system may also determine the outcomes of the disease. The beneficial effects from anti-platelet, anticoagulation and anti-thrombotic therapies in prevention and treatment of ACS proved that hypercoagulable state should be controlled to avoid its harmful effects in coronary artery disease.

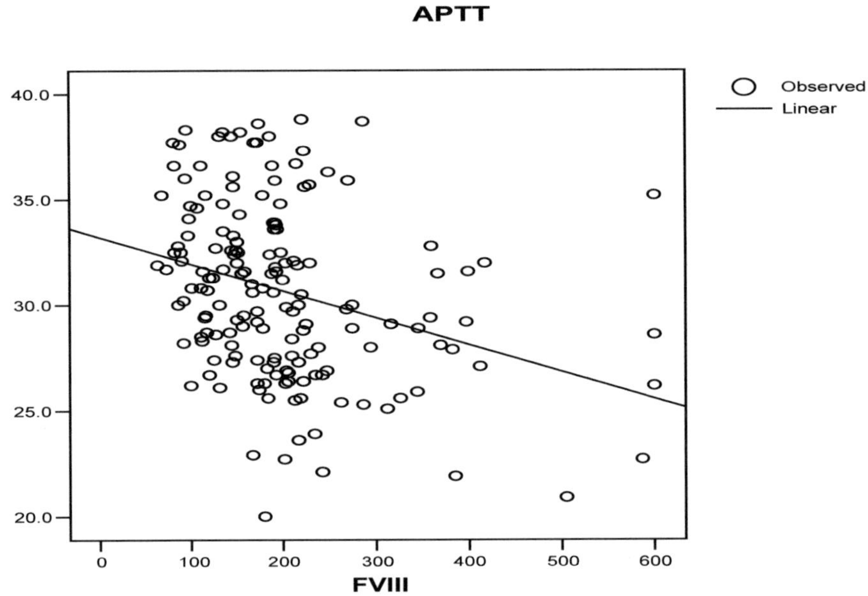

Fig. 2. The correlation between FVIII and APTT among coronary heart disease patients.

Variable	β(S.E)	(95% CI)	*p* value*
FVIII	-0.013(0.003)	(-0.019,-0.007)	**< 0.0001**

(R square = 0.097 (10%), predictor = FVIII, dependent variable = APTT. **p* value is significant when ≤ 0.05)

Table 1. The correlation between FVIII level and APTT among coronary heart disease patients.

4. Consequences of hypercoagulable state following ACS

The after effect of acute coronary thrombosis may further complicate both the local coronary artery and systemic circulation by the burden of this hypercoagulable state. This condition can be harmful and leads to an imbalance state between the natural anticoagulant and procoagulant activities. Hypercoagulable state potentially caused repeated episodes of vascular thrombosis and may lead to increased in morbidity and mortality. This is especially true if this state is not controlled adequately with the given treatment, especially the anticoagulant and antiplatelet therapy. Resistance to certain anti-platelet drugs have been reported and extensively discussed in the literatures, which partly explained why some patients developed repeated thrombotic event despite on adequate therapy (Flaherty MP., et al 2011).

5. Conclusion

ACS by definition is a hypercoagulable state and shortened APTT is a useful haemostatic marker. Shortened APTT is associated with increased coagulation factors for example fibrinogen and FVIII. Previous studies have shown a consistent association of increased haemostatic factors in acute coronary artery thrombosis. It is now understood that hypercoagulable state is likely to be present before or after this event. Limited investigation is recommended pertaining to haemostatic tests in coronary artery thrombosis.

Haemostatic activities for example thrombin generation, platelet activation and abnormal fibrinolysis may significantly influence the outcomes of patients with this disease. In patients with risk factors of coronary artery disease, the presence of shortened APTT at the onset of acute clinical presentation is associated with higher chance of ACS. There is a relationship of shortened APTT and hypercoagulable state during acute thrombotic episodes, although the possibility remains that an acute phase responses (increase fibrinogen and FVIII) present at a wide range of time since the initial onset of vascular injury during the atherosclerotic process.

6. References

Abdullah, WZ.; Moufak, SK.; Yusof, Z.; Mohamad, M.S.; Kamarul, I.M. (2010). Shortened activated partial thromboplastin time, a hemostatic marker for hypercoagulable state during acute coronary event. *Translational Research,* Vol. 155, No. 6, (June 2010), pp. 315-319, ISSN 1931-5244

Abdullah,WZ.; Moufak, SK.; Yusof, Z. (2011). *Haemostatic markers and prothrombotic genes,* VDM Verlag, ISBN 978-3-639-35969-5, Saarbrucken, Germany

Cushman, M.; Rosendaal, F. R.; Psaty, B. M.; Cook, E. F.; Valliere, J.; Kuller, L. H. & Tracy, R. P. (1998). Factor V Leiden is not a risk factor for arterial vascular disease in the elderly: results from the Cardiovascular Health Study. *Thrombosis Haemostasis,* Vol. 79, No.5, pp.912-5, ISSN 0340-6245

Cooper, J. A.; Miller, G. J.; Bauer, K. A.; Morrissey, J. H.; Meade, T. W.; Howarth, D. J.; Barzegar, S.; Mitchell, J. P. & Rosenberg, R. D. (2000). Comparison of novel hemostatic factors and conventional risk factors for prediction of coronary heart disease. *Circulation,* Vol. 102, No.23, pp.2816-22, ISSN 0009- 7322

Fareed, J.; Hoppensteadt, D. A.; Leya, F.; Iqbal, O.; Wolf, H. & Bick, R. (1998). Useful laboratory tests for studying thrombogenesis in acute cardiac syndromes. *Clinical Chemistry,* Vol.44, No. 8, pp. 1845- 53, ISSN 0009-9147

Flaherty, MP.; Johnston, PV.; Rade, JJ. (2011) Subacute stent thrombosis owing to complete clopidogrel resistance successfully managed with prasugrel. *Journal of Invasive Cardiology,* Vol.23, No.7, pp.300-4, ISSN 1042-3931

Fuster, V.; Moreno, P. R.; Fayad, Z. A.; Corti, R. & Badimon, J. J. (2005). Atherothrombosis and high-risk plaque: part I: evolving concepts. *Journal of the American College of Cardiology,* Vol. 46, No.6, pp.937-54, ISSN 0735-1097

Legnani, C.; Mattarozzi, S.; Cini, M.; Cosmi, B.; Favaretto, E.; Palareti, G. (2006). Abnormally short activated partial thromboplastin time values are associated with increased risk of recurrence of venous thromboembolism after oral anticoagulation withdrawal. *British Journal Haematology*, Vol.134 No.2, pp.227-32, ISSN 0007-1048

McCrath, D. J.; Cerboni, E.; Frumento, R. J.; Hirsh, AL.; Bennett-Guerrero E. (2005). Thromboelastography maximum amplitude predicts postoperative thrombotic complications including myocardial infarction. *Anaesthesia Analgesia*, Vol.100, No.6, pp.1576-83, ISSN 0003-2999

McKenna, R.; Bachmann, F. & Miro-Quesada, M. (1977). Thrombo-embolism in patients with abnormally short activated partial thromboplastin time. *Thrombosis Haemostasis,* Vol.38, No.4, pp.893-9, ISSN 0340-6245

Rosenrberg, R. D & Aird, W. C. (1999). Mechanism of disease: Vascular-bed-specific haemostasis and hypercoagulable states. *New England Journal of Medicine*, Vol. 340, No. 22, pp. 1555 - 1564, ISSN 0028-4793

Ten Boekel, E. & Bartels, P. (2002). Abnormally short activated partial thromboplastin times are related to elevated plasma levels of TAT, F1+2, D-dimer and FVIII:C. *Pathophysiology Haemostasis and Thrombosis,* Vol.32, No. 3, pp.137-42, ISSN 1424-8832

Thomas, D. P. & Roberts, H. R. (1997). Hypercoagulability in venous and arterial thrombosis. *Annals of Internal Medicine,* Vol. 126, No.8, pp. 638-44, ISSN 0003-4819

Tripodi, A.; Chantarangkul, V.; Martinelli, I.; Bucciarelli, P.; Mannucci, PM. A shortened activated partial thromboplastin time is associated with the risk of venous thromboembolism. *Blood,* Vol.104,No.12, (December 2004), pp.3631-4, ISSN 0006-4971

Part 3

Cardiovascular Prevention

9

Individualized Cardiovascular Risk Assessment

Eva Szabóová
4th Department of Internal Medicine, Faculty of Medicine,
PJ Šafárik University in Košice
Slovakia

1. Introduction

Cardiovascular diseases (CVD) are the main cause of death and disease burden in Europe. 48% of all deaths are from CVD: 54% of deaths in women and 43% of death in men. CVD is the main cause of death for women in Europe and also for men except France, the Netherlands and Spain (Allender et al., 2009) (Figure l). Coronary heart disease (CHD) itself is the single most common cause of death in Europe, which is followed by stroke. Overall CVD is estimated to cost EU economy €192 billion a year (Allender et al., 2009).

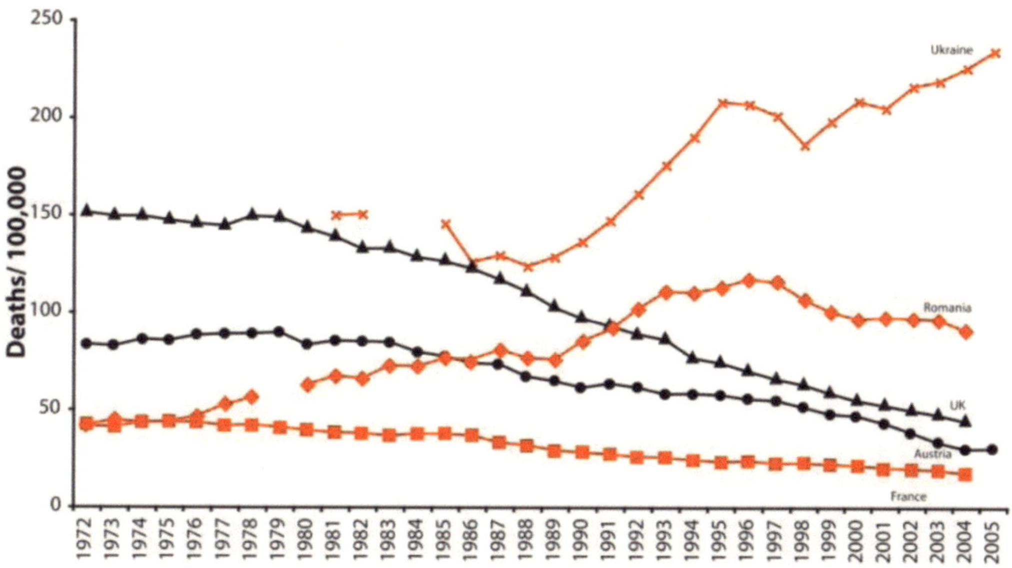

Fig. 1. Death rates from CHD, men aged under 65, 1972 to 2005, selected countries. European cardiovascular disease statistics 2008 edition (Allender et al., 2009)

Mortality rate from CHD in various countries underwent profound changes during the 20th century. While there is a trend to rapid fall in mortality rate from CHD over the past 30 years in higher-income countries, such as most Northern, Western and Southern Europe, the United States, Canada and parts of the Western Pacific, in regions with lower income, including Central and Eastern Europe, mortality, incidence, and case fatality of CVD either not falling as fast or rising (Allender et al., 2009). Different therapeutic and preventive approaches including lifestyle changes may explain this state.

In Finland, where CHD mortality among Finnish men was the highest in the world in the late 1960s, over the 35-year period - as a result of the North Carelia Project - an 80% decline in coronary mortality in middle-aged men was observed. In this Finish model risk factor modifications (total cholesterol, blood pressure, smoking) explained a 60% reduction in CHD mortality, further 20% decline was a result of improved therapy (Vartainen et al., 2010). Similarly in Sweden, over the period of 4 decades risk factor modifications in 50-year-old men demonstrated a >50% decline in myocardial infarction (MI) rate (Wilhelmssen et al., 2008). An increased prevalence of obesity in both countries and also diabetes mellitus (DM) was observed in Swedish population over the observational period (Vartainen et al., 2010; Wilhelmssen et al., 2008), surprisingly with no influence on CVD outcome. This "obesity paradox" is probably caused by compensation of obesity associated risk with reduced overall risk due to higher rate of nonsmoking, normotension and normocholesterolaemia in population achieved by large community-based preventive and health promotion activities (Rosengren et al., 2009).

In the U.S. after peaking around 1968, over the period of 2 decades, the age-adjusted CHD death rate were cut in half (Ford et al., 2007). Approximately 44% of decline was attributed to reductions in major risk factors, including high total cholesterol, blood pressure, smoking, and physical inactivity (Hajjar & Kotchen, 2003; Johnson et al., 1993), although these reductions were partially offset by increases in the body-mass index (BMI) and the prevalence of DM (Harris et al., 1998; Hedley et al., 2004). Further 47% of this decrease was explained by evidence-based therapies including secondary preventive therapies after MI or revascularization, initial treatments for acute myocardial infarction (AMI) or unstable angina, treatments for heart failure, revascularization for chronic angina and other therapies. However, 9% of decline was unexplained (Ford et al., 2007). Similar conclusion was also found in analysis of the CHD mortality decline over the last 20-year period in UK (Unal et al., 2004). The WHO MONICA Project results (1980-1990) from 37 populations worldwide showed aorund 2/3 decline in CHD mortality by the decline in CHD incidence rates and the remaining 1/3 by the survival improvements due to better treatment (Tunstall-Pedoe et al., 1999).

Current statistical data over the past 3 decades clearly show the decline in incidence of CHD in patients aged<65 years in Europe. Alarmingly, among subjects who developed CHD <45 years, the incidence is unchanged, which may predict stagnation in CHD treatment and prevention in this population (Allender et al., 2009).

2. Active approach to the prevention of CVD: The European Heart Health Charter – The European perspective. America´s plan for better health and wellness. Action plan for non-communicable diseases

An active approach to the prevention of CHD in Europe was firstly declared in 1994 (Pyörälä et al., 1994), with the latest revision and extension to other atherosclerotic (AS) CVD in the „Fourth Task Force of the European guidelines on CVD prevention in clinical practice" (Graham et al., 2007). The current guidelines implement the previous initiatives of major international organizations and declarations (the Osaka Declaration, 2001; the Luxembourg Declaration, 2005) regarding the necessity to achieve cardiovascular (CV) health. These guidelines do not serve as a rigid rule, they are always open for modification and should be interpreted in the clinician´s judgement with regard to national guidelines and regional differences. This document underlines the importance of preventive strategies, because: CVD mortality, morbidity, and disability is still high, their contribution to the costs of health care is escalating as well as there is increasing evidence when and how to effectively reduce CVD mortality and morbidity.

Documented secular changes in CV risk factors in high-income countries (Ford et al., 2007; O´Flaherty et al., 2008; Vartainen et al., 2010; Wilhelmsen et al., 2008) and their positive influence on CHD mortality clearly demonstrate the crucial role of risk factor modification in CV prevention. The multinational (52 countries) INTERHEART study identified the 9 major modifiable CHD risk factors associated with MI. The raised apolipoprotein B/apolipoprotein A-I ratio (ApoB/ApoA-I), smoking, hypertension, DM, abdominal obesity, combined psychosocial stressors, avoidance of any regular exercise physical activity, irregular consumption of fruits and vegetables as well as no alcohol intake accounted for 90% of MI risk worldwide in both sexes and at all ages in all regions. In this study, abnormal lipid levels showed the strongest association with MI, while daily consumption of fruits or vegetables, moderate or strenuous physical exercise ≥4 hours a week, and consumption of alcohol ≥3 times per week seemed to be protective in MI risk (Yusuf et al., 2004). The importance of modifying risk factors is supported by data from other randomised trials [blood-pressure lowering (Mancia et al., 2009), lipid lowering (CTT Collaborators, 2005; CTT Collaborators, 2008; HPS Study, 2003; Jupiter Study, 2008), dietary and life style modification (DASH Study, 2006; de Lorgeril et al., 1999; Stampfer et al., 2000)] or from observational studies (Doll et al., 2004). Some investigators have suggested that a pill that combines a statin, antihypertensive drugs, and aspirin, together with avoidance of smoking, could potentially reduce the risk of MI by 80%-90% (Wald & Law, 2003).

In spite of the improvements of CV outcome by risk factor modification, the EUROASPIRE III survey (2009) from 22 European countries showed that large proportions of coronary patients do not achieve the lifestyle, risk factor and therapeutic targets for CVD prevention: 56% had a blood pressure ≥140/90 mmHg, 53% were centrally obese, 17% of patients smoked cigarettes, 51% had a suboptimal serum total cholesterol level, and only 35% of diabetics had glycated haemoglobin A1C <6.5%. There is still considerable potential throughout Europe to raise standards of preventive care.

This findings underline the important role of lifestyle and risk factor management in CVD prevention and suggest why **to prefer primary prevention in CVD management**. Moreover, prevention of CVD should go beyond the concept of primary prevention, towards a „primordial prevention“, to prevent the penetration of risk factors into the population by intervening to stop the appearance of the risk factors. The realisation of such strategic goals in everyday clinical practice requires an active approach to the CVD prevention. **The European Health Charter,** declared in 2007 in Brussels, advocates the development and implementation of comprehensive health strategies, measures and policies at European, national, regional and local level that promote cardiovascular health and prevent CHD by the assistance of guidelines on CVD prevention (Graham et al., 2007). In June, 2011, the U.S.´s first ever **National Prevention and Health Promotion Strategy** was declared: America´s plan for better health and wellness. An active and preventive approach is postulated in several points: active living, healthy eating, tobacco as well as injury and violence free living, preventing drug and excessive alcohol use, strengthening reproductive and sexual health as well as mental and emotional well-being. The America´s National Prevention Strategy indicates a 20% reduction of both CHD and stroke mortality by 2020. Novel, global effort to promote uniform approach to risk factor reduction provides **the Non Communicable Diseases (NCD) Alliance,** launched in 2009 in Geneva as a formal alliance of four international federations representing the four main NCDs - cardiovascular disease, diabetes, cancer, and chronic respiratory disease. These conditions share common risk factors and also share common solutions.

There is a real, world-wide research network for study determinants of lifestyle and its impact on risk factors and disease progression as well as to develop realistic, cost-effective strategies to reduce global burden of CVD and to face new challenges for prevention such as: a) increase of CVD in low- and middle-income countries, b) increase of diabetes and obesity, c) flattening of CHD mortality trends in the young, d) maintenance of high heart failure-incidence after MI, e) stroke.

3. Risk stratification and identification of persons at high risk of CVD has a crucial role in cardiovascular prevention

Current management of patients everywhere should provide complex program focusing on all aspects of care, including environment and lifestyle, psychosocial factors, management of risk factors, adherence to up-to-date treatment. Preventive strategies are the most effective and achievable means for improving health and may form the basis for a prevention-oriented society and health care. Preventive strategies are generally based on primordial, primary, secondary, tertiary and quaternary concepts. Due to continuous character of CVD progression, primordial, primary, and secondary preventive strategies should be implemented jointly. CV preventive strategies focus on: a) population at high risk, to reduce their morbidity and mortality, b) on the whole population at lower CVD risk, to maintain their state lifelong. Both approaches must be complementary. Paradoxically, high risk subjects develop fewer deaths compared with subjects at low risk, because they are more numerous (Rose, 1981).

Estimation of total CVD risk has been a crucial recommendation in patient management in European CVD Prevention guidelines since 1994 (Pyörälä et al., 1994). Such model assists to promote management of patients with CVD towards individual approach. **The rationale for the risk assessment is based on the following arguments**: a) risk factors are strongly associated with CVD morbidity and mortality, b) CVD is usually the product of several interacting risk factors, which may multiply the global risk, c) the possibility to reduce a risk, d) the need to treat the whole patients, not only one risk factor, e) the need for CV risk threshold to optimally manage patients, f) epidemiological data allow to estimate a global risk, g) identification of patients at high risk with most benefit from risk factor modification/treatment.

4. CVD risk assessment. Framingham risk scoring – Establishment of the 10-year absolute total risk for coronary events (fatal and non-fatal). The SCORE project – Establishment of the 10-year absolute risk for fatal CVD

The initiation of CVD prevention as well as the intensity of treatment of the individual patient depends on the patient´s risk status. Different multifactorial risk scoring systems have been developed: Framingham CHD Prediction Score 1976, Joint British Societies Coronary Risk Prediction Charts 1998, Framingham Risk Score 2002, Euroscore 2003, Procam Risk Score 2004, Progetto Cuore 2007, Qrisk 2007, Assign 2007, Framingham General CV Risk Score 2008, Predict 2008, and other systems (Lenz & Mühlhauser, 2004). A variety of risk calculators is available as charts, tables, computer programs, and web based tools. **Risk charts are intended to facilitate risk estimation in apparently healthy persons with no signs of clinical or preclinical disease.**

Because CVD is usually a result of a multiple risk factors interaction, the CVD risk should be calculated as a **global risk**, considering the global assessment of all major risk factors rather than the identification of the strength of each risk factor individually (Graham et al., 2007). Therefore, global risk is neither based on the simple summation of risk factors' values (risk score) nor on counting risk factors (Haq et al., 1999; Palmieri et al., 2004). One aim of primary prevention is to reduce **long-term risk** (>10 years) as well as **short-term risk** (≤10 years). Current practice in primary prevention of CVD involves estimation of short-term (typically 10-year) risk for developing CVD to identify individuals at high risk. Therapeutic goals in primary prevention depend on **absolute risk** of persons for AS CVD (i.e. the percentage chance of developing a CVD event over a given period of time). **Relative risk** is the ratio of the absolute risk of a given patient to that of a lower risk.

Equations derived from the American Framingham Heart Study are most widely used in the U.S. and have been used for many years in European countries too. Based on NCEP-ATP I and II documents, since 1988, risk stratification was provided by counting risk factors. **Framingham risk scoring** for determining the 10-year absolute total risk for developing hard coronary events (fatal - CHD death, non-fatal - myocardial infarction) was firstly used in NCEP-ATP III Recommendations (2001). To calculate risk, it used classical Framingham risk factors: age, sex, smoking, systolic blood pressure, total cholesterol, and HDL cholesterol. NCEP-ATP III defined individual absolute risk and metabolic syndrome, classified 4 patient categories: low, moderate, moderately high, and high risk as well as introduced the category of "**high CV risk**" individuals. At present, the National Heart, Lung, and Blood Institute Adult Cardiovascular Risk Reduction Guidelines effort includes both a shorter-term strategy of updating the existing guidelines for blood cholesterol, high blood pressure, and obesity as well as a longer-term strategy of developing an integrated CV risk reduction guideline. Two strategies are being undertaken because identification and management of individual risk factors, as well as a comprehensive integrated CV risk reduction approach to patients, are both important. Expected release date is 2012.

The first set of recommendations for prevention of CHD in clinical practice in Europe from 1994 included a new "risk chart" of classical Framingham risk factors for 10-year risk assessment of any CHD event, developed by Anderson et al. (1991). A 10-year ≥20% risk was used arbitrarily as a threshold for intensified risk factor intervention.

Endorsed by the Third Joint Task Force in 2003, a new risk chart was constructed: the **SCORE project** (Systematic COronary Risk Evaluation). 12 European cohort studies provided a scientific background to the development of this model for the estimation of a 10-year absolute fatal CVD in population based on the following risk factors: age, gender, smoking, systolic blood pressure, and either total cholesterol or total cholesterol/HDL cholesterol ratio. Separate charts were produced for total cholesterol/HDL cholesterol ratio as well as for low (Belgium, France, Greece, Italy, Luxembourg, Spain, Switzerland, Portugal, and countries with recently experienced substantial lowering of the CV mortality rates) and high risk regions (all other European countries). **The Third Joint Task Force** shifted the prevention from CHD to CVD, introduced the multifactorial SCORE model for risk assessment, continued in CV prevention focusing to determine high risk subjects, identified subclinical AS and other conditions as higher CV risk than indicated in the chart. Changing mortality trends in various countries required the recalibration of risk chart, which resulted in construction of national guidance enforced by **Fourth Joint Task Force** in 2007. Introduction of relative risk chart, its use in conjunction with the absolute SCORE chart, revised approach to the effect of other risk factors and organ damage on total CV events and mortality, the nomenclature of increased risk instead of high risk as well as introduction of fatal and nonfatal instead of only fatal risk estimation were other new features in the latest Task Force. SCORE model allows the estimation of absolute CVD death risk, its extrapolation to age 60 years as well as the estimation of a relative risk. The following risk categories can be differentiated by SCORE model: low, moderate, increased, and markedly increased. Risk ≥5% is considered increased/high (Figure 2, 3).

An update version of this latest guidelines will become available in 2012, but at the present time the new **ESC/EAS guidelines on management of dyslipidaemias** modify in several ways the current CVD risk assessment (Reiner et al., 2011): redefine risk categories; introduce very high risk category; determine persons at automatically high or very high CV risk adding chronic kidney disease and documented CVD by invasive or non-invasive methods to the previously automatically determined diseases; modify the relative risk of diabetes; indicate multipliers to convert fatal to total (fatal + non-fatal) CVD risk; refine the HeartScore by entering actual HDL cholesterol level instead of the combined HDL/LDL cholesterol level (www.escardio.org/guidelines), "fast track" calculator of BMI in the unavailability of blood pressure and cholesterol inputs as well as „risk age" function to determine the theoretical age of a person. **The primacy of managing total risk rather than focusing on individual risk factors is stressed in all latest European preventive documents with definition of desirable levels of individual risk factors. The threshold for high total CVD risk is arbitrary, but targets to initiate pharmacological interventions are open** because the risk is a continuum and there is a need for continuous up-to-date modification.

The main difference between the 2 major scoring systems - Framingham Risk Score vs. SCORE - is expressed in some aspects: a) population based: 5000 Americans vs. 200,000 Europeans, b) prediction: coronary events vs. AS CVD, c) end points: composite including also non-fatal events vs. fatal events, d) adjustment: impossibility for national variations vs. possibility to be customized using national statistics.

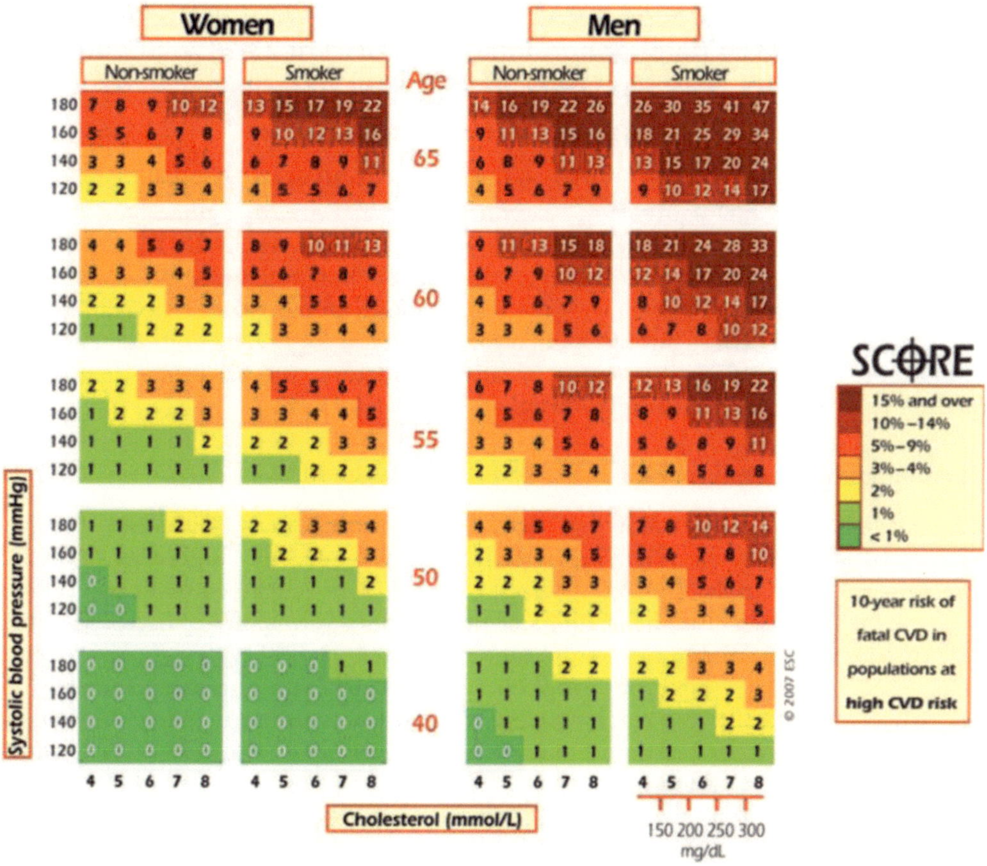

Fig. 2. SCORE chart: 10-year risk of fatal CVD in populations at high CVD risk based on the following risk factors: age, gender, smoking, systolic blood pressure, and total cholesterol. ©The European Society of Cardiology

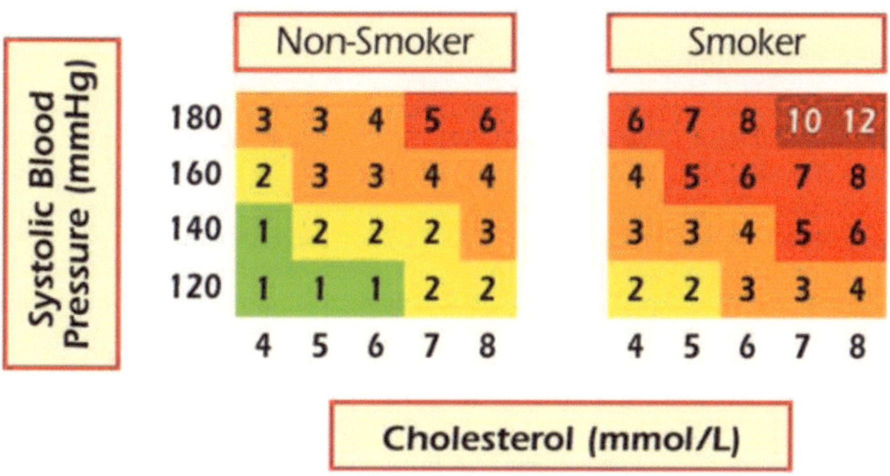

Fig. 3. Relative risk chart. ©The European Society of Cardiology

5. High /very high risk groups. FRAMINGHAM (NCEP-ATP III Update, 2004) high risk: 10-year total (fatal or non-fatal) hard CHD risk >20%. SCORE (ESC/EAS 2011) high /very high risk: 10-year fatal CVD risk ≥5%/10%

5.1 Determined high /very high risk groups (without estimation)

NCEP-ATP III described the high CV risk individuals with 10-year risk >20%: those with the presence of CHD or CHD equivalent. According to ESC/EAS 2011 guidelines, subjects at high or very high risk are as follows: a) subjects with known CVD, b) asymptomatic patients: with DM2, DM1 with target organ damage such as microalbuminuria, markedly elevated level of individual risk factors with /without target organ damage, c) chronic kidney disease (CKD). **These subjects are automatically at high/very high total/fatal CVD risk and need intensive management of all risk factors, for all other people a risk estimation is recommended using Framingham/SCORE system.**

5.2 Framingham risk categories

NCEP-ATP III identified the following 10-year CV risk categories: a) low risk: (<10%: 0-1 risk factor, b) moderate risk: (<10%): ≥2 risk factors, c) moderately high risk: (10-20%): ≥2 risk factors, d) high risk: (>20%): presence of CHD or CHD equivalent. CHD risk equivalents include clinical manifestations of noncoronary forms of AS disease [peripheral arterial disease (PAD), abdominal aortic aneurysm, and carotid artery disease (transient ischemic attacks or stroke of carotid origin or >50% obstruction of a carotid artery)], DM, and ≥2 risk factors with 10-year risk for hard CHD >20%. According to NCEP-ATP III panel, major risk factors (exclusive of high LDL cholesterol) modifying the risk include: cigarette smoking, hypertension [blood pressure (BP) ≥140/90 mmHg or antihypertensive medication], low HDL cholesterol (<40 mg/dl), family history of premature CHD (CHD in male first-degree relative <55 years of age; CHD in female first-degree relative <65 years of age), and age (men ≥45 years; women ≥55 years). The NCEP-ATP III Update document introduced the "very high risk" category, i.e. patients with acute coronary syndromes (ACS) or with CVD and a) DM, b) severe and poorly controlled risk factors, c) metabolic syndrome (MS).

5.3 SCORE risk categories

According to SCORE chart, the 10-year absolute total risk of CVD death ≥5% is considered as high/increased risk. **The European Third Joint Task Force Guidelines on CVD Prevention** (De Backer et al., 2003) determined high risk patients as follows: 1) patients with established AS CVD, 2) asymptomatic subjects at high risk for AS CVD because of: a) multiple risk factors with a 10-year risk ≥5%, b) markedly increased levels of single risk factors: cholesterol ≥8 mmol/l (320 mg/dl), LDL cholesterol ≥6 mmol/l (240 mg/dl), BP ≥180/110 mmHg, c) DM type 2 or DM type 1 with microalbuminuria, 3) close relatives of a) patients with early onset AS disease, b) asymptomatic subjects at particularly high risk. **The Fourth Joint Task Force** (Graham et al., 2007) selected four 10-year fatal CVD risk categories: a) low (<1%); b) moderate (1-4%); c) increased (5-9%); d) very increased risk (≥10%). It confirmed the same high-risk patient groups as the Third Task Force, but reclassified they as increased-risk groups as well as endorsed an increased risk in those subjects with markedly elevated level of single risk factors, especially in association with end-organ damage.

The new **ESC/EAS guidelines on management of dyslipidaemias** classify the following risk categories (Reiner et al., 2011): 1) very high risk: patients with any of the following: a) documented CVD by invasive or non-invasive testing (such as coronary angiography, nuclear imaging, stress echocardiography, carotid plaque on ultrasound), previous MI, ACS, coronary revascularization (percutaneous coronary intervention, coronary artery bypass graft) and other arterial revascularizations, ischaemic stroke, PAD, b) patients with DM2, DM1 with target organ damage such as microalbuminuria, c) patients with moderate to severe CKD [glomerular filtration rate (GFR) <60 ml/min/1.73 m^2], d) calculated 10-year risk SCORE ≥10%, 2) high risk: subjects with markedly elevated single risk factor with /without target organ damage or a calculated risk ≥5% SCORE <10%, 3) moderate risk: subjects with ≥1% SCORE <5%, 4) low risk: subjects with SCORE <1%. Calculated risk may underestimate the real risk in various conditions.

The 10-year fatal CVD risk ≥5% (high/increased risk) is equated approximately to 10-year total (fatal and non-fatal) CHD risk ≥20% according to previous European risk charts based on the Framingham Heart Study results (De Backer et al., 2003) and to 10-year total fatal and non-fatal CVD risk about ≥15% according to the latest ESC/EAS guidelines, considering also data from FINRISK MONICA; the multiplier is slightly higher in women and lower in older persons (Reiner et al., 2011; Vartiainen et al., 2000).

6. Limitations of a current system. Underestimation of a real 10-year CHD/CVD risk in various clinical conditions

The most frequently used risk models (Framingham, SCORE) have also limitations such as: 1) may overestimate the risk in low risk regions or in countries with a falling CVD mortality rate and underestimate it in high risk ones or if the risk is rising, 2) may underestimate the individual risk, 3) at any given age, the estimated risk is lower in women than men because it is deferred by 10 years, 4) the risk algorithms do not include several risk factors strongly associated with CVD mortality with higher real than calculated CV risk, 5) short-term risk prediction.

Despite the availability of several validated risk prediction algorithms, their use has lagged in primary care. One potential reason for physician inertia in using risk prediction instruments is the multiplicity of such algorithms, each for predicting an individual CVD component, e.g. hard coronary event, stroke, fatal CVD, etc. There is a need in primary care for risk scoring of developing any major AS CVD event using a single, general CVD risk assessment tool, enabling physicians to identify high-risk candidates for any and all initial AS CVD events using measurements readily available. A sex-specific multivariable risk factor algorithm (D´Agostino et al., 2008) can be conveniently used to assess absolute general CVD risk and risk of individual CVD events (coronary, cerebrovascular, PAD, and heart failure).

Current practice in primary prevention of CVD involves estimation of short-term (typically 10-year) risk for developing CVD to identify individuals at high risk, resulting in treatment only for older individuals with substantial risk factor burden. Younger and middle-age individuals with clearly adverse risk factor levels may have low short-term but substantial lifetime risks for development of CVD. The estimated lifetime risks for CVD and median survival are associated with different clinical strata of individual risk factors and with aggregate risk factor burden at 50 years of age. Compared with participants with ≥2 major risk factors at 50 years of age, those with optimal levels had substantially lower lifetime risks (5.2% vs. 68.9% in men, 8.2% vs. 50.2% in women) and markedly longer median survivals (>39 vs. 28 years in men, >39 vs. 31 years in women). The presence of diabetes at 50 years of age conferred the highest lifetime risk for CVD of any single risk factor (Lloyd-Jones et al., 2006) (Figure 4).

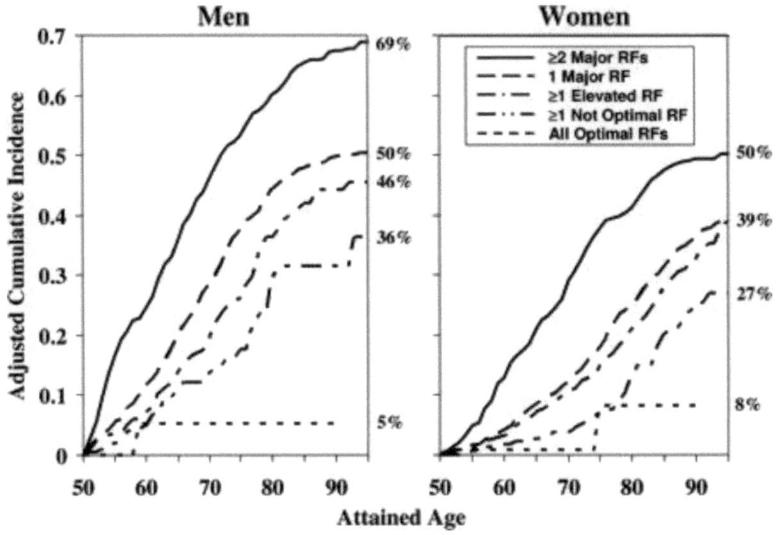

Fig. 4. Lifetime risk. Prediction of lifetime risk for CVD by risk factor burden at 50 years of age (Lloyd-Jones et al., 2006)

7. Population groups with increasing evidence of high CV risk (similarly to those with automatically determined high risk according to NCEP-ATP III 2004 and ESC/EAS 2011 guidelines)

7.1 Subjects with established subclinical atherosclerosis

The total CVD risk may be higher than indicated in the Framingham/SCORE chart (Reiner et al., 2011) **mainly in the following situations (qualifiers):** a) preclinical AS, particularly evidence of vascular wall morphological abnormalities detected by imagine methods such as ultrasonography [(plaques, increased carotid intima-media thickness (CIMT)], CT scanning, assessment of coronary artery calcium, etc., as well as detection of functional abnormalities of vascular wall, for example, ankle-brachial index (ABI), decreased flow mediated vasodilation (FMD), etc.; increasing role in detection of preclinical AS is attributed to biochemical markers of preclinical AS, mainly high sensitivity C-reactive protein (hs-CRP) (Greenland et al., 2010), b) renal impairment, c) DM, d) severe abnormalities of single risk factors, e) obesity, especially with central type (waist circumference [International Diabetes Federation (IDF), 2005]: ≥94 cm in men and ≥80 cm in women), physical inactivity, unhealthy diet, f) social deprivation, g) low HDL cholesterol or apoA-I in SCORE, increased triglycerides (TG), fibrinogen, homocysteine, apoB, lipoprotein(a) (Lp(a)), familial hypercholesterolaemia, increased hs-CRP; these factors indicate a higher level of risk in both genders, all age groups and at all levels of risk, h) strong positive family history of premature CVD. From these, **renal impairment, DM, and severe abnormalities of single risk factors are classified similarly to documented CVD as determined high/very high risk condition, without need to calculate it.**

DM is associated with 5x higher CVD risk in women and 3x higher in men in comparison with those without DM. Epidemiological data documented progressive rise (20-30x) of CVD risk from microalbuminuria with preserved GFR to end-stage renal disease. Recently a KDIGO report has suggested a new global guideline to assess all-cause and CV mortality, end-stage renal disease, acute kidney injury, and progressive chronic kidney disease based on estimated GFR (eGFR) and level of albuminuria. As the data have indicated, those at lower level of eGFR and higher levels of albuminuria were at increased risk for all outcomes, including CV (Levey et al., 2010).

7.2 Subjects with elevated heart rate

Beyond qualifiers recommended by the European guidelines to check while calculating the 10-year fatal CVD risk, another clinical conditions have been shown to be associated with high CV risk, e.g. elevated heart rate. Elevated heart rate (>70/min) is strongly, gradually, and independently of other factors associated with increased risk of all-cause and CV mortality as well as development of CVD in general population, hypertensives, diabetics, and those with pre-existing CHD (Diaz et al., 2005; INVEST Study, 2008; Kannel et al., 1987; OPERA registry, 2007; TNT Study, 2006; WOSCOPS Study, 1995). Risk of sudden death in men is particularly associated with elevated resting heart rate, but in women and the elderly this association is not so strong (Shaper et al., 1993). Arterial hypertension (AH) in conjunction with elevated heart rate is associated with the worst prognosis (Levy, 1945). Heart rate >80/min, left ventricular mass >270 g, and increased pulse pressure are considered as negative prognostic markers of plaque rupture. Elevated heart rate is a frequent symptom of physical inactivity and associated obesity, diabetes and MS, excessive use of psychostimulants, psychological stress and associated hypertension as well as smoking. Up-to now, elevated heart rate as a part of a pathophysiological pathway of most traditional modifiable risk factors is declared neither as a separate high CV risk state nor as a qualifier. Pharmacological reduction of heart rate is not recommended in asymptomatic population.

8. Personalized CV prevention. Identification of subjects at high CV risk among those without determined or calculated high risk

To identify patients at high risk with most benefit from risk factor modification or specific pharmacological treatment is a crucial step in primary prevention. Current guidelines based on the most frequently used Framingham and SCORE model determine subjects at high/very high 10-year total CHD/fatal CVD risk without necessity to calculate it. To identify other subjects at high risk, risk stratification is recommended. The AS CV continuum is a multiple interaction of a wide spectrum of risk factors, but **available risk charts based on the set of a few risk factors have limitations to asses a real CVD risk, thus sometimes the calculated risk underestimates the real one.** Epidemiological data from studies (Belcaro et al., 1996; Postley et al., 2009), which failed in prediction CV risk assessed by risk charts, based on classical risk factors. Only 40% of patients with high risk developed CV event, while 70% of those with low risk. **To document high risk condition in those**

without determined or calculated high risk is a target for individualized risk stratification. According to the latest guidelines, **two main subclinical CV pathologies are strongly associated with the increased CV risk: a) subclinical AS** (either early or advanced stage), **and b) end-organ damage.** Thus personalized prevention aims to focus on active search for these conditions. Sometimes a physician would like to target risk assessment and preventive measures to a specific CV end point such as MI or stroke depending, for example, on an individual patient's family history, age, diabetic status, or predisposition to a particular outcome by valve disease. If calculation does not indicate high risk, the individual risk assessment is recommended.

Up to now there is no strict recommendation for individual risk assessment: whom, when, and how to investigate. Because screening of the whole population is extremely time-consuming, expensive, and ineffective, much more effective way with better cost/benefit ratio might be the selection of either subjects, time, or screening tools for individualized risk stratification. **Personalized CV prevention may be useful mainly at the time of expected acceleration of AS** (age risk, in the onset of multiple risk factors with multiplicative interactions, in various comorbidities). We do not know with certainty what changes are typical for accelerated AS (dynamics of morphological changes, presence of specific markers, highly increased level of some markers, etc.). Identification of AS acceleration could serve as an indicator to start with pharmacotherapy in asymptomatic patients in whom benefits of treatment could outweigh its adverse effects, cost, burden of staff, and stress from "health loss".

9. Beyond the SCORE chart. Personalized risk assessment in Europe. Whom, when, and how?

9.1 Whom?

Persons, who are not classified automatically as high CV risk and are not at high but moderate calculated risk with the presence of:

1. obesity, dyslipoproteinaemia (low HDL cholesterol or apoA-I, high TG, fibrinogen, homocysteine, apoB, Lp(a), hs-CRP),
2. positive family history,
3. psychosocial factors,
4. multiple risk factors (mostly modifiable),
5. specific comorbidities, mainly associated with inflammation, but also with cardiometabolic risk: (autoimmune chronic inflammatory diseases: rheumatic diseases, vasculitides, psoriasis; infections associated with AS; organ transplantations; sleep apnoea, chronic obstructive lung disease; some endocrinopaties, hormonal substitution; etc.).

Certain clinical states are recognized at higher 10-year fatal CVD risk than indicated in the SCORE chart (with rationale for individualized risk stratification): sedentary or obese subjects, especially with central obesity, with low HDL cholesterol or apoA-I, raised TG, fibrinogen, homocysteine, apoB, Lp(a), hs-CRP, with strong family history of premature CVD, in social deprivation, but increasing data suggest the need for screening also in the setting of multiple risk factors with <5% 10-year fatal CVD risk as well as in the presence of specific comorbidities.

9.1.1 Sedentary lifestyle and associated risk factors

Sedentary lifestyle doubles the risk of premature death and increases the risk for CVD (Paffenbarger et al., 1993; Rosengren & Wilhelmsen, 1997). Obesity, a worldwide epidemic in both children and adults (Poirier et al., 2006) is considered as an insulin resistant, pro-inflammatory, and prothrombotic state. Fat is associated with hypersecretion of free fatty acids, hyperinsulinaemia, insulin resistance, hypertension and dyslipidaemia (Carr & Brunzell, 2004; Wajchenberg, 2000). Excess central fat is strongly associated with metabolic and CVD risk (Despres et al., 1990). It has been shown that body weight increases CV risk by its adverse effect on many risk factors such as blood pressure, total, LDL, and HDL cholesterol, waist circumference, sleep apnoea, etc. (Graham et al., 2007). The association between increasing BMI, waist circumference as well as waist-to hip ratio (WHR) and greater CVD risk has been also demonstrated (Larsson et al., 1984). Taking into account known associations between increasing waist circumference/WHR and other cardiometabolic risk factors and cost/benefit relations, screening for the presence of preclinical AS or end-organ damage is highly indicated in patients with MS. In spite of the fact that MS represents an increased risk of developing CVD and DM type 2, it does not indicate a priori high risk similar to those with CVD and diabetes.

The causal relationship between total and LDL cholesterol and CVD risk is generally known, beyond the "standard risk assessment" there is no recommendation for further risk screening (CTT Collaborators, 2005). While treatment goals are clearly declared for total and LDL cholesterol, no specific ones are documented for HDL cholesterol and triglycerides. The benefits of statins are proven for both genders and age except for in healthy, asymptomatic women (HPS Study, 2003). Current ESC/EAS guidelines modify indications for lipid analysis (Reiner et al., 2011).

9.1.2 Positive family history for early CHD

A positive family history of early CHD is an independent risk factor for CHD. The risk of CHD increases in a first, second, and third degree relatives, as the number of family members with CHD increases and the younger the age at which family members develop CHD (Graham et al., 2007). Impact of risk factors on the development of AS is influenced by environmental and genetic factors. Relatively high level of heritability for many CHD phenotypes may partially explain a strong genetic determination (Pankow et al., 2001; Worns et al., 2006). The identification of **new genetic polymorphisms** associated with CV phenotypes opened novel perspectives in AS research. Polymorphisms of chromosomal loci (9p21, 1p13, 1q41, 10q11, 21q22, 6p24, 2q33 and 3q22) were associated with development of AS and its complications in genome wide association studies (GWAS) published in 2007-2009. 9p21 locus showed the strongest association with stroke, peripheral artery disease, aortic and cerebral artery aneurysm and sudden cardiac death. Significant but relatively low effect on CV risk is documented for variants of genes involved in lipid metabolism, coagulation, and various aspects of endothelial function (Pankow et al., 2001; Worns et al., 2006).

In spite of the suggestive results, population screening for genetic polymorphism is currently not yet realistic (Casas et al., 2006; Purcell et al., 2003). Individual stratification of CVR could be an alternative bridging tool between use of risk algorithm based on classical risk factors with low predictive value and population screening for presence of genetic polymorphisms. Genetic screening may promote in the future search for individuals at high CVD risk as well as individual therapeutic approaches according to the individual genetic make-up. Subjects with positive family history may gain from further risk stratification.

9.1.3 Psychosocial factors

Psychosocial factors increase the risk of the first event and also a worsening of CHD prognosis (Rozanski et al., 2005). Besides the presence of smoking and unhealthy diet as risk factors, endocrine, autonomic and inflammatory changes contribute in promoting CHD. Beyond the CHD risk they show problematic management and no active approach of subjects to lifestyle modification. The following types are involved in CHD risk: low socio-economic status, social isolation and lack of social support, stress at work and in family life, negative emotions including depression and hostility. For non-compliance there is no strict rule for screening these patients for subclinical AS or end-organ damage.

9.1.4 Multiple risk factors

Markedly increased levels of single risk factors: total cholesterol ≥8 mmol/l (320 mg/dl), LDL cholesterol ≥6 mmol/l (240 mg/dl), BP ≥180/110 mmHg, severe continuous smoking are automatically high risk conditions.

Management of patients with **arterial hypertension**, particularly the initiation of pharmacological treatment, depends not only on the BP level but also on total CV risk assessment, including identification of a) associated clinical condition: established CVD, renal impairment (plasma creatinine >133 umol/l in men, >124 umol/l in women, proteinuria >300 mg/24h), as well as advanced retinopathy (haemorrhages, exudates or papilloedema), b) coexistence of other CV risk factors, i.e. high pulse pressure, c) the presence of subclinical end-organ damage such as: electrocardiographic or echocardiographic left ventricular hypertrophy, carotid-wall thickening (CIMT ≥0.9 mm) or plaque, abnormal pulse-wave velocity (carotid-femoral ≥12 m/s), pathological ankle-brachial index (ABI <0.9), slight increase of plasma creatinine (115-133 umol/l in men, 107-124 umol/l in women), low eGFR (<60 ml/min/1.73m^2 MDRD; <60ml/min Cockroft-Gault) or microalbuminuria (30-300 mg/24h). Associated clinical condition represents a very high and subclinical organ damage a high CV risk (Graham et al., 2007). ESH Task Force (Mancia et al., 2009) recommends a search for subclinical organ damage in hypertension. **Active and passive smoking** increase the risk of CHD and smoking-related diseases. The adverse effect of smoking is related to the amount of tobacco smoked daily and to the duration of smoking. Smoking interact synergistically in the presence of other CVD risk factors such as age gender, AH, and DM (Law et al., 1997; US Department of Health and Human Services, 2004). Individualized risk stratification in smoking is of great importance in a cluster with other risk factors.

9.1.5 Specific comorbidities associated with inflammation or cardiometabolic risk

Evidence suggests that enhanced AS causes premature CV events in some autoimmune diseases. Patients with **rheumatoid arthritis** (RA) have a 2-5 times increased risk of developing premature CV event that shortens life expectancy by 5-10 years. Indeed, low-grade inflammation and endothelial dysfunction play pivotal roles in enhanced atherogenesis in rheumatic diseases. The joint influence of CV risk factors and inflammation causes expression of adhesion molecules [selectins, vascular cell and intracellular adhesion molecules (VCAM-1, ICAM-1)] induced by pro-inflammatory cytokines [interleukin (IL)-1β and tumor necrosis factor-α (TNF-α)] as well as by CRP and CD40/CD40 ligand interactions that promote the adherence of monocytes (Gasparyan et al., 2010). In addition, coagulation factors [increased levels of tissue factor, van Willebrand factor (vWF), and plasminogen activator inhibitor-1 (PAI-1)] as well as proteolytic enzymes [matrix metalloproteinases (MMPs)] with their role in destruction, destabilization, and rupture of vulnerable atherosclerotic plaques are also important (Hürlimann et al., 2004). Advanced glycation end-products (AGE), their receptors (RAGE) as well as antiphospholipid antibodies and other inflammation propagating factors may be contributed to accelerated AS during the course of different systemic inflammatory diseases.

Remarkably, relatively few studies have been published on the occurrence of accelerated AS in patients with **vasculitis**. In giant cell arteritis, mortality because of ischaemic heart disease is not increased. During active stage of Takayasu arteritis (large vessel vasculitis), Kawasaki disease (medium-sized vessel vasculitis) as well as in small vessel vasculitis (anti-neutrophil cytoplasmic autoantibodies-associated) accelerated AS has been well documented. Several risk factors, such as DM and AH are present more often in patients with vasculitis in comparison with healthy controls. In addition, steroid therapy, impaired renal function, persistent proteinuria, increased levels of CRP and autoantibodies, enhanced oxidation processes, activated T-cells as well as inhibited regulatory T-cells documented in these patients are well-known risk factors for acceleration of AS (Tervaert, 2009).

According to various authors, the hypothesis of a **relationship between infection and AS** is still alive, recently an answer is required about whether the atherogenic process is triggered, accelerated, or both by infection (Gurfinkel, 2006). The association of Chlamydia pneumoniae, Helicobacter pylori, cytomegalovirus, Epstein-Barr virus as well as other viruses and parasites with AS lesions are generally known. Infective agents act through the tool like receptors, having crucial role in natural defence against microbial pathogens (Ekesbo et al., 2001). Human immunodeficiency virus **(HIV)-infected patients** are at a significantly higher risk from CHD and MI compared to gender- and age-matched non-infected individuals. Antiretroviral therapy induces metabolic abnormalities in HIV-infected patients that are linked to inflammation, probably also via visceral adipose tissue activation affecting the liver function, followed by pro-atherogenic dyslipidaemia. Pro-inflammatory cytokines released by adipocytes are responsible for worsening insulin sensitivity and hyperglycaemia. As a result of nuclear factor-kappa B (NFκB) activation, hs-CRP up-regulates cytokines that contribute to MI by recruiting leukocytes and promoting thrombosis (De Lorenzo et al., 2008).

Both CRP (marker of systemic inflammation) and asymmetric dimethylarginine (ADMA - endogenous inhibitor of NO-synthase) have been shown to be associated with increased incidence and progression of AS lesions in carotid arteries as well as to be important risk factors for CVD and mortality in the **end-stage renal disease** population (Rattazzi et al., 2003).

The accelerated AS in **transplanted kidneys and hearts** has a complex pathogenesis, which includes both immunological and nonimmunological factors. Hypertension is one such factor, which has been claimed to be an independent risk factor for chronic renal transplant dysfunction, usually characterised by transplant AS (Fellström et al., 1989). Recent experimental and clinical data suggest accelerated AS occurs following bone marrow mobilisation or intracoronary haematopoietic stem cell therapy (Vanderheyden et al., 2005).

Obstructive sleep apnoea (OSA) may accelerate AS by exacerbating key atherogenic risk factors (secondary hypertension, insulin resistance, diabetes, dyslipidaemia) (Szabóová et al., 2008). In addition, clinical data and experimental evidence in animal models suggest that OSA can have direct proatherogenic effects inducing systemic inflammation, oxidative stress, vascular smooth cell activation, increased adhesion molecule expression, monocyte/lymphocyte activation, increased lipid loading in macrophages, lipid peroxidation, and endothelial dysfunction (Drager et al., 2011). Several cross-sectional studies have shown consistently that OSA is independently associated with surrogate markers of premature AS, most of them in the carotid bed (Szabóová et al., 2007). Moreover, OSA treatment with continuous positive airway pressure may attenuate carotid AS, as has been shown in a randomized clinical trial. High prevalence of CIMT and increased CVD risk as assessed by carotid ultrasonography in **chronic obstructive pulmonary diseases** with a broad spectrum of airway obstruction severity has been shown in a recent study (Pobeha et al., 2011).

It is generally known, that some **endocrinopaties** may increase the cardiometabolic risk (e.g. acromegaly, thyreopathies, hyperparathyreosis, adrenal hyperfunction as well as hormonal treatment associated with cardiometabolic and thrombogenic risk such as corticosteroid therapy, hormone substitution/replacement therapy, oral contraceptive use, etc.). Because of high incidence, the greatest clinical significance is linked to hypothyreosis as well as hormone replacement therapy in perimenopausal women.

Active risk screening in above-mentioned clinical conditions may add to the overall precision of CV risk quantification.

9.1.6 Personal opinion

A. Patients are a priori at high/very high risk, no additional testing, but aggressive management is recommended in:

1. known CVD,
2. DM type 2/DM type 1 with end-organ damage (microalbuminuria),
3. renal impairment,
4. very high level of single risk factor with /without target organ damage,
5. presence of multiple risk factors with calculated 10-year risk ≥5%.

B. Individual stratification seems to be useful for identification of other high-risk patients, particularly, in those at moderate calculated risk with:

1. metabolic syndrome (involving obesity and dyslipoproteinaemia),
2. arterial hypertension,
3. positive family history,
4. presence of ≥2 risk factors, especially smoking in cluster with other risk factors,
5. specific comorbidities with suspected acceleration of AS.

9.2 When?

The probability to detect preclinical AS/end-organ damage is higher at the time with possible acceleration of AS:

1. risky age,
2. the onset of multiple risk factors,
3. the onset of specific comorbidity.

9.2.1 Risky age

Age ≥45 years in men and ≥55 years in women is considered as non-modifiable risk factor. CVD risk in women is deferred by 10 years. More older women die than men from CVD. The actual incidence of CVD is increased in older women, which further support the specific age-related risk for CVD in women (Stramba-Badiale et al., 2006). The age-related worsening of classical risk factors in women may be explained by: increased incidence of systolic hypertension, cholesterol peak, obesity, diabetes, oral contraceptive use in combination with smoking.

9.2.2 The onset of multiple risk factors

Detectability of following markers for accelerated AS is extremely important: biochemical (classical, novel: specific vascular proteomes, combination of various cell, tissue, and plasma proteomes), functional, and morphological markers. Various emerging risk factors are involved in the regulation of crucial pathways of AS development such as endothelial dysfunction, inflammation, lipid metabolism, haemostasis, etc. Multiple risk factors may accelerate the development of AS. **In diabetics** a cluster of potent CV risk factors is present, which explains an extremely high risk for future CV event. Well documented is a specific role of inflammation in the development of macrovascular (AS) complications of DM. The following pathophysiological steps are stressed: a) activation of NFκB (potent pro-inflammatory and pro-atherosclerotic mediator), b) expression of AGE, reactive oxygen species with promoting AS, c) hyperglycaemia-induced vascular cell changes (loss of non-adhesivity of endothelial cells, adhesion of monocytes to endothelial surface, promotion of oxidative stress, decreased expression of NO, activation of matrix metalloproteinases (involved in plaque rupture and vascular remodeling) in smooth muscle cells, stimulation of smooth muscle cells to proliferation/migration/changed reactivity, d) hyperglycaemia-induced vascular inflammation by activation of cytokines from monocytes (IL-1β, IL-6, etc.) and lymphocytes resulting in acceleration of AS.

A strong association was documented between **inflammatory markers** and **obesity** as well as **insulin resistance** (TNF-α, adiponectin) (Rask-Madsen et al., 2003; Tsuchiya et al., 2007), between inflammatory markers, haemostasis, and the development of MI as well as between haemostatic factors and incidence of CHD (Ridker et al., 2000; Scarabin et al., 2003).

Lower HDL cholesterol levels, positive family history of CHD, and elevated fibrinogen concentrations were found as independent predictors for future CV events in a recent study (Rizzo et al., 2008). Lower HDL cholesterol levels may potentially accelerate the progression from subclinical lesions [CIMT, asymptomatic atherosclerotic carotid plaque (ACP)] to clinical events. Fibrinogen as a glycoprotein is involved in a number of mechanisms with a crucial role of early formation and growth of atheroma (Coppola et al., 2006; Maresca et al., 1999; Wilhelmsen et al., 1984; Woodward et al., 1997). In a recent study a significant inverse correlation between HDL cholesterol levels and fibrinogen concentrations has been shown, suggesting a possible "synergistic" role of low HDL cholesterol and inflammation on the atherosclerotic disease progression from subclinical lesions to clinical events (Rizzo et al., 2008). **The presence of subclinical carotid AS together with low HDL cholesterol concentrations points to a category of subjects at "high" CV risk**. This effect could be due to the up-regulation of the inflammatory pathway: HDL cholesterol may promote inflammation in the acute phase.

9.2.3 The onset of specific comorbidity

Histologically is well documented a vascular AS calcification in most patients with **severe CKD** as part of cholesterol crystallization within AS lesions. Prominent AS medial calcification has been previously identified as Mönckeberg's sclerosis. A unifying concept supported by the preponderance of pathologic evidence contends that Mönckeberg's sclerosis is a manifestation of accelerated AS in patients with CKD. Factors that seem to promote the osteoblastic transformation of vascular smooth muscle cells and enhance deposition of calcium hydroxyapatite crystals include phosphorus activation of the Pit-1 receptor, bone morphogenic proteins 2 and 4, leptin, endogenous 1,25 dihydroxyvitamin D, vascular calcification activating factor, and oxidative stress (McCullough et al., 2008).

9.3 How?

Detection of preclinical AS increases the CV risk. Preclinical markers of AS are related to the presence of AS risk factors, to multifocal AS, and to the severity of coronary artery stenosis assessed by intravascular ultrasound (IVUS) or angiographically (Amato et al., 2007). They are classified as:

1. biochemical,
2. genetic,
3. functional,
4. morphological markers.

In assessing risk is recommended to follow standard diagnostic steps: history taking including family history, physical examination (blood pressure, heart and lung examination, heart rate, foot pulses, BMI, waist circumference), laboratory tests (urine for glucose and protein, total, HDL, LDL cholesterol, triglycerides, glucose, creatinine, eGFR), ECG and exercise ECG if angina suspected, ECG/echocardiogram in young or severely hypertensive persons, hsCRP, Lp(a), fibrinogen, or homocysteine in positive family history (Graham et al., 2007).

9.3.1 Biochemical markers of preclinical AS

A. Markers of endothelial dysfunction

- **adhesion molecules:** ICAM-1, VCAM-1, E-selectin, P-selectin, platelet-endothelial cell adhesion molecule PECAM-1, endoglin, vascular endothelial (VE)-Cadherin, S-Endo-1 antigen, CD40 L,

- **cytokines:** IL-6, IL-18, TNF-α, 8-iso-prostaglandin F2α, endothelin-1 (ET-1), metalloproteinases,
- **others**: endothelial-derived microparticles, progenitor cells, glycocalyx measurements (invasively, non-invasively), microalbuminuria (Nieuwdorp et al., 2006; Romanens et al., 2010).

B. Inflammatory markers: hs-CRP, fibrinogen, serum amyloid A, dimethylamine (DMA), asymmetrical dimethylarginine (ADMA), oxLDL, lipoprotein-associated phospholipase A2.

C. Factors of haemostasis: vWf, tissue plasminogen activator (t-PA), PAI-1, factor VII (F VII), F V, prothrombin, plasminogen, D-dimers, Lp(a).

Endothelial dysfunction is consistently associated with CV risk factors and predicts higher risk of CV event. Endothelial dysfunction is the first, functionally important stage of AS, detected far before the structural changes of arterial wall. Any endothelial damage may trigger inflammatory response involving endothelial cells by several mechanisms: expression of adhesion molecules, production of cytokines, transmigration of leukocytes, and angiogenesis. Microalbuminuria as a biochemical parameter of endothelial dysfunction is recommended in hypertesives and diabetics to detect end-organ damage as well as to predict overall and CV risk in chronic kidney disease. Increasing evidence is for its role in the population screening in the future (Kalaitzidis & Bakris, 2009; Levey et al., 2010).

A strong correlation has been detected between **hs-CRP** and CV risk, moreover hs-CRP predicts destabilisation of the AS plaque (Burke et al., 2002; Ridker, 2001). The rationale for incorporation of biochemical markers (especially CRP) into prediction risk model is accentuated with findings from recent trials (JUPITER, 2008; MARS, 2010), where CRP level ≥2 mg/l appears as an effective tool for identification of subjects with increased risk independently from LDL cholesterol. The utility of hs-CRP in risk assessment is weakened by: a possible reverse causality and findings from recent genetic analysis, which failed to support association between CRP genotypes coding higher CRP levels with CVD or risk factors. Interestingly, genetic analysis of haemostatic factors documented an moderate association of factor V gene and prothrombin gene with CHD risk (Ye et al., 2006). In spite of strong arguments based on numerous meta-analyses from epidemiological trials **there is still no joint consensus on the use of inflammatory markers (especially CRP) in risk evaluation in Europe, but not so in the U.S.**

Biochemical markers of haemostasis. High Lp(a) predicts risk of early AS similar to high level of LDL cholesterol. Lp(a) is a risk factor for advanced AS independent of LDL cholesterol that indicates a risk for plaque thrombosis. High heritability may signalize its role in person with positive family history and with high risk for sudden cardiac death (Nordestgaard et al., 2010). Fibrinogen has been identified in large prospective studies as an independent risk factor for CHD (Wilhelmsen et al., 1984; Woodward et al., 1997) and strong predictor for CV events (Coppola et al., 2006; Maresca et al., 1999). There is no joint consensus on the use of haemostatic markers in risk evaluation, except some specific indications mainly in subjects with positive family history.

9.3.2 Genetic markers of subclinical AS

A. Markers of lipid metabolism: apolipoprotein E, B, B-100 (ApoE, ApoB, ApoB-100), lipoprotein lipase (LPL), cholesterol-ester transferprotein, PCSK9 for proprotein convertase subtilisin/kexin type 9, USF-1 for upstream transcription factor-1, Lp(a), LDL-receptor for familial defective ApoB-100 (FDB).

B. Markers of coagulation: PAI-1, t-PA, glycoprotein IIb/IIIa, F V, vWF, methylene-tetrahydropholate reductase, homocysteine, prothrombin.

C. Markers of endothelial function: endothelial nitric oxid synthase (eNOS), angiotensin converting enzyme (ACE), preproendothelin-1 (PPET-1), endothelin converting enzyme-1 (ECE-1), endothelin B receptor, NFκB, ICAM-1, VCAM-1, E-selectin, adrenomedullin, C-type natriuretic peptide (CNP), p22phox for NAD(P)H oxidase, superoxide dismutase, leptin receptor, a-adducin, caveolin, MEF2A (15q26.3) for myocyte-specific enhancer factor 2A, LTA (6p21.3) for lymphotoxin alpha, LGALS2 (22q12-q13) for galectin-2, ALOX5AP for 5-lipoxygenase, PDE4D (5q12) for phosphodiesterase 4D (Casas et al., 2006; Purcell et al., 2003).

Population screening for genetic polymorphism is currently not yet realistic.

9.3.3 Functional changes of the vascular wall (Lekakis et al., 2011)

Diagnostic modalities of endothelial dysfunction include assessment of epicardial and microvascular coronary endothelial function, local vasodilation by venous occlusion plethysmography, flow-mediated dilatation, arterial pulse wave analysis and pulse amplitude tonometry as well as microvascular blood flow assessment by laser Doppler flowmetry. Asymptomatic but advanced AS may be detected by ankle-brachial index (ABI). **These methods are widely used for identification of preclicnial AS in different studies, but only some of them seem to be recommended as screening tool (ABI for subclinical AS, parameters of arterial stiffness for end-organ damage).**

Quantitative coronary angiography (QCA) measures epicardial coronary vasodilatation either invasively [after intracoronary pharmacological stimuli, such as acetylcholine (ACh), metacholine, or papaverine] or non-invasively [using computed tomography (CT) or magnetic resonance imaging (MRI)] (Husmann et al., 2008). **Microvascular coronary endothelial function** is assessed by non-invasive methods, such as MRI and positron emission tomography (PET).

Venous occlusion plethysmography estimates the dose–response forearm blood flow (FBF) due to the local endothelium-dependent vasodilation (Joyner et al., 2001). An impaired endothelium-dependent relaxation (low ACh-induced FBF) has been documented in patients with CV risk factors at the level of microcirculation (Chowienczyk et al., 1992; Panza et al., 1990). **Brachial artery flow-mediated dilatation (FMD)** is evaluated through an ultrasound assessment of brachial artery diameter in basal condition and after 5 minutes of suprasystolic occlusion determined reactive hyperaemia, causing vasodilation. FMD is associated with a traditional risk factors for AS, it predicts CV risk and seems to be an independent prognostic marker of advanced AS. A low FMD is a marker of multifocal AS and disease extension (Coretti et al., 2002; Landmesser et al., 2004; Schroeder et al., 1999). Due to high interindividual variations of measurements, time-consuming character, and complicated technique, FMD is not recommended for population screening.

Parameters of arterial stiffness [aortic pulse wave velocity (PWV), augmentation index of a. brachialis (Aix)] are also associated with traditional risk factors for AS as well as are independent predictors of CV risk, mainly in patients with AH, DM, end-stage chronic renal failure, and in the elderly hospitalized patients (Hansen al., 2006; Safar &, O´ Rourke, 2006). Abnormal values of arterial stiffness identify early AS and according to some authors may confirm endothelial dysfunction. Pulse wave registration is performed by various methods using different principles, such as piezoelectric, oscillometry, or applanation tonometry.

Measurement of peripheral vasodilator response with fingertip **peripheral arterial tonometry** (PAT) technology is emerging as a useful method for assessing endothelium-dependent vascular function (Kuvin et al., 2003). In response to hyperaemic flow, the digital pulse amplitude increases (Nohria et al., 2006). Patients at low Framingham Risk Score but with endothelial dysfunction are at a higher actual risk than patients with high Framingham Risk Score but normal endothelial function. Furthermore, endothelial dysfunction was found to be an independent risk factor for a future major adverse cardiovascular event (Rubinshtein et al., 2010).

Non-invasive **laser doppler flowmetry** enables the monitoring of skin microvascular blood flow, a window towards the responses that should be observed in other vascular beds, using various techniques (i.e. direct delivery of Ach, adrenaline, insuline, sodium nitroprusside, etc.) through iontophoresis, micro-dialysis, post-occlusive hyperaemia, or local skin heating (Fredriksson et al., 2009; Ozbebit et al., 2004).

Ankle-brachial systolic pressure index can reflect altered pressure values in PAO, most frequently of AS origin (Hirsh et al., 2001). Some authors define 5 ABI categories (McDermott et al., 2005): a) definite peripheral PAD: ABI <0.90, b) borderline ABI: 0.90–0.99, c) low-normal ABI: 1.00–1.09, d) normal ABI: 1.10–1.29, e) high ABI (possibly indicative of medial arterial calcinosis): >1.30. The optimal upper limit of normal ABI is unknown, recently ABI >1.30 has been suggested as the upper limit of normal for ABI (Hiatt, 2001). ABI is a marker of subclinical and advanced AS and correlates well with risk factors for AS. A strong correlation between decreased ABI, carotid or coronary AS and future cardiac or cerebrovascular events was demonstrated in different studies (Diehm et al., 2006; Dormandy & Creager, 1999; Fowkes et al., 1991; Ostergren et al., 2004). ABI <0.9 is linked with 2-4 fold increase of relative risk of CV events and mortality (Ankle Brachial Index Collaboration, 2008). Recently, an association had been found between ABI >1.4 and CV mortality (Resnick et al., 2004).

9.3.4 Morphological changes of the vascular wall

Morphological changes of the vascular wall are mostly detected by imaging techniques, such as ultrasound (IMT, AS plaque), IVUS, multiple detector-row (MDCT) coronarography, coronary Ca-scoring, MRI, PET, selective coronarography, etc. **AS changes of the arterial wall detected by any imaging techniques** (except for pathological ABI, "functional abnormality", that may prone also asymptomatic but advanced changes of peripheral arteries) clearly **confirm preclinical AS as a condition with increased CVD risk** (Graham et al., 2007).

Diagnosis of **coronary artery disease** is based generally on the confirmation of ischaemia by non-invasive functional tests (exercise ECG testing, stress echocardiography, or radionuclide scintigraphy), which are not suitable for population screening. Selective coronarography is a gold standard for visualization of coronary artery morphology, but cost-benefit relations do not favour its use as screening tool. Nowadays, new imaging techniques are available (MRI, multi-slice CT for detecting coronary artery lesions and coronary calcium, as well as IVUS capable to provide a virtual histology from the coronary artery wall). Up to now, they have little significance as screening tools.

Due to the correlation between the severity of AS in one arterial territory and involvement of other arteries, it appears logical to examine non-invasively **peripheral arteries** (carotid) instead of coronary or intra-cerebral arteries. Ultrasound is relatively cheep, widely available, low-cost, and non-invasive method with good reproducibility. It may serve as a screening tool for morphological assessment of arterial wall (IMT or presence of AS plaque). IMT (carotid, femoral) shows a remarkable correlation with traditional RF, as well as their number, intensity, or duration. Moreover, IMT is associated with endothelial dysfunction (Corrado et al., 2006; Corrado et al., 2005; Novo et al., 1997). CIMT indicates multifocal AS as well as predicts target organ damage (CIMT ≥0.9 mm) and coronary artery disease (CIMT ≥0.85 mm) (Touboul et al., 2005). CIMT is also an independent predictor of future stroke and MI (ARIC Study, 2000; Rotterdam Study, 1997). A recent meta-analysis of 8 population studies [ARIC Study, 2000; Cardiovascular Health Study (CHS), 1999; Carotid Atherosclerosis Progression Study (CAPS), 2006; Kitamura Study, 2004; Kuopio Ischemic Heart Disease Risk Factor Study (KIHD RF), 1993; Longitudinal Investigation for the Longevity and Aging in Hokkaido Country (LILAC), 2005; Malmo Diet and Cancer Study (MDCS), 2005; Rotterdam Study, 1997] registered an increased rate of myocardial infarction (15%) and stroke (18%) for every increase of 0.1 mm in the CIMT value (Matthias et al., 2007). According to this data, IMT may be a "more powerful" predictor than other traditional risk factors. Significant carotid artery stenosis increases coronary risk about 6 times to those without AS lesion. Plaque characteristics appear to be crucial in prediction of cerebrovascular events (The ACSRS Study, 2005). Complex ultrasound evaluation of vascular wall morphology (carotid, femoral, and popliteal) has a higher predictive value for future CV in comparison with IMT (Belcaro et al., 1996). Detection of AS by ultrasound or other imaging methods indicates a high-risk condition.

10. Personalized CV risk assessment – Cost/benefit relations

Personalized CV risk assessment means identification of subjects with accelerated AS by evidence-based, non-invasive, widely available, cheap, and preferably objective method with good reproducibility. CVD risk should be known in every subject.

If there is a known CHD or CHD equivalent (Framingham), as well as CVD, type 2 DM or type 1 DM with end-organ damage such as microalbuminuria, renal impairment, or very high levels of individual risk factors with/without end-organ damage (SCORE), the risk estimation is not necessary, because patients are already in high/increased CVD risk and need aggressive management of all risk factors.

If the risk in not evident, should be estimated:

1. in countries using Framingham score, dominantly if ≥2 risk factors are present,
2. in European countries using ScoreCard, in every other patient.

If the calculated risk is ≤20% (Framingham) or <5% (SCORE), an individual risk assessment should be considered.

How to assess the absolute CVD risk quickly and easily?

ATP III Update:

1. patients with acute coronary syndromes or with CVD + DM are at very high risk,
2. patients with CHD or CHD equivalents are at high risk,
3. in every other patient - count the risk factors (see further a. and b.):
   3.1. calculate the number of points for each risk factor,
   3.2. estimate the global risk score by adding together the points for each risk factor,
   3.3. assess for each score the corresponding total risk for suffering a hard (fatal or nonfatal) CHD event within the next 10 years.
   a. if ≤1 risk factor is present, Framingham scoring is not necessary, patient is at low risk,
   b. if ≥2 risk factors are present, according to the Framingham Global Risk Point Score, 3 categories of CHD risk are possible: high (>20%), moderately high (10-20%), and moderate (<10%).

SCORE chart (table) (the risk can be read directly without any calculation):

1. choose a low or high risk chart,
2. in a table for one´s gender, smoking status, and age find the cell nearest to the ones´s systolic blood pressure and total cholesterol, use the HDL cholesterol table to refine the risk,
3. read directly the 10-year risk from the chart without any calculation,
4. to establish individual risk, check qualifiers listed in the latest preventive guidelines,
5. to project the risk to higher age, simply shift the found table cell upward to the desired age,
6. to project the relative risk, shift the found cell within the gender-age table downward and to the left to find the corresponding normal systolic BP and total cholesterol level, finally, shift this relative cell to the non-smoking table,
7. estimating the relative risk is simpler by using the relative risk chart,
8. to convert the risk for fatal CVD to the risk for total (fatal+nonfatal) hard CVD, multiply by 3 in men, and 4 in women, and slightly <3 in old people (ESC/EAS Guidelines, 2011).

There are no strictly recommended methods for population screening. No data are available about the validity of different methods in screening for subclinical AS. They should be evidence-based, non-invasive, objective, widely available, reproducible, cheap, and quick (Criqui et al., 2008). A recent paper has documented a 42% prevalence of functional markers of subclinical AS in a sample of primary prevention subjects from a high-risk Eastern region of Central Europe (Szabóová et al., 2010). Rigorous expert analysis of the available data documenting benefits and risks of therapies and procedures can improve the effectiveness of care, optimize patient outcomes, and favourably affect the cost of care by focusing resources on the most effective strategies.

11. Current guidelines modifying CV risk assessment. ACCF/AHA Guideline, 2010; ESH Task Force Document, 2009; ESC/EAS Guidelines, 2011

ACCF/AHA guideline (Greenland et al., 2010) for assessment of CV risk in asymptomatic adults differs from those used in Europe and recommend:

1. Risk assessment in all asymptomatic adults without a clinical history of CHD,
2. Family history of atherothrombotic CVD should be obtained in all asymptomatic adults,
3. CRP measurement is indicated:
   a. in the selection of patients for statin therapy: in men aged ≥50 years or women aged ≥60 years with LDL cholesterol <130 mg/dl (not on lipid-lowering, hormone replacement, or immunosuppressant therapy; without clinical CHD, DM, chronic kidney disease, severe inflammatory conditions, or contraindications to statins),
   b. in asymptomatic intermediate-risk men aged ≤50 years or women aged ≤60 years,
4. Hemoglobin A1C in patients with/without DM,
5. Microalbuminuria in asymptomatic hypertensives or diabetics as well as in asymptomatic adults at intermediate risk without AH or DM,
6. Lipoprotein-associated phospholipase A2 in intermediate-risk,
7. A resting ECG in asymptomatic adults with/without AH or DM,
8. Echocardiography to detect left ventricular hypertrophy in asymptomatic adults with AH,
9. Measurement of carotid artery IMT at intermediate risk,
10. Measurement of ABI at intermediate risk,
11. Exercise ECG in intermediate risk,
12. Stress myocardial perfusion imaging (MPI) in diabetics or asymptomatic adults with a strong family history of CHD or when previous risk assessment testing suggests high risk of CHD, such as a coronary artery calcium (CAC) score of ≥ 400,
13. Measurement of CAC at intermediate (10-20%) as well as low to intermediate risk (6-10%) 10-year risk,
14. In asymptomatic adults with DM aged ≥40 years: measurement of CAC,
15. Hemoglobin A1C may be considered for CV risk assessment in asymptomatic diabetics,
16. Stress MPI in asymptomatic adults with DM or when previous risk assessment testing suggests a high risk of CHD, such as a CAC score of ≥400.

ACCF/AHA guideline in asymptomatic adults does not recommend:

a) genotype testing for CHD risk, b) measurement of lipid parameters beyond a standard fasting lipid profile, c) natriuretic peptides, d) CRP neither in asymptomatic high-, nor low-risk men aged <50 years or women aged <60 years, e) FMD, arterial stiffness, stress echocardiography in low- or intermediate-risk, echocardiography without hypertension, stress MPI in low- or intermediate-risk, measurement of CAC in low-risk, coronary CT angiography, MRI coronary angiography.

Reappraisal of European guidelines on hypertension management (2009) modify the CV risk assessment in hypertension:

1. Total CV risk assessment must include a search for subclinical organ damage (SOD),
2. The presence of SOD in hypertension represents a high CV risk,
3. Simple, widely available, and low-cost measures are suitable for routine use: urinary protein excretion (including microalbuminuria), eGFR [Modification of Diet in Renal Disease (MDRD) formula], and ECG; cardiac and vascular ultrasound are more and more encouraged in Europe,
4. SOD should be assessed in screening and during the treatment.

ESC/EAS guidelines for the management of dyslipidaemias (2011) recommend the following evaluation of laboratory lipid and apolipoprotein parameters:

Lipid profile may be considered in:

1. Type2 DM, established CVD, hypertension, smoking, BMI ≥30 kg/m^2, waist circumference >94 (90 cm for Asian) males or 80 cm for women, family history of premature CVD or familial dyslipidaemia, chronic inflammatory diseases, chronic kidney disease,
2. Adult men ≥40 years and women ≥50 years of age or post-menopausal, particularly in the presence of other risk factor.

Recommendations for lipid analyses for screening for CVD risk:

1. Total cholesterol (TC), LDL cholesterol (LDL-C), HDL cholesterol (HDL-C), TG (I/C),
2. Non-HDL-C as well as apoB as alternative risk markers in combined hyperlipidaemias, DM, MS, or CKD; Lp(a) in selected cases at high risk and in subjects with a positive family history of CVD (IIa/C),
3. apoB/apoA-1 ratio as well as non-HDL-C/HDL-C ratio as alternative parameters for risk analysis (IIIb/C).

Recommendations for lipid analyses of dyslipidaemias before treatment:

1. LDL-C, HDL-C, TG (I/C),
2. Non-HDL-C as well as apoB in combined hyperlipidaemias, DM, MS, CKD; Lp(a) in selected cases at high risk and in subjects with a positive family history of CVD (IIa/C),
3. TC may be considered but is usually not enough (IIb/C) before initiation of treatment.

Recommendations for lipid analyses as treatment target in the CVD prevention:

1. LDL-C (I/A),
2. TC if other analysis is not available; TG in hypertriglyceridaemias; non-HDL-C as well as apoB as secondary target in combined hyperlipidaemias, DM, MS, CKD (IIa/B),
3. HDL-C, apoB/apoA-1 ratio are not recommended (III/C).

12. Management of patients at high CVD risk

The management of patients, including type and intensity of treatment, is based on the CVD risk category. Persons at low risk do not require further testing for risk assessment, those already documented to be at high/very high risk are already candidates for intensive preventive interventions, so that added testing will not provide benefit.

Aggressive control of risk factors:

Epidemiological data suggest that eating fruit and vegetables, taking exercise, and avoiding smoking could lead to about 80% lower relative risk for myocardial infarction (Yusuf et al., 2004). Thus, lifestyle modification is of substantial importance in both men and women, at all ages, in individuals from all geographic regions of the world. **Luxembourg Declaration defined the characteristics for achievement of CV health as follows: 0-3-5-140-90-5-3-0** (avoidance of tobacco - adequate physical activity avoiding overweight (3 km walking at least 30 min per day) - 5 daily portions of fruit and vegetables - BP <140/90 mmHg - total cholesterol <5 mmol/l - LDL cholesterol <3 mmol/l) (Ryden et al., 2007). Among individuals with ≥1 intermediate or major risk factors at 50 years of age, data suggest that aggressive global risk factor modification should be considered, given the associated high lifetime risks for CVD. Much more intensive lifestyle changes and aggressive risk factor modifications are needed in subjects at high risk (Yusuf et al., 2004).

Current recommendations of the European guidelines on disease prevention in clinical practice: Fourth Joint Task Force (Graham et al., 2007**) for management of patients at high risk,** updated according to Reappraisal of European guidelines on hypertension management (Mancia et al., 2009) and ESC/EAS guidelines for the management of dyslipidaemias (2011) underline the need for achievement of most rigorous risk factor control:

1. blood pressure 130-139/80-85 mmHg for all hypertensive patients, if possible, close or slightly below to lower values in this range for very high risk category,
2. total cholesterol <4.5 mmol/l (175 mg/dl) with an option of <4 mmol/l (155 mg/dl), if possible,
3. LDL-C <1.8 mmol/l (70 mg/dl) and/or ≥50% LDL-C reduction when target level cannot be reached in very high risk; LDL-C <2.5 mmol/l (100 mg/dl) in high risk; LDL-C <3.0 mmol/l (115 mg/dl) in moderate risk,
4. fasting glucose <6 mmol/l (110 mg/dl) and HbA1C <6.5%, if possible,
5. hs-CRP as a secondary target is not recommended for everybody, may be useful in people close to high risk category, for those hs-CRP <2mg/l.

The use of cardioprotective drugs (aspirin, ACE inhibitors, statins, beta-blockers, anticoagulants) mainly depends on the type and severity of organ involvement and is guided by evidence-based recommendations.

13. Further studies are needed to achieve an optimal approach to CV risk assessment in communities

Implementation of novel biomarkers and new methods into clinical practice will further promote the CV research and thus the assessment of CV risk. Based on new data from ongoing trials and scientific research, guidelines are continuously modified. In the near future, proteomic and genetic analyses may help to target vulnerable patients and monitor the beneficial effects of pharmacologic agents.

14. References

ACSRS Study. Nicolaides, A., N., Kakkos, S., K., Griffin, M., Sabetai, M., Dhanjil, S., Tegos, T., Thomas, D., J., Giannoukas, A., Geroulakos, G., Georgiou, N., Francis, S., Ioannidou, E., & Dorè, C., J. for the Asymptomatic Carotid Stenosis and Risk of Stroke (ACSRS) Study Group. (2005). Severity of asymptomatic carotid stenosis and risk of ipsilateral hemispheric ischemic events: results from the ACSRS Study. *Eur J Vasc Endovasc Surg,* Vol. 30, No. 3, pp. 275-284

Allender, S., Scarborough, P., Peto, V., Rayner, M., Leal, J., Luengo-Fernandez, R., & Gray, A. (2009). *European cardiovascular disease statistics 2008* (third edition), European Health Network AISBL, Brussels, Belgium

Amato, M., Montorsi, P., Rafani, A., Oldani, E., Galli, S., Ravagnani, P., M., Tremoli, E., & and Baldassarre, D. (2007). Carotid intima-media thickness by B-mode ultrasound as surrogate of coronary atherosclerosis: correlation with quantitative coronary angiography and coronary intravascular ultrasound findings. *European Heart Journal*, Vol. 28, No. 17, pp. 2094-2101

Ankle Brachial Index Collaboration. (2008). Ankle brachial index combined with Framingham risk score to predict cardiovascular events and mortality. A meta-analysis. *JAMA*, Vol. 300, No. 2, pp. 197-208

Anderson, K., M., Wilson, P., W., Odell, P., M., & Kannel, W., B. (1991). An updated coronary risk profile. A statement for health professionals. *Circulation*, Vol. 83, No. 1, pp. 356-362

ARIC Study. The Atherosclerosis Risk in Communities Study. Chambless, L., E. (2000). Carotid wall thickness is predictive of incident clinical stroke. *Am J Epidemiol*, Vol. 151, No. 5, pp. 478-487

Belcaro, G., Nicolaides, A., N., Laurora, G., Cesarone, M., R., De Sanctis, M., Lucrezia-Incandela, L., & Barsotti, A. (1996). Ultrasound Morphology Classification of the Arterial Wall and Cardiovascular Events in a 6-Year Follow-up Study. *Arteriosclerosis, Thrombosis, and Vascular Biology*, Vol. 16, No. 7, pp. 851-856

Burke, A., P., Tracy, R., P., Kolodgie, F., Malcom, G., T., Zieske, A., Kutys, R., Pestaner, J., Smialek, J., & Virmanie, R. (2002). Elevated C-reactive protein values and atherosclerosis in sudden coronary death: association with different pathologies. *Circulation*, Vol. 105, No. 17, pp. 2019-2023

Carr, M., & Brunzell, J., D. (2004). Abdominal obesity and dyslipidemia in the metabolic syndrome: importance of type 2 diabetes and familial combined hyperlipidemia in coronary artery disease risk. *J Clin Endocrinol Metab*, Vol. 89, No. 6, pp. 2601-2607

Casas, J., Cooper, J., Miller, G., J., Hingorani, A., D., & Humpries, S., E. (2006). Investigating the genetic determinants of cardiovascular disease using candidate genes and meta – analysis of association studies. *Ann Hum Genet*, Vol. 70, No. 2, Pt. 2, pp. 145-169

Cholesterol Treatment Trialists' (CTT) Collaborators. Baigent, C., Keech, A., Kearmey, P., M., Blackwell, L., Buck, G., Pollicino, C., Kirby, A., Sourjina, T., Peto, R., Collins, R., & Simes, R. (2005). Efficacy and safety of cholesterol lowering treatment: prospective meta – analysis of data from 90,056 participants in 14 randomised trials of statins. *Lancet*, Vol. 366, No. 9463, pp. 1267-1278

Cholesterol Treatment Trialists' (CTT) Collaborators. Downs, J., R., Gotto, A., Clearfield, M., Holdaas, H., Gordon, D., Davis, B., Koren, M., Dahlof, B., Poulter, N., Sever, P., Wedel, H., Braunwald, E., Cannon, C., Goldbourt, U., & Kaplinsky, E. (2008). Efficacy of cholesterol-lowering therapy in 18, 686 people with diabetes in 14 randomised trials of statins: a meta-analysis. *Lancet*, Vol. 371, No. 9607, pp. 117-125

Chowienczyk, P., J., Watts, G., F., Cockcroft, J., R., & Ritter, J., M. (1992). Impaired endothelium-dependent vasodilation of forearm resistance vessels in hypercholesterolaemia. *Lancet*, Vol. 340, No. 8833, pp. 1430–1432

Coppola, G., Corrado, E., Muratori, I., Tantillo, R., Vitale, G., Lo Coco, L., & Novo, S. (2006). Increased levels of C-reactive protein and fibrinogen influence the risk of vascular events in patients with NIDDM. *Int J Card*, Vol. 106, No. 1, pp. 16-20

Corrado, E., Bonura, F., Tantillo, R., Muratori, I., Rizzo, M., Vitale, G., Mansueto, S., & Novo, S. (2006). Markers of infection and inflammation influence the outcome of patients with baseline asymptomatic carotid lesions in a 5 years follow-up. *Stroke,* Vol. 37, No. 2, pp. 482-486

Corrado, E., Muratori, I., Tantillo, R., Contorno, F., Coppola, G., Strano, A., & Novo, S. (2005). Relationship between endothelial dysfunction, intima media thickness and cardiovascular risk factors in asymptomatic subjects. *Int Angiol,* Vol. 24, No. 1, pp. 52-58

Coretti, M., C., Anderson, T., J., Benjamin, E., J., Celermajer, D., Charbonneau, F., & Creager, M., A. (2002). Guidelines for ultrasound assessment of Endothelial-Dependent Flow-mediated Vasodilatation of Brachial Artery. *J Am Coll Cardiol,* Vol. 39, No. 2, pp. 257-265

Criqui, M., H., Alberts, M., J., Gerald, F., Fowkes, F., G., R., Hirsch, A., T., O'Gara, P., T., & Olin, J., W. for Writing Group 2. (2008). Atheroslerotic peripheral vascular symposium II. AHA conference proceedings. *Circulation,* Vol. 118, No. 25, pp. 2830-2836

D´Agostino, R., B., Sr., Vasan, R., S., Pencina, M., J., Wolf, Ph., A., Cobain, M., Massaro, J. M., & Kannel, W., B. (2008). General Cardiovascular Risk Profile for Use in Primary Care. The Framingham Heart Study. *Circulation,* Vol. 117, No. 6, pp. 743-753

DASH Study. Appel, L., J., Brands, M., W., Daniels, S., R., Karanja, N., Elmer, P., J., & Sacks, F., M. (2006). Dietary Approaches to Prevent and Treat Hypertension. A Scientific Statement From the American Heart Association. *Hypertension,* Vol. 47, No. 2, pp. 296-308

De Lorenzo, F., Collot-Teixeira, S., Boffito, M., Feher, M., Gazzard, B., & McGregor, J., L. (2008). Metabolic-inflammatory changes and accelerated atherosclerosis in HIV patients: rationale for preventive measures. *Curr Med Chem,* Vol. 15, No. 28, pp. 2991-2299

De Lorgeril, M., Salen, P., Martin, J., L., Monjaud, I., & Delaye, J. (1999). Mediterranean diet, traditional risk factors, and the rate of cardiovascular complications after myocardial infarction: final report of the Lyon Diet Heart Study. *Circulation,* Vol. 99, No. 6, pp. 779-785

Despres, J., Moorjani, S., Lupien, P., J., Tremblay, A., Nadeau, A., & Bouchard, C. (1990). Regional distribution of body fat, plasma lipoprotein, and cardiovascular disease. *Arteriosclerosis,* Vol. 10, No. 4. pp. 497-511

Diaz, A., Bourassa, M., Guertin, M., & Tardiff, J. (2005). Long – term prognostic value of resting heart rate in patients with suspected or proven coronary artery disease. *Eur Heart J,* Vol. 26, No. 10, pp. 967-974

Diehm, C., Lange, S., Darius, H., Pittrow, D., von Stritzky, B., Tepohl, G., Haberl, R., L., Allenberg, J., R., Dasch, B., & Trampisch, H., J. (2006). Association of low ankle brachial index with high mortality in primary care. *Eur Heart J,* Vol. 27, No. 14, pp. 1743-1749

Doll, R., Peto, R., Boreham, J., & Sutherland, I. (2004). Mortality in relation to smoking: 50 years' observations on male British doctors. *BMJ,* Vol. 328, No. 7455, pp. 1519-1528

Dormandy, J., A., & Creager, M., A. (1999). Ankle:arm blood pressure index as a predictor of atherothrombotic events: evidence from CAPRIE (Abstract). *Cerebrovasc Dis,* Vol. 9, (Suppl. 1), pp. 1-128

Drager, L., F., Polotsky, V., Y., & Lorenzi-Filho, G. (2011). Obstructive Sleep Apnea an Emerging Risk Factor for Atherosclerosis. *Chest,* Vol. 140, No. 2, pp. 2534-2542

Ekesbo, R., Nillson, P., M., Lindholm, L., H., Persson, K., & Wadström, T. (2000). Combined seropositivity for H. pylori and C. pneumoniae is associated with age, obesity, and social factors. *J Cardiovasc Risk,* Vol. 7, No. 3, pp. 191-195

ESC/EAS Guidelines for the management of dyslipideamias. Reiner, Ž., Catapano, A., L., De Backer, G., Graham, J., Taskinen, M., R., Wiklund, O., Agewall, S., Alergria, E., Chapman, M., J., Durrington, P., Erdine, S., Halcox, J., Hobbs, R., Kjekshus, J., Filaardi, P., P., Riccardi, G., Storery, R., F., & Wood, D. (2011). The Task Force for the management of dyslipidaemias of the ESC and EAS. *EHJ,* Vol. 32, No. 14, pp. 1769-1818

'EUROSPIRE III. Kotseva, K., Wood, D., Backer, G., D., Bacquer, D., D., Pyöräalä, K., Keil, U., & Goup, E., S. (2009). EUROSPIRE III: a survey on the lifestyle, risk factors, and use of cardioprotective drug therapies in coronary patients from 52 European countries. *European Journal of Cardiovascular Prevention & Rehabilitation,* Vol. 16, No. 2, pp. 121-137

Fellström, B., Backman, U., Larsson, E., & Wahlberg, J. (1989). Accelerated atherosclerosis in the transplant recipient: role of hypertension. *J Hum Hypertens,* Vol. 12, No. 12, pp. 851-854

Ford, E., S., Ajani, U., A., Croft, J., B., Critchley, J., A., Labarthe, D., R., Kottke, T., E., Giles, W., H., & Capewell, S. (2007), 'Explaining the Decrease in U.S. Deaths from Coronary Disease, 1980/2000'. *New England Journal of Medicine,* Vol. 356, No. 23, pp. 2388-2398

Fourth Joint Task Force of the European Society of Cardiology and Other Societies on Cardiovascular Disease Prevention in Clinical Practice. Graham, I., Atar, D., Borch-Johnsen, K., Boysen, G., Burell, G., Cifkova, R., Dallongeville, J., De Backer, G., Ebrahim, S., Gjelsvik, B., Herrmann-Lingen, C., Hoes, A., Humphries, S., Knapton, M., Perk, J., Priori, S., G., Pyorala, K., Reiner, Z., Ruilope, L., Sans-Menendez, S., Scholte, O., P., Reimer, W., Weissberg, P., Wood, D., Yarnell, J., & Zamorano, J., L. (2007). European guidelines on cardiovascular disease prevention in clinical practice: executive summary. *Eur Heart J,* Vol. 28, No. 19, pp. 2375-2414

Fowkes, F., G., Housley, E., Cawood, E., H., Macintyre, C., C., Ruckley, C., V., & Prescott, R., J. (1991). Edinburgh Artery Study: prevalence of asymptomatic and symptomatic peripheral arterial disease in the general population. *Int J Epidemiol,* Vol. 20, No. 2, pp. 384-392

Fredriksson, I., Larsson, M., & Stromberg, T. (2009). Measurement depth and volume in laser doppler flowmetry. *Microvasc Res,* Vol. 78, No. 1, pp. 4-13

Gasparyan, A., Y., Stavropoulos-Kalinoglou, A., Mikhailidis, D., P., Toms, T., E., Douglas, K., M., & Kitas, G., D. (2010). The rationale for comparative studies of accelerated atherosclerosis in rheumatic diseases. *Curr Vas. Pharmacol,* Vol. 8, No. 4, pp. 437-449

Greenland, Ph., Joseph, S., Alpert, J., S., Beller, G., A., Benjamin, E., J., Budoff, M., J., Fayad, Z., A., Foster, E., Hlatky, M., A., Hodgson, J., Mc., B., Kushner, F., G., Lauer, M., S., Shaw, L., J., Sidney, C., Smith, S., C., Allen, J., Taylor, A., J., Weintraub, W., S., Nanette, K., & Wenger, N., K. (2010). ACCF/AHA Guideline for Assessment of Cardiovascular Risk in Asymptomatic Adults: Executive Summary Report of the American College of Cardiology Foundation/American Heart Association Task Force on Practice Guidelines Writing Committee Members, ACCF/AHA Task Force Members. *J Am Coll Cardiol,* Vol. 56, No. 25, pp. 2182-2199

Gurfinkel, E. (2006). Infection and atherosclerosis: is this hypothesis still alive? *Nature Clinical Practice Cardiovascular Medicine,* Vol. 3, No. 1, pp. 1

Hajjar, I., & Kotchen, T., A. (2003). Trends in prevalence, awareness, treatment, and control of hypertension in the United States, 1988-2000. *JAMA*, Vol. 290, No. 2, pp. 199-206

Hansen, T., W., Staessen, J., A., Torp-Pedersen, Ch., Rasmussen, S., Thijs, L., Ibsen, H., & Jeppesen, J. (2006). Prognostic Value of Aortic Pulse Wave Velocity as Index of Arterial Stiffness in the General Population. *Circulation*, Vol. 113, No. 5, pp. 664-670

Harris, M., I., Flegal, K., M., Cowie, C., C., Eberhardt, M., S., Goldstein, D., E., Little, R., R., Wiedmeyer, H., M., & Byrd-Holtet, D., D. (1998). Prevalence of diabetes, impaired fasting glucose, and impaired glucose tolerance in U.S. adults: the Third National Health and Nutrition Examination Survey, 1988-1994. *Diabetes Care*, Vol. 21, No 4, pp. 518-524

Haq, I., U., Ramsay, L., E., Jackson, P., R., & Wallis, E., J. (1999). Prediction of coronary risk for primary prevention of coronary heart disease: a comparison of methods. *QJM*, Vol. 92, No. 7, pp. 379-385

Heart Protection Study Collaborative Group. Collins, R., Armitage, J., Parish, S., Sleigh, P., & Peto, R. (2003). MRC/BHF Heart Protection Study of cholesterol-lowering with simvastatin in 5963 people with diabetes: a randomised placebo-controlled trial. *Lancet*, Vol. 361, No. 9374, pp. 2005-2016

Hedley, A., A., Ogden, C., L., Johnson, C., L., Carroll, M., D., Curtin, L., R., & Flegal, K., M. (2004). Prevalence of overweight and obesity among US children, adolescents, and adults, 1999-2002. *JAMA*, Vol. 291, No. 23, pp. 2847-2850

Hiatt, W., R. (2001). Medical treatment of peripheral arterial disease and claudication. *N Engl J Med*, Vol. 344, No. 21, pp.1608-1621

Hirsh, A., T., Hiatt, W., R., Treat-Jacobson, D., Regensteiner, J., G., Creager, M., A., Olin, J., W., Krook, S., H., Hunninghake, D., B., Comerota, A., J., Walsh, M., E., McDermott, M., M., & Criqui, M., H. (2001). PARTNERS Study - Peripheral Arterial Disease Detection, Awareness, and Treatment in Primary Care. *JAMA*, Vol. 286, No. 11, pp. 1317-1324

Husmann, L, Gaemperli, O., Schepis, T., Scheffel, H., Valenta, I., Hoefflinghaus, T., Stolzmann, P., Desbiolles, L., Herzog, B., A., Leschka, S., Marincek, B., Alkadhi, H., & Kaufmann, P., A. (2008). Accuracy of quantitative coronary angiography with computed tomography and its dependency on plaque composition: plaque composition and accuracy of cardiac CT. *Int J Cardiovascular Imaging,* Vol. 24, No. 8, pp. 895-904

Hürlimann, D., Enseleit, F., & Ruschitzka, F. (2004). Rheumatoid arthritis, inflammation, and atherosclerosis. *Herz,* Vol. 29, No. 8, pp. 760-768

INVEST Study. Kolloch, R., Legler, U., F., Champion, A., Cooper-Dehoff, R., M., Handberg, E., Zhou, Q., & Pepine, C., J. (2008). Impact of resting heart rate on outcomes in hypertensive patients with coronary artery disease: findings from the International VErapamil-SR/trandolapril Study (INVEST). *Eur Heart J*, Vol. 29, No. 10, pp. 1327-1334

Johnson, C., L., Rifkind, B., M., Sempos, C., T., Carroll, M., D., Bachorik, P., S., Briefel, R., R., Gordon, D., J., Burt, V., L., Brown, C., D., & Lippel, K. (1993). Declining serum total cholesterol levels among US adults: the National Health and Nutrition Examination Surveys. *JAMA*, Vol. 269, No. 23, pp. 3002-3008

Joyner, M., J., Dietz, N., M., & Shepherd, J., T. (2001). From Belfast to Mayo and beyond: the use and future of plethysmography to study blood flow in human limbs. *J Appl Physiol*, Vol. 91, No. 6, pp. 2431–2441

Jupiter Study Group. Ridker, P., M., Danielson, E., Fonseca, F., A., Genest, J., Gotto, A., M., Jr., Kastelein, J., J., Koenig, W., Libby, P., Lorenzatti, A., J., MacFadyen, J., G., Nodestgaard, B., G., Shepherd, J., Willerson, J., T., & Glynn, R., J. (2008). Rosuvastatin to prevent vascular events in men and women with elevated C reactive protein. *N Engl J Med*, Vol. 359, No. 21, pp. 2195-2207

Kalaitzidis, R., & Bakris, G. (2009). Pathogenesis and treatment of microalbuminuria in patients with diabetes: The road ahead. *J Clin Hypert*, Vol. 11, No. 11, pp. 636-643

Kannel, W., Kannel, C., Paffenbarger, R., S., & Cupples, L., A. (1987). Heart rate and cardiovascular mortality: the Framingham Study. *Am Heart J*, Vol. 113, No. 6, pp. 1489-1494

Kuvin, J., T., Patel, A., R., Sliney, K., A., Pandian, N., G., Sheffy, J., Schnall, R., P., Karas, R., H., & Udelson, J., E. (2003). Assessment of peripheral vascular endothelial function with finger arterial pulse wave amplitude. *Am Heart J*, Vol. 146, No. 1, pp. 168-174

Landmesser, U., Hornig, B., & Drexler, H. (2004). Endothelium Function: A Critical Determinant in Atherosclerosis. *Circulation*, Vol. 109, No. 21, Suppl. I, pp. 1127-1133

Larsson, B., Svardsudd, K., Welin, L., Wileklmsen, L., Bjomtorp, P., & Tibblin, G. (1984). Abdominal adipose tissue distribution, obesity and risk of cardiovascular disease and death: 13-year follow up of participants in the study of men born in 1913. *BMJ*, Vol. 288, No. 6428, pp. 1401-1411

Law, M., Morris, J., K., & Wald, N., J. (1997). Environmental tobacco smoke exposure and ischaemic heart disease: an evaluation of the evidence. *BMJ*, Vol. 315, No. 7144, pp. 973-980

Lekakis, J., Abraham, P., Balbarini, A., Blann, A., Boulanger, Ch., M., Cockcroft, J., Cosentino, F., Deanfield, J., Gallino, A., Ikonomidis, I., Kremastinos, D., Landmesser, U., Protogerou, A., Stefanadis, Ch., Tousoulis, D., Vassalli, G., Vink, H., Werner, N., Wilkinson, I., & Vlachopoulos, Ch. (2011). Methods for evaluating endothelial function: a position statement from the European Society of Cardiology. *Eur J Cardiovasc Prev Rehabil*, Vol. 18, No. 6, pp. 775-789

Lenz, M., & Mühlhauser, I. (2004). Kardiovaskuläre Risikoschätzung für eine informierte Patientenentscheidung. Wie valide sind die Prognoseinstrumente? *Med Klinik*, Vol. 99, No. 11, pp. 651-661

Levey, A., S., Jong, P., E., Coresh, J., El Nahas, M., Astor, B., C., Matsushita, K., Gansevoort, R., T., Kasiske, B., & Eckardt,. K., U. (2010). The definition, classification, and prognosis of chronic kidney disease: a KDIGO Controversies Conference report. *Kidney Int,* Vol. 80, No. 1, pp. 17-28

Levy, R., L., White, P., D., Stroud, W., D., & Hillman, Ch., C. (1945). Transient tachycardia: prognostic significance alone and in association with transient hypertension. *JAMA,* Vol. 129, No. 9, pp. 585-588

Lloyd-Jones D., M., Leip, E., P., Larson, M., G., Ralph, B., D'Agostino, R., B., Beiser, A., Wilson, P., W., F., Philip, A., Wolf, Ph., A., & Levy, D. (2006). Prediction of Lifetime Risk for Cardiovascular Disease by Risk Factor Burden at 50 Years of Age. *Circulation,* Vol. 113, No. 6, pp. 791-798

Mancia, G., Laurent, S., Agabiti-Rosei, E., Ambrosioni, E., Burnier, M., Caulfield, M., J., Cifkova, R., Clément, D., Coca, A., Dominiczak, A., Erdine, S., Fagard, R., Farsang, Cs., Grassi, G., Haller, H., Heagerty, A., Kjeldsen, S., E., Kiowski, W., Mallion, J., M., Manolis, A., Narkiewicz, K., Nilsson, P., Olsen, M., H., Rahn, K., H., Redon, J., Rodicio, J., Ruilope, L., Schmieder, R., E., Struijker-Boudier, H., A., J., van Zwieten, P., A., Viigimaa, M., & Zanchetti, A. (2009). 'Reappraisal of European guidelines on hypertension management. European Society of Hypertension Task Force document'. *Journal of Hypertension,* Vol. 27, No. 11, pp. 2121-2158

Maresca, G., Di Blasio, A., Marchioli, R., & Di Minno, G. (1999). Measuring Plasma Fibrinogen to Predict Stroke and Myocardial Infarction. *Arteriosclerosis, Thrombosis, and Vascular Biology,* Vol. 19, No. 6, pp. 1368-1377

MARS Study. Terentes-Printzios, D., Vlachopoulos, Ch., Vyssoulis, G., Xaplanteris, P., Alexopoulos, N., Pietri, P., Ioakeimidis, N., Samentzas, A., Siama, A., & Stefanadis, Ch. (2010). From JUPITER to MARS (Major Arterial Stiffness Study): clinical implications in hypertensives, Abstract Book of ESC Congress 2010, P. 4694, Stockholm, Sweden, 28 Aug-01 Sep, 2010

Matthias, W., Lorenz, Hugh, S., Michiel, L., Rosvall, M., & Sitzer, M. (2007). Prediction of clinical cardiovascular events with carotid intima-media thickness. A systematic review and meta-analysis. *Circulation,* Vol. 115, No. 4, pp. 459-467

McCullough, P., A., Agrawal, V., Danielewicz, E., & Abela, G., S. (2008). Accelerated Atherosclerotic Calcification and Mönckeberg's Sclerosis: A Continuum of Advanced Vascular Pathology in Chronic Kidney Disease. *Clin J Am Soc Nephrol,* Vol. 3, No. 6, pp. 1585-1598

McDermott, M., M., Liu, K., Criqui, M., H., Ruth, K., Goff, D., Saad, M., F., Wu, K., Homma, S., & Sharrett, A., R. (2005). Ankle-Brachial Index and Subclinical Cardiac and Carotid Disease. The Multi-Ethnic Study of Atherosclerosis. *Amer J Epidemiol,* Vol. 162, No. 1, pp. 33-41

National Cholesterol Education Program (NCEP). Report. Goodman, D., S., Hulley, S., B., Clark, L., T., Davis, C., E., Fuster, V., LaRosa, J., C., Oberman, A., Schaefer, E., J., Steinberg, D., Brown, W., V., Grundy, S., M., Becker, D., Bierman, E., Sooter-Bochenek, J., Mullis, R., Stone, N., Hunninghake, D., B., Dunbar, J., M., Ginsberg, H., N., Illingworth, D., R., Sadin, H., C., Schonfeld, G., Cleeman, J., I., Brewer, Jr., H., B., Ernst, N., Friedewald, W., Hoeg, J., M., Rifkind, B., & Gordon, D. (1988). Expert Panel on Detection, Evaluation, and Treatment of High Blood Cholesterol in Adults. The expert panel. *Arch Intern Med,* Vol. 148, No. 1, pp. 36-69

National Cholesterol Education Program (NCEP). Adult Treatment Panel II (ATP II). Grundy, S., Bilheimer, D., Chait, A., Clark, L., T., Denke, M., A., Havel, R., J., Hazzard, W., R., Hulley, S., B., Hunninghake, D., B., Kresiberg, R., A., Kris-Etherton, P., McKenney, J., M., Newman, M., A., Schaefer, E., J., Sobel, B., E., Somelofski, C., & Weinstein, M., C. (1993). Summary of the Second Report of NCEP Expert Panel on Detection, Evaluation, and Treatment of High Blood Cholesterol in Adults (ATP II). *JAMA,* Vol. 269, No. 23, pp. 3015-3023

National Cholesterol Education Program (NCEP). Adult Treatment Panel III (ATP III). Grundy, S., M., Becker, D., Clark, L., T., Cooper, T., S., Denke, M., A., Howard, W., J., Hunninghake, D., B., Illingworth, D., R., Luepker, R., V., McBride, P., McKenney, J., M., Pasternak, R., C., Stone, N., J., & Van Horn, L. (2001). Summary of the Third Report of NCEP Expert Panel on Detection, Evaluation, and Treatment of High Blood Cholesterol in Adults (ATP III). *JAMA,* Vol. 285, No. 19, pp. 2486-2497

National Cholesterol Education Program (NCEP). ATP III Update. Grundy, S., M., Cleeman, J., I., Merz, N., B., Brewer, H., B., Clark, L., T., Hunninghake, D., B., Pasternak, R., C., Smith, S., C., & Stone, N., J. (2004). Implications of Recent Clinical Trials for the National Cholesterol Education Program Adult Treatment Panel III Guidelines. *Circulation,* Vol. 110, No. 2, pp. 227-239

National Prevention Council. (2011). *National Prevention Strategy. America´s plan for better health and wellness.* U.S. Department of Health and Human Services, Office of the Surgeon General, Washington, DC

Nieuwdorp, M., van Haeften, T., W., Gouverneur, M., C., Mooij, H., L., van Lieshout, M., H., Levi, M., Meijers, J., C., Holleman, F., Hoekstra, J., B., Vink, H., Kastelein, J., J., & Stroes, E., S. (2006). Loss of endothelial glycocalyx during acute hyperglycemia coincides with endothelial dysfunction and coagulation activation in vivo. *Diabetes,* Vol. 55, No. 2, pp. 480-486

Nohria, A., Gerhard-Herman, M., Creager, M., A., Hurley, S., Mitra, D. & Ganz, P. (2006). Role of nitric oxide in the regulation of digital pulse volume amplitude in humans. *J Appl Physiol,* Vol. 101, No. 2, pp. 545-548

Nordestgaard, B., G., Chapman, M., J., Ray, K., Borén, J., Andreotti, F., Watts, G., F., Ginsberg, H., Amarenco, P., Catapano, A., Descamps, O., S., Fisher, E., Kovanen, P., T., Kuivenhoven, J., A., Lesnik, Ph., Masana, L., Reiner, Z., Taskinen, M., Tokgözoglu, L., & Tybjærg-Hansen, A. (2010). Lipoprotein(a) as cardiovascular risk factor: current status. *Eur Heart J,* Vol. 31, No. 23, pp. 2844-2853

Novo, S., Pernice, C., Barbagallo, C., M., Tantillo, R., Caruso, R., & Longo, B. (1997). Influence of risk factors and aging on asymptomatic carotid lesions, In: *Advances in Vascular Pathology,* Nicolaides, A., N., & Novo, S. (Eds.), pp. 33-44, Elsevier Science, Excerpta Medica, Amsterdam

O'Flaherty, M., Ford, E., S., Allender, S., Scarborough, P., & Capewell, S. (2008). Coronary heart disease trends in England and Wales from 1984 to 2004: concealed levelling of mortality rates among young adults. *Heart,* Vol. 94, No. 2, pp. 178-181

OPERA registry. Montalescot, G., Dallongeville, J., Van Belle, E., Rouanet, S., Baulac, C., Degrandsart, & Vicaut, E. for the OPERA Investigators (2007). STEMI and NSTEMI: are they so different? 1 year outcomes in acute myocardial infarction as defined by the ESC/ACC definition. *Eur Heart J,* Vol. 28, No. 12, pp. 1409-1417

Ostergren, J., B., Sleight, P., Dagenais, G., Danisa, K., Bosch, J., Qilong, Y., & Yusuf, S. for the HOPE study investigators. (2004). Impact of ramipril in patients with evidence of clinical or subclinical peripheral arterial disease. *Eur Heart J,* Vol. 25, No.1, pp. 17-24

Ozbebit, F., Y., Esen, F, Gulec, S., & Esen, H. (2004). Evaluation of forearm microvascular blood flow regulation by laser doppler flowmetry, iontophoresis, and curve analysis: contribution of axon reflex. *Microvasc Res,* Vol. 67, No. 3, pp. 207-214

Paffenbarger, R., Hyde, R., T., Wing, A., L., Jung, D., L., & Kampret, J., B. (1993). The association of changes in physical - activity level and other lifestyle characteristics with mortality among men. *N Engl J Med,* Vol. 328, No. 8, pp. 538-545

Palmieri, L., Panico, S., Vanuzzo, D., Ferrario, M., Pilotto, L., Sega, R., Cesana, G., & Giampaoli, S. Gruppo di Ricerca del Progetto CUORE. (2004). Evaluation of the global cardiovascular absolute risk: the Progetto CUORE individual score. *Ann 1st Super Sanita,* Vol. 40, No. 4, pp. 393-399

Pankow, J., Folsom, A., R., Cushman, M., Borecki, I., B., Hopkins, P., N., Eckfeldt, J., H., & Tracy, R., P. (2001). Familial and genetic determinants of systemic markers of inflammation: the NHLBI family heart study. *Atherosclerosis,* Vol. 154, No. 3, pp. 681-689

Panza, J., A., Quyyumi, A., A., Brush, Jr., J., E., & Epstein, S., E. (1990). Abnormal endothelium-dependent vascular relaxation in patients with essential hypertension. *N Engl J Med,* Vol. 323, No. 1, pp. 22-27

Pobeha, P., Skyba, P., Joppa, P., Kluchová, Z., Szabóová, E., Tkáč, I., & Tkáčová, R. (2011). Carotid intima-media thickness in patients with chronic obstructive pulmonary disease. *Bratisl Lek Listy,* Vol. 112, No. 1, pp. 24-28

Poirier, P., Giles, T., D., Bray, G., A., Hong, Y., Stem, J., S., Pi-Sunyer, F., X., & Eckel, R., H. (2006). Obesity and cardiovascular disease: pathophysiology, evaluation, and effect of weight loss: an update of the 1997 American Heart Association Scientific Statement on Obesity and Hearth Disease from the Obesity Committee of the Council on Nutrition, Physical Activity, and Metabolism. *Circulation,* Vol. 113, No. 6, pp. 898-918

Postley, J., E., Perez, A., Wronmg, N., D., & Gardin, J., M. (2009). Prevalence and distribution of subclinical atherosclerosis by screening vascular ultrasound in low and intermediate risk adults: The New York Physicians Study. *J Am Soc Echocardiogr,* Vol. 22, No. 10, pp. 1145-1151

Purcell, S., Cherny, S., S., & Sham, P., C. (2003). Genetic Power calculator: design of linkage and association genetic mapping studies of complex traits. *Bioinformatics,* Vol. 19, No. 1, pp. 149-150

Pyörälä, K., Backer, G., D., Graham, I., Poole-Wilson, P., & Wood, D. (1994). 'Prevention of coronary heart disease in clinical practice. Recommendations of the Task Force of the European Society of Cardiology, European Atherosclerosis Society, and European Society of Hypertension.' *Eur Heart J,* Vol. 15, No. 10, pp. 1300-1331

Rask-Madsen, C., Dominguez, H., Ihlemann, N., Hermann, T., Kober, L., & Torp-Pedersen, C. (2003). Tumor necrosis factor-alpha inhibits insulin´s stimulating effect on glucose uptake and endothelium-dependent vasodilatation in humans. *Circulation,* Vol. 108, No. 15, pp. 1815-1821

Rattazzi, M., Puato, M., Faggin, E., Bertipaglia, B., Grego, F., & Pauletto, P. (2003). New markers of accelerated atherosclerosis in end-stage renal disease. *J Nephrol,* Vol. 16, No. 1, pp. 11-20

Resnick, H., E., Lindsay, R., S., McDermott, M., M., Devereux, R., B., Jones, K., L., Fabsitz, R., R., & Howard, B., V. (2004). Relationship of High and Low Ankle Brachial Index to All-Cause and Cardiovascular Disease Mortality. The Strong Heart Study. *Circulation,* Vol. 109, No. 6, pp. 733-739

Ridker, P., M. (2001). High-sensitivity C-reactive protein: potential adjunct to global risk assessment in primary prevention of cardiovascular disease. *Circulation,* Vol. 103, No. 13, pp. 1813-1818

Ridker, P., M., Hennekens, C., H., Buring, J., E., & Rifai, N. (2000). C-reactive protein and other markers of inflammation in the prediction of cardiovascular disease in women. *N Engl J Med,* Vol. 342, No. 12, pp. 836-843

Rizzo, M., Corrado, E., Coppola, G., Muratori, I., Novo, G., & Novo, S. (2008). Prediction of cardio- and cerebrovascular events in patients with subclinical carotid atherosclerosis and low HDL-cholesterol. *Atherosclerosis,* Vol. 200, No. 2, pp. 389-395

Romanens, M., Ackermann, F., Spence, J., D., Darioli, R., Rodondi, N., Corti, R., Noll, G., Schwenkglenks, M., & Pencina, M. (2010). Improvement of cardiovascular risk prediction: Time to review current knowledge, debates, and fundamentals on how to assess test characteristics. *Eur J Cardiovasc Prev Rehabil,* Vol. 17, No. 1, pp. 18-23

Rose, G. (1981). The strategy of prevention: lessons from cardiovascular disease. *BMJ,* Vol. 282, No. 6279, pp. 1847-1851

Rosengren, A., Eriksson, H., Hansson, P., O., Svärdsudd, K., Wilhelmsen, L., Johansson, S., & Welin, C. (2009), 'Obesity and trends in cardiovascular risk factors over 40 years in Swedish men aged 50'. *Journal of Internal Medicine,* Vol. 266, No. 3, pp. 268-276

Rosengren, A., & Wilhelmsen, L. (1997). Physical activity protects against coronary death and deaths from all causes in middle aged men. Evidence from a 20-year follow up of primary prevention study in Goteburg. *Ann Epidemiol,* Vol. 7, No. 1, pp. 69 -75

Rotterdam Study. Bots, M., L. (1997). Tissue plasminogen activator and risk of myocardial infarction. *Circulation,* Vol. 96, No. 5, pp. 1432-1437

Rozanski, A., Blumenthal, J., A., Davidson, K., W., Saab, P., G., & Kubzansky, L. (2005). The epidemiology, pathophysiology, and management of psychosocial risk factors in cardiac practice: the emerging field of behavioral cardiology. *J Am Coll Cardiol,* Vol. 45, No. 5, pp. 637-651

Rubinshtein, R., Kuvin, J., T., Soffler, M., Lennon, R., J., Lavi, S., Nelson, R., E., Pumper, G., M., Lerman, L., O. & Lerman, A. (2010). Assessment of endothelial function by non-invasive peripheral arterial tonometry predicts late cardiovascular adverse events. *Eur Heart J,* Vol. 31, No. 9, pp. 1142-1148

Rydén, L., Martin, J., & Volqvartz, S. (2007). The European Heart Health Charter: towards a healthier Europe. *Eur J Cardiovasc Prev Rehabil,* Vol. 14, No. 3, pp. 354-356

Safar, M., E., & O´Rourke, M., F. (2006). *Arterial Stiffness in Hypertension, Handbook of hypertension,* Elsevier, Amsterdam

Scarabin, P., Arveiler, D., Amouyel, P., Dis Santos, C., Evans, A., Luc, G., Ferrieres, J., & Juhan-Vague, I. (2003). Prospective Epidemiological Study of Myocardial Infarction. Plasma fibrinogen explains much of the difference in risk of coronary heart disease between France and Northern Ireland. The PRIME Study. *Atherosclerosis,* Vol. 166, No. 1, pp. 103-109

Schroeder, S., Enderle, M., D., Ossen, R., Meisner, C., Baumbach, A., Pfhol, M., Herdeg, C., Oberhoff, M., Haering, H., U., & Karsch, K., R. (1999). Noninvasive determination of endothelium-mediated vasodilation as a screening test for coronary artery disease: pilot study to assess the predictive value in comparison with angina pectoris, exercise electrocardiography and myocardial infarction perfusion imaging. *Am Heart J*, Vol. 138, No. 4, pp. 731-739

Shaper, A., Wannamethee, G., Macfarlane, P., & Walker, M. (1993). Heart rate, ischaemic heart disease, and sudden death in middle - aged British men. *Br Heart J*, Vol. 70, No. 1, pp. 49-55

Stampfer, M., J., Hu, F., B., Manson, J., E., Rimm, E., B., & Willett, W., C. (2000). Primary prevention of coronary heart disease in women through diet and lifestyle. *N Engl J Med*, Vol. 343, No. 1, pp. 16-22

Stramba-Badiale, M., Fox, K., M., Priroi, S., G., Collins, P., Daly, C., Graham, I.., Johnson, B., Schenk-Gustaffson, K., & Tendera, M. (2006). Cardiovascular disease in women: a statement from the policy conference of the European Society of Cardiology. *Eur Heart J*, Vol. 27, No. 8, pp. 994-1005

Szabóová, E., Donič, V., Petrovičová, J., Szabó, P., & Tomori, Z. (2007). Sleep apnoea inducing hypoxemia is associated with early signs of carotid atherosclerosis in males. *Respiratory Physiology & Neurobiology*, Vol. 155, No. 2, pp. 121-127

Szabóová, E., Tomori, Z., Gonsorčík, J., & Petrovičová, J. (2008). Tradičné rizikové faktory aterosklerózy u pacientov so syndrómom obštrukčného spánkového apnoe-hypopnoe. *Vnitřní lékařství*, Vol. 54 , No. 4, pp. 352-360 (In Slovak)

Szabóová, E., Kozárová, M., Kmecová, D., & Tkáč, I. (2010). Skríning subklinickej aterosklerózy na vzorke jedincov bez kardiovaskulárneho postihnutia na východnom Slovensku. *Interná medicína*, Vol. 10, No. 5, pp. 292-296 (In Slovak)

Tervaert, J., W. (2009). Translational mini-review series on immunology of vascular disease: accelerated atherosclerosis in vasculitis. *Clin Exp Immunol*, Vol. 156, No. 3, pp. 377-385

Third Joint Task Force of the European and other Societies on Cardiovascular Disease Prevention in Clinical Practice. De Backer., G., Ambrosioni, E., Borch-Johnsen, K., Brotons, C., Cifkova, R., Dallongeville, J., Ebrahim, Sh., Faergeman, O., Graham, I., Mancia, G., Cats, V., M., Orth-Gomer, K., Perk, J., Pyorala, K., Rodicio, J., L., Sans, S., Sansoy, V., Dechtem, U., Silber, S., Thomsen, T., Wood, D., & others. (2003). European guidelines on cardiovascular disease prevention in clinical practice. *Eur J Cardiovasc Prev Rehabil*, Vol. 10, Suppl. 1, pp. S1-78

TNT Study. Shepherd, J., Barter, P., Carmena, R., Deedwania, P., Fruchart, J., C., Haffner, S., Hsia, J., Breazna, A., LaRosa, J., Grundy, S., & Waters, D. (2006). Effect of lowering LDL cholesterol substantially below currently recommended levels in patients with coronary heart disease and diabetes: the Treating to New Targets (TNT) study. *Diabetes Care*, Vol. 29, No. 6, pp. 1220-1226

Touboul, P., J., Vicaut, E., Labreuche, J, Belliard, J., P., Cohen, S., Kownator, S., Portal, J., J., Pithois-Merli, I., & Amarenco, P. on behalf of the Paroi Artérielle et Risque Cardiovasculaire Study Investigators. (2005). Design, Baseline Characteristics, and Carotid Intima-Media Thickness Reproducibility in the PARC Study. *Cerebrovasc Dis, Vol.* 19, No. 1, pp. 57-63

Tsuchiya, K., Nakayama, C., Iwashima, F., Sakai, H., Izumiyama, H., Doi, M., & Hirata, Y. (2007). Advanced endothelial dysfunction in diabetic patients with multiple risk factors; importance of insulin resistance. *J Atheroscler Thromb,* Vol. 14, No. 6, pp. 303-309

Tunstall-Pedoe, H., Kuulasmaa, K., Mähönen, M., Tolonen, H., Ruokokoski, E., & Amouyel, P. for the WHO MONICA Project. (1999). 'Contribution of trends in survival and coronary-event rates to changes in coronary heart disease mortality: 10-year results from 37 WHO MONICA Project populations. Monitoring trends and determinants in cardiovascular disease.' *Lancet, Vol.* 353, No. 1547, pp. 1547-1557

Unal, B., Critchley, J., & Capewell, S. (2004), 'Explaining the decline in coronary heart disease mortality in England and Wales between 1981 and 2000'. *Circulation,* Vol. 109, No. 9, pp. 1101-1107

US Department of Health and Human Services, Washington, D.C. (2004). The health consequences of smoking: a report of the Surgeon General, N.d., available from www.surgeongeneral.gov/library/smokingconsequences/

Vanderheyden, M., Mansour, S., & Bartunek J. (2005). Accelerated atherosclerosis following intracoronary haematopoetic stem cell administration. *Heart,* Vol. 91, No. 4, pp. 448

Vartiainen, E., Jousilahti, P., Alfthan, G., Sundvall, J., Pietinen, P., & Puska, P. (2000). Cardiovascular risk factor changes in Finland I. 1972-1997. *Int J. Epidemiol,* Vol. 29, No. 1, pp. 49-56

Vartiainen, E., Laatikainen, T., Peltonen, M., Juolevi, A., Männistö, S., Sundvall, J., Jousilahtu, P., Salomaa, V., Vaslta, L., & Puska, P. (2010). Thirty-five-year trends in cardiovascular risk factors in Finland. *Int J Epidemiol,* Vol. 39, No. 2, pp. 504-518

Wajchenberg, B. (2000). Subcutaneous and visceral adipose tissue: their relation to the metabolic syndrome. *Endocr Rev,* Vol. 21, No. 6, pp. 697-738

Wald, N., J., & Law, M., R. (2003). A strategy to reduce cardiovascular disease by more than 80%. *BMJ,* Vol. 326, No. 7404, pp. 1419-1423

Wilhelmsen, L., Svardsudd, K., Korsan-Bengtsen, K., Larsson, B., Welin, L., & Tibblin, G. (1984). Fibrinogen as a risk factor for stroke and myocardial infarction. *N Engl J Med,* Vol. 311, No. 8, pp. 501-505

Wilhelmsen, L., Welin, L., Svärdsudd, K., Wedel, H., Eriksson, H., Hansson, P., & Rosengren, A. (2008). Secular changes in cardiovascular risk factors and attack rate of myocardial infarction among men aged 50 in Gothenburg, Sweden. Accurate prediction using risk models. *Journal of Internal Medicine,* Vol. 263, No. 6, pp. 636-643

Woodward, M., Lowe, G., D., Rumley, A., Tunstall-Pedoe, H., Philippou, H., Lane, D., A., & Morrison, C., E. (1997). Epidemiology of coagulation factors, inhibitors and activation markers: The Third Glasgow MONICA Survey. II. Relationships to cardiovascular risk factors and prevalent cardiovascular disease. *Br J Haematol,* Vol. 97, No. 4, pp. 785-797

Worns, M., Victor, A., Galle, P., R., & Hohler, T. (2006). Genetic and environmental contributions to plasma C-reactive protein and interleukin-6 levels - a study in twins. *Genes Immun,* Vol. 7, No. 7, pp. 600-605

WOSCOPS Study. Shepherd, J., Cobbe, S., M., Ford, I., Isles, C., G., Lorimer, A., R., MacFarlane, P., W., McKillopp, J., H., & Packard, C., J. for the West of Scotland Coronary Prevention Study Group. (1995). Prevention of coronary heart disease with pravastatin in men with hypercholesterolemia. *New Engl J Med,* Vol. 333, No. 20, pp. 1301-1307

Ye, Z., Liu, E., H., Higgins, J., P., Keavney, B., D., Lowe, G., D., Collins, R., & Danesh, J. (2006). Seven haemostatic gene polymorphisms in coronary disease: meta - analysis of 66, 155 cases and 91,307 controls. *Lancet,* Vol. 367, No. 511, pp. 651-658

Yusuf, S., Hawken, S., Oupuu, S., Dans, T., Avezum, A., Lanas, F., McQueen, M., Budaj, A., Pais, P., Varigos, J., & Lisheng, L. (2004). Effect of potentially modifiable risk factor associated with myocardial infarction in 52 countries (The INTERHEART study): case- control study. *Lancet,* Vol. 364, No. 9438, pp. 937-952

10

Metabolomics in Cardiovascular Disease: Towards Clinical Application

Ignasi Barba and David Garcia-Dorado
Institut de Recerca, Àrea del Cor, Hospital Universitari Vall d'Hebron, Universitat Autònoma de Barcelona, Barcelona, Spain

1. Introduction

Metabolomics were initially defined as the global analysis of all metabolites present in a sample (metabolomics) and the analysis of metabolic responses to drugs and diseases (metabonomics) [Nicholson et al., 1999, Fiehn 2002, Weckwerth and Morgenthal 2005]. These two definitions have an historical origin, while metabolomics has its foundations in microbial and plant sciences metabonomics originated in toxicology studies of mamalian systems. Today the two terms are becoming synonyms [Nicholson and Lindon 2008]. Other useful definitions have appeared in the literature [Ellis et al., 2007, Dunn et al., 2011] Table 1. In the particular setting of disease diagnosis it is relevant to talk about metabolic fingerprinting and metabonomics, both strategies aimed mainly at differentiating between two or more sets of data (i.e., disease/healthy) in a quantitative (metabonomics) or qualitative approach (fingerprinting).

As with other 'omics' technologies metabolomics aims to measure metabolite dynamics in an unbiased manner; the advent of analytical and statistical methods has made possible to apply metabolic analysis to a wide range of applications. 'Omics' technologies allows the simultaneous measure of thousands of parameters from a single sample; together with new statistical methods able to tackle very large databases and systems or network approaches we should be able to extract the knowledge in order to better phenotype disease and help in the diagnostic process. Being able to apply all this newly found knowledge to the clinic is the next big challenge at the beginning of the 21st century.

Genomics, proteomics and metabolomics are closely related approaches as they are all aimed at the quantitative, non-biased study of biological systems although not at the same level. Genomics was the first to appear, the relative chemical simplicity of DNA allowed the implementation of high throughput approaches first; it was followed by proteomics and finally metabolomics. Although there is a continuum between genomics and metabolomics with multiple interactions between genes, proteins and metabolites (Figure 1) the study of the metabolome is relevant because the it is downstream of the genome it is thereby amplified both in theory [Mendes et al., 1996] and in practice [Raamsdonk et al., 2001]. It has also been shown that small changes in the concentration of enzymes have only small effects on the fluxes through metabolic pathways but the changes in metabolite intermediates may be substantial [Cascante et al., 2002].

Term	Definition
Metabolomics	The nonbiased identification and quantification of all the metabolites present in a biological system
Metabolome	The complete set of low-molecular-weight metabolites present in a biological sample (i.e., biofluid, organism, bacterial community)
Metabolic profiling	Identification and quantification of a selective number of metabolites, usually related to a specific metabolic pathway.
Metabolic fingerprint	Global, high-throughput analysis aimed at sample classification. Also used as a screening tool.
Metabolic footprint	Analysis of the metabolites secreted/excreted by an organism; it may include environmental and growth substances.
Metabolite target analysis	Qualitative and quantitative analysis of one, or several, metabolites related to a specific metabolic reaction.
Metabonomics	Quantitative analysis of metabolites in response of biological perturbations or genetic modification.
Lipidomics	Analysis of all lipids, and the molecules with they interact, and their function within a biological system.
Metabolite flux analysis	Also known as fluxomics. Labeled metabolites are fed into a biosystem and the destination of the label is assessed, usually in a time-dependent manner.
Metabotype	The metabolic phenotype.

Table 1. Definitions of terms used in metabolomics. Modified from [Ellis et al 2007, Goodacre 2007].

Metabolism is downstream of the genome, transcriptome and proteome leading to an amplification of the signal. Only 2766 metabolites are estimated to be derived from man [Duarte et al., 2007], compared with 31896 genes [http://eugenes.org] and 10^6 different proteins estimated from gene expression, alternative splicing and post-translational modifications [Oh 2004, Goodacre 2007] makes the metabolome relatively simple.

Also, another characteristic of the metabolome is that it is affected by disease and external perturbations, such as age [Fredman et al., 2004, Athertorn et al., 2009], nutrition, disease, gut microflora, toxins and drugs [Bollard et al., 2005]. This favours the study of the metabolome as a relevant representation of the phenotype [Ellis et al., 2007]. While the genome does provide information about the future (for example, the probability of suffering a disease) the metabolome reflects what is actually happening to the system (i.e. is it diseased? How is responding to treatment?).

Metabolism is organized as a scale-free network [Jeong et al., 2000]. These networks are composed of highly interconnected nodes (metabolites) that link together the various parts of the network making them are very robust against random errors [Albert et al., 2000]. Also, any perturbation will be rapidly and widely spread throughout the network, thus, the detection of a few highly interconnected nodes allows to detect differences originating in distant parts of the metabolic network [Brindle KM 2003] (Figure 2). The way metabolic networks spread perturbations allow for an easy detection but it is difficult to retrace the steps back to the origin unless there is some prior knowledge as in the case of the FANCY approach [Raamsdonk et al., 2001].

The properties of a system are different from those of its individual components; systems biology aims to study all the components of a systems and their interaction; according to Sauer and cols. [2007], complex biological networks are "better addressed by observing, through quantitative measures, multiple components simultaneously, and by rigorous data integration with mathematical models" [Sauer et al., 2007]. Accordingly, the integration of all the information obtained from the 'omics' approaches will be essential when trying to understand how biological networks change during disease; a new field of network analysis is emerging in oder to tackle the integration of various 'omics technologies and *in silico* models [Loscalzo et al., 2007].

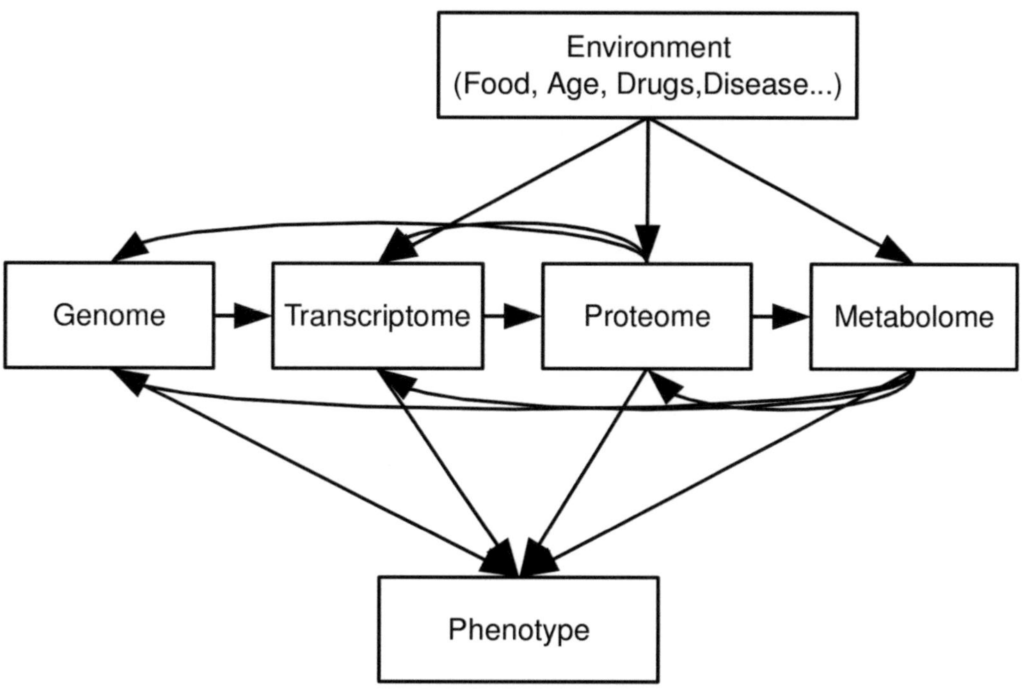

Fig. 1. Schematic representation of the interaction between different 'omes'. The metabolome or metabolic phenotype is both downstream of the genome, proteome and trasciptome and also affected by the environment including disease and drug treatments; it is thus well suited as a diagnostic and treatment follow-up tool.

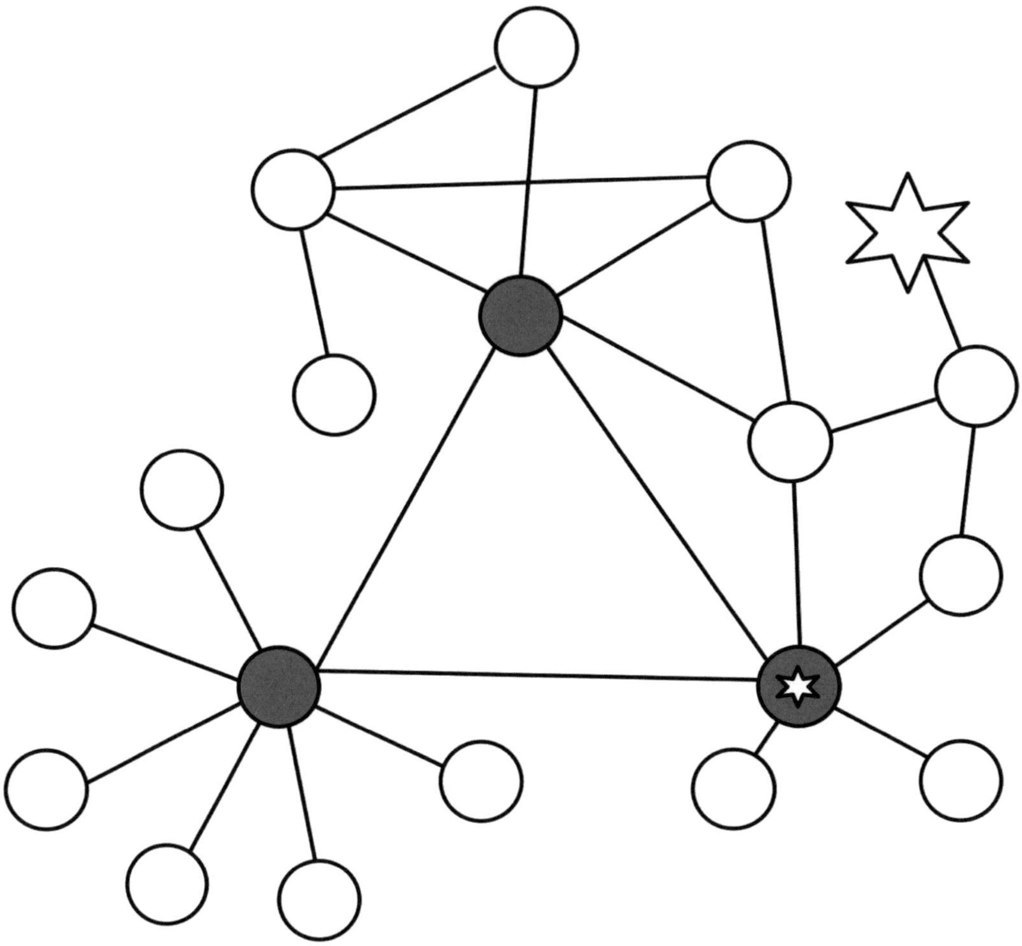

Fig. 2. Organization of scale free networks, perturbations (marked here as star) in the network are transferred to the central hubs of metabolism (Gray circles) allowing the detection of many different situations even though the metabolites directly responsible for them are beyond the limits of technical detection. Once a change in one or more hubs is detected, knowing the metabolic reactions ultimately responsible for them may not be straight forward unless there is some prior knowledge as in the FANCY approach [Raamsdonk et al., 2001].

1.1 Methodologies

The chemical diversity of metabolites has promoted the use of various analytical methods (Table 2), the most common ones being NMR spectroscopy and Mass spectrometry. There are other analytical methods including infrared, visible, and Raman spectroscopy reviewed elsewhere [Ellis et al., 2007].

Mass spectrometry operates by forming ions (positively or negatively charged) and separating them according to their mass to charge ratio (m/z). It is a high sensitivity method that allows high mass accuracy and resolution thus allowing chemical identification of metabolites; it has been proposed as the real metabolomic approach [Kell 2004]. Mass spectrometer detectors are usually placed after a chromatography (gas or liquid) step; this introduces a bias as there will be some metabolites that will not be able to reach the detector. If there is prior knowledge of which group of metabolites may be affected the bias may turn to be an advantage and mass spectra the ideal tool to use as it is possible to focus interest in a group of metabolites (Figure 3A).

NMR spectroscopy looks into magnetic properties of atomic nuclei when placed in a magnetic field; the molecular environment (electronic cloud) is able modify the magnetic field thus each nuclei within a molecule will sense a slightly different magnetic field that in turn allow to differentiate between them in a spectra (Figure 3B). A more detailed description of the applications of biological NMR spectroscopy can be found elsewhere [Bothwell and Griffin 2011]

When sample classification, as in the case of disease diagnosis, is the primary objective, metabonomics or metabolic fingerprinting is the desired approach. In this case, NMR spectroscopy is the preferred analytical technique because it is fast, reproducible and cheap on a per-sample basis. NMR spectroscopy is only able to detect a limited number of metabolites but it is able to pick metabolic differences arising from very different parts of the metabolic network; the reason behind this lies on the fact that most of the central hubs of metabolic networks are 'NMR visible', by monitoring these hubs it is possible to indirectly detect a huge number of metabolic alterations [Griffin 2003].

Mass and NMR spectroscopy can be performed on easy to obtain biofluids (serum, urine, saliva, etc) that integrate metabolites from various processes and organs thus providing an integrative metabolic snapshot.

1.2 Data analysis

Metabolomic, and other 'omic' technical advances has been mirrored by advances in data processing, statistical methods able to work with large data sets comprising many more variables than subjects under study. The objective of the various pattern recognition techniques is two-fold; on the one hand they aim at classification between two or more groups of samples but also to extract information about which variables (metabolites) are relevant for each classification.

To investigate the innate variation in a dataset, unsupervised techniques such as principal component analysis (PCA) [Hotellin 1933] could be used. In this approach, the sources of variation within the dataset are organized as orthogonal, thus independent, vectors in a descending manner so the first principal component (PC) is the one that explains more variation, followed by the second, third, etc. It is possible that the condition under study, for example a disease, is one of the main sources of metabolic variation; then one of the first PCs will be related to the effect of disease to the metabolic profile and allow for a discrimination between healthy and diseased samples. The great advantage of unsupervised techniques is that they don't require prior knowledge of the condition under study. Also, unsupervised approaches are useful in removing out-layers from the dataset.

However, when unsupervised approaches are not sufficient, supervised techniques may be better suited to answer specific questions. These approaches require the input of the group of each sample in order to create a statistical model that maximizes the differences between groups and minimizes inter-group variation. In the case of supervised models, it is necessary to test the robustness and predictability of the models produced in order to avoid creating models that will only fit the data used to create them. The ideal situation is when two different datasets are used, one to create the model and an independent one to test it; when the number of samples is limited, internal validation protocols like 'leave-one-out' may be used.

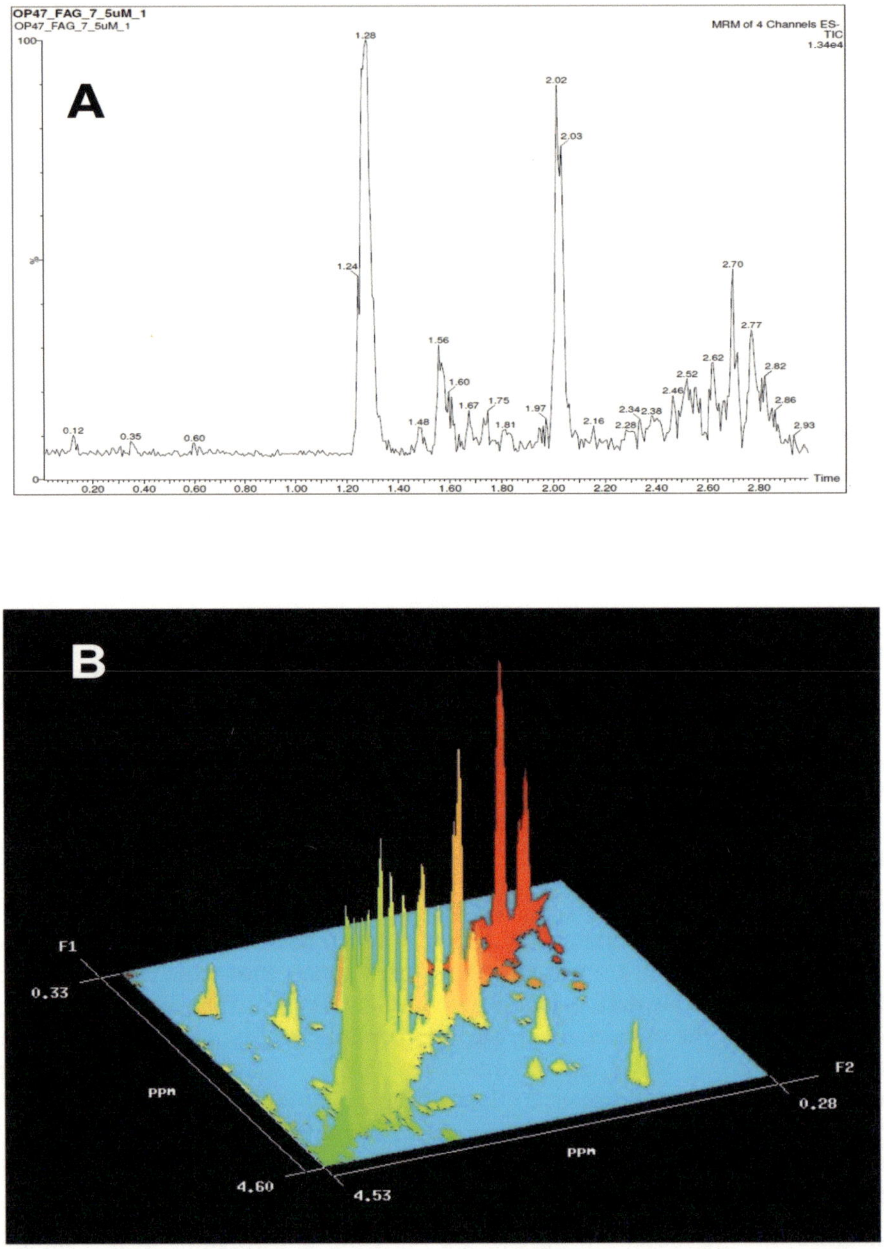

Fig. 3. Examples of UPLC MS-MS spectra (A) from rat urine treated with phenilacelilglutamine where each peak corresponds to an ion and an ^{1}H-^{1}H COSY NMR spectra of human serum (B) showing the correlation between close (three bond) protons in a molecule.

1.3 Metabolic profiling

Sample classification is one of the main targets of any 'omics' technology, when the groups of samples include a healty (control) and at least one diseased group (case) the method can be used directly as a diagnostic tool.

Metabolite levels, at least some of them, change between healthy and diseased states and may respond to therapeutic intervention (Figure 4). Perturbations in the metabolic pathways may occur prior to clinical symptoms, those would be the early prognostic markers. It is likely that at the early stage of disease a few metabolites may be slightly altered but not far away from normal values; in this case fingerprinting (Figure 5A), measuring a variety of metabolites, may be the tool to use in order to detect early markers of diagnosis. On the other hand, as a disease progresses it is more likely that one (or more) metabolites alter their concentration significantly, consequently looking for individual metabolites associated to a disease may be the better choice.

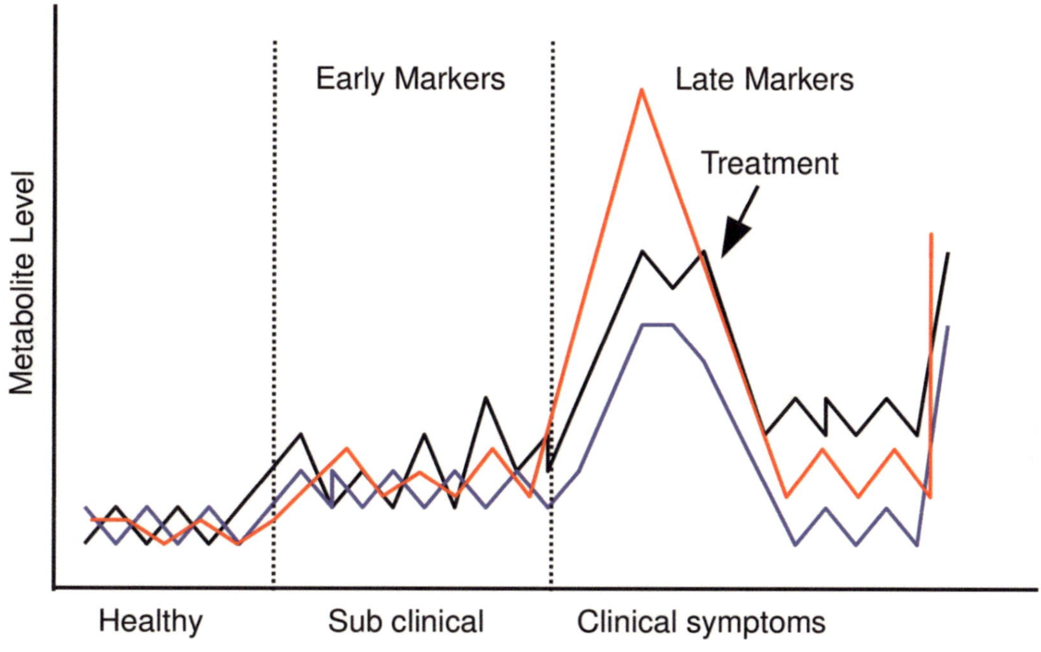

Fig. 4. Metabolite levels during disease evolution. In the pre-clinical stage some metabolites may be altered but likely within the normal deviation of the population, in this setting metabolic profiling of various metabolites may be a good approach towards finding discriminant models; on the other hand in the clinical stages it is possible that one or a few metabolites are highly modified from their normal values in this case looking for biomarkers would be relevant. Some metabolites may change after treatment allowing for unbiased follow-up and pre-treatment metabolomic pattern may also be useful to predict treatment response.

1.4 Biomarker discovery

On top of sample classification, metabolomic analysis is able to provide information regarding which metabolites are more relevant for a classification. It is thus possible to identify individual metabolites that could be used as biomarkers and use metabolomic analysis can be used as a tool for biomarker discovery. Once a metabolite is identified (Figure 5A) as a biomarker using high throughoutput metabolomic methodologies it may be detected by classical analytical methods for clinical practice. For example, Sreekumar and cols. [2009] were able to identify sarcosine in urine as potentially important metabolic intermediary of cancer cell invasion and aggressiveness after profiling 1126 metabolites from 262 clinical samples.

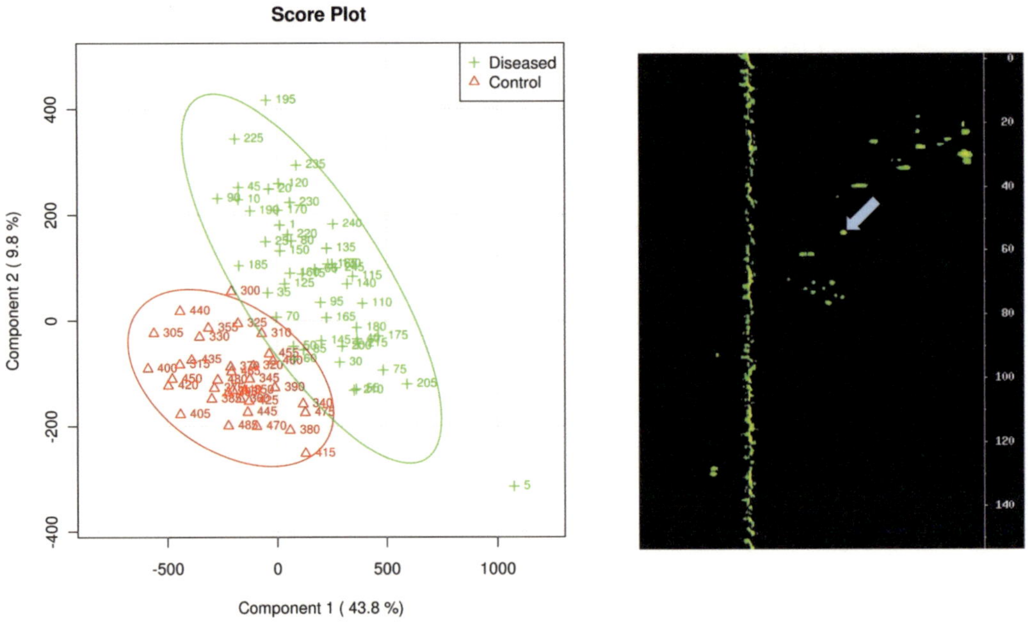

Fig. 5. Metabolomics in clinical applications. Panel A shows the result of a discriminant analysis of NMR spectra from serum obtained from patients in the coronary unit and healthy controls. Circles correspond to 95% confidence intervals. Note that dispersion in samples from patients is higher that that of controls. Pattern recognition analysis allows to identify the most relevant variables in an analysis and it is possible to identify the metabolite responsible. Panel B shows a ^{1}H-^{13}C HSQC NMR spectra; a useful approach to identify metabolites. Processing shown in panel A was obtained using Metaboanalyst software [Xia et al., 2009].

Once a variable in the analysis is found to be relevant in a classification model it can be associated to a metabolite because mass to charge ratio and chemical shift are specific for each metabolite. There are public databases that help metabolite identification http://www.hmdb.ca/. In order to obtain an absolute identification, though, it is important to perform co-resonance or co-elution experiments.

Figure 6 shows a typical metabolomic experimental design aimed at disease diagnosis. Metabolic profiling and biomarker discovery are not excluding strategies; moreover there is a synergy between them and also with the use of metabolic and pathway information that are not directly associated to diagnostic applications.

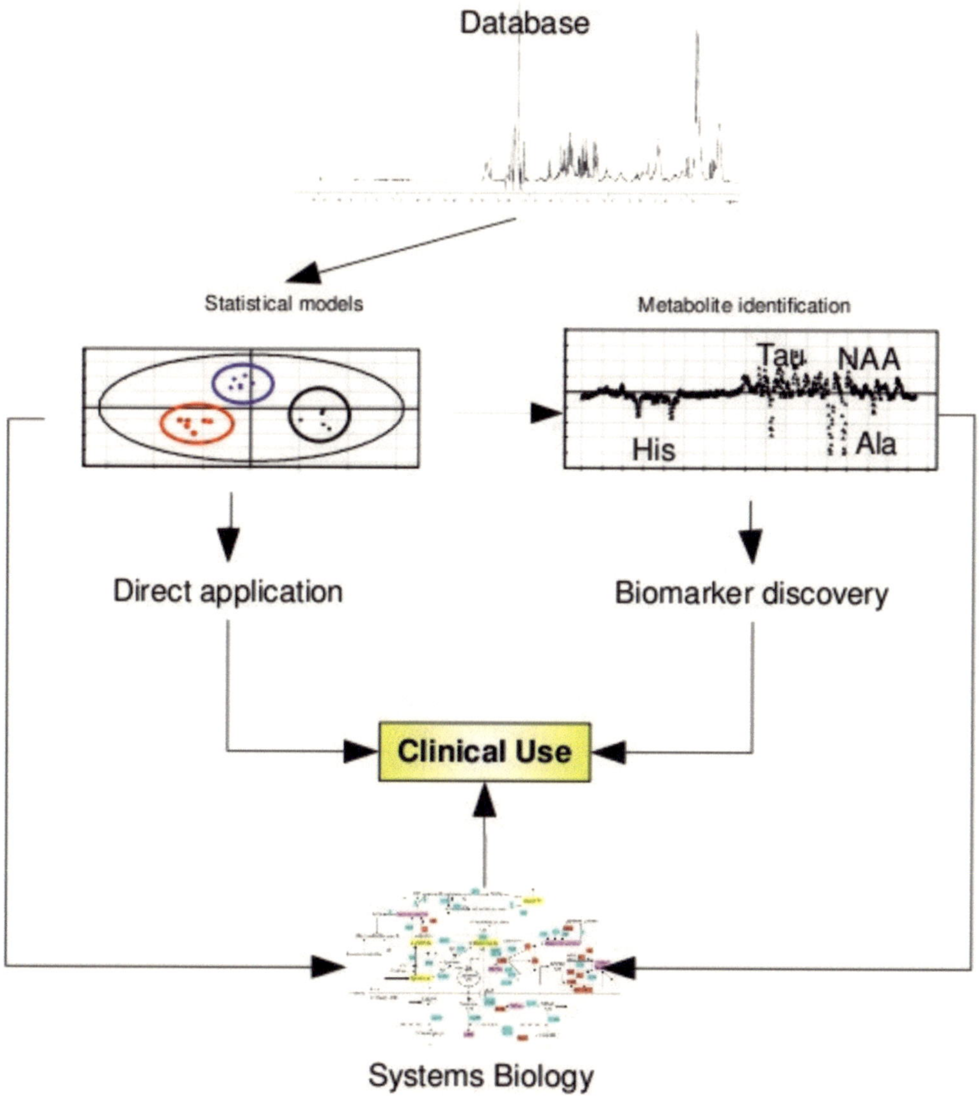

Fig. 6. Typical work-flow in a metabolomic study aimed at disease diagnosis. Once the database is obtained, supervised and unsupervised statistical methods are applied to obtain discriminant models that could be applied directly in the clinic or to find biomarkers. The future of metabolomics will be the implementation of information obtained at different stages of the analysis, particularly relating to metabolites and metabolic pathways into systems biology approaches.

2. Metabolomic applications in cardiovascular diseases

2.1 Basic research applications/metabolic phenotyping

Metabolic analysis has been widely used in laboratory research applications. One of the main uses in this field was the metabolic phenotyping of mouse models of cardiovascular diseases; this approach was pioneered by the group of Julian Griffin mainly using models of Duchenne muscular distrophy where they were able to show different metabolic profiles associated with the expression of dystrophin and utrophin in heart muscle [Griffin et al., 2002, Griffin and Des Rosiers 2009]. In a later work the same group applied the FANCY approach (Functional Analysis by Co-responses in Yeast) to mouse models of cardiac diseases and showed that although the background strain of mice was an important source of metabolic variation, multivariate statistics were able to separate each disease model from the control strain [Jones et al., 2005].

Another mouse model well characterized form the metabolic point of view is the PPAR-α null mouse where authors demonstrate that age exacerbates the changes associated with genotype in this mouse model lacking the peroxisome proliferator activated receptor-a [Athertorn et al., 2009]. Recent reports describing the phenotype of genetically modified mouse models tend to include data regarding the metabolism [Inserte et al., 2009, Rodriguez-Sinovas et al., 2010, Ashrafian et al., 2010]. This is a trend that will become increasingly popular as it becomes clear that the the metabotype is a relevant part of the phenotype.

In 2003 a method to hyperpolarize ^{13}C and increase the signal to noise ratio 10000 times was described [Ardenkjaer-Larsen et al., 2003], this opened the possibility of following metabolism *in vivo* through ^{13}C NMR spectroscopy. It has been possible to measure energy production, particularly the Krebs cycle turnover, by following the label in 1-^{13}C-pyruvate [Golman et al., 2008, Schroeder et al., 2009, 2010] in animal models. Also, pH can be monitored in vivo by measuring hyperpolarised bicarbonate signals [Gallagher et al., 2008, Schroeder et al., 2010]. This extremely sensitive method may play a great role in clinical practice, specially in heart failure where metabolism and its modification through medical treatment is relevant [Lee et al., 2005, Abozguia et al., 2006]

Because NMR is non-invasive, there is the possibility of obtaining localized spectra. While this is technically feasible in brain [Sundgren et al., 2009] it is more complex in the case of heart due mainly to cardio-respiratory motion. However, we were able to differentiate between necrotic, at risk and control areas in an animal model using high resolution magic angle spinning NMR (HR-MAS) [Barba et al., 2007], in consequence, if chemical shift imaging becomes feasible it would be possible to necrosis and at risk areas after myocardial infarction.

2.2 Treatement monitoring and follow up

One of the key areas of metabolomics application is treatment monitoring and follow-up; actually the term metabonomics was introduced by Nicholson and cols [Nicholson et al., 1999] as a toxicology tool to evaluate the effect of drugs. A decade later the same authors have introduced the term 'pharmacometabonomics' in drug treatment defined as an approach "which uses metabolite profiling and chemometrics to model and predict responses of individual subjects" [Clayton et al., 2006, Nicholson et al., 2011]

A great variety of studies have been published in the literature, mostly in the field of cancer [Spratlin et al., 2009]. But in the area of cardiovascular diseases the amount of reports has been very limited, possibly associated to the few new drug treatments appearing for cardiovascular diseases as compared to, for example, cancer.

So far, reports regarding heart disease and drug treatments in the literature are focused on animal models either studying drug toxicity [Perrine et al., 2009, Andreadou et al., 2009] or the effect of antioxidant intervention [Constantinou et al., 2009]. This relative lack of reports may be due to the fact that the number of new drugs under development in the cardiovascular area is not as high as in other fields such as oncology.

2.3 Clinical application of metabolomics

Since the beginning of the 21st century the term 'personalized medicine' has continuously gained popularity and is now considered an essential trait of present and future medicine. For personalized medicine to be successful, it is necessary to properly identify subjects at increased risk of developing a disease, which patients will respond to a given therapy or how a disease will evolve in each case. In other words it is important to genotype and or phenotype the individual patient so that its individual response to disease and treatment can be predicted.

Metabolomics is a promising technology for personalized medicine, it is fast, reproducible, easy to automate and not very expensive on a per sample basis. Most important, unlike the genome, the metabolome is modified by external factors such as disease. Today the only field where personalized medicine is flourishing is cancer; by definition cancer does imply modifications of the genome and genomics is technically more advanced than metabolomics. For diseases that does not imply the modification of the genome, such as cardiovascular pathology, metabolomics may be the tool of choice and extensive research has been conducted in recent years towards achieving this goal.

In 2002, Brindle and cols. published a paper in which they describe "a techniques capable of providing an accurate, noninvasive and rapid diagnosis of coronary heart disease" [Brindle et al., 2002]. ^{1}H NMR spectra from serum samples from patients diagnosed with no coronary artery disease or with one, two or three vessel disease was used to create discriminant models able to differentiate the severity of coronary artery disease. Unfortunately, the authors did not take into account the effects of medical treatments (particularly statins) and patient gender in their analysis and was later demonstrated that those two factors have a strong influence in the NMR pattern. As a result, the specificity and sensitivity first predicted of above 90% was reduced, once corrected by gender and statin use to approximately 60% [Kirschenlohr et al., 2006]. Also, age has also been described as a differential factor regarding lipoprotein subclasses measured by NMR spectroscopy [Freedman 2004]. Nevertheless, the paper by Brindle and cols [Brindle et al., 2002] has been extremely important in the field because it quick started pre-clinical metabolomic studies.

Sabatine and cols [Sabatine et al., 2005] showed that it was possible to apply metabolomic analysis in a carefully characterized cohort of patients undergoing exercise stress testing and to differentiate between patients that developed inducible ischemia from the ones that did not [Sabatine et al., 2005]. This work was done by analyzing serum samples obtained before, during and after stress testing by high performance liquid chromatography coupled to mass spectroscopy; ischaemic patients had higher circulating levels of metabolites belonging to the citric acid pathway. Later, we were able to show that it was possible to predict which patients would suffer from a positive stress test by analyzing serum samples obtained before the stress test using ^{1}H NMR spectroscopy [Barba et al., 2008]. Ischemic patients had relatively higher lactate levels than non ischemic suggesting an underlying ischemic process although it could not be directly related to myocardial ischemia. Differences between the two groups were seen in samples obtained prior to the stress test thus, at least in theory, it would be possible to use metabolic profiling instead of stress testing but, unfortunately, the accuracy of the predictions was around 85%, clearly not high enough as to be used in the clinical setting. Searching for early markers of ischemia, Lewis and cols [Lewis et al., 2008] studied patients undergoing planed alcohol septal ablation and were able to detect several metabolites that changed early after myocardial injury and report a ROC curve for a composite metabolite score with an area under the curve of 0,88 ± 0,07.

It has been known for a time that patients with heart failure (HF) have an altered heart metabolism [Clark et al., 1996] and that metabolic modulation (shifting the main substrate from free fatty acids to glucose) improved VO2max, left ventricular ejection fraction, symptoms, resting and peak stress myocardial function, and skeletal muscle energetics [Lee et al., 2005]. Metabolic modulation as a tool to treat patients with heart failure has attracted interest [Abozguia et al., 2006] but the metabolomic analysis has not followed suit until recently when Kang and cols showed by profiling urine by NMR spectroscopy that it was possible to detect changes between HF patients and controls [Kang et al., 2011]. It could be interesting to evaluate possible changes in the urine metabolic profile of patients treated with drugs targeting heart metabolism for example, perhexiline or trimetazidine.

Metabolomics have been used to study diseases related to the cardiovascular system like diabetes [Wang et al., 2011], and obesity [van de Woestinje et al., 2011] reviewed in [Griffin and Nichols 2006, Muller 2010] but this is beyond the scope of the present work.

3. Future directions

3.1 Next hurdles before clinical application

There has been interest to apply metabolomic analysis to the clinical setting and it has been shown in the literature that various cardiovascular-related pathologies could be differentiated using metabolic analysis [Lee et al., 2005, Lewis et al., 2008, Barba et al., 2008, Kang et al., 2011] but there is still some work to be done for metabolomics in order becoming a clinical reality.

There are two main problems to solve before metabolomics becomes a widespread clinical reality; the first is to make metabolomics technically easy from both data acquisition and processing point of view as to be used in daily routine by non-specialists. The second problem will be more difficult to solve and it relates to population variation; so far studies have focused in small, controlled populations; studies with large cohorts of patients are not yet present in the literature.

Technical problems will be solved soon, there are new advances in automation procedures, mainly in the NMR field, that will allow to use metabolomics routinely for screening purposes in the near future. Moreover, once metabolic biomarkers are found using any of the hypothesis free metabolomics approaches their detection may be done using standard analytical methodologies already implemented in the clinical laboratory; in this case the application of metabolomics derived results would be straight forward.

Solving problems related to population variability is much more challenging; first of all 'omics' data processing is focused on finding sources of variation that can be later correlated with disease, treatment response, etc. Adding sources of variation to the dataset makes it difficult to identify specific patterns. Studies at population level should provide evidence for the background variation in metabolic profile and, thus tell how well metabolomics can perform in the clinical setting.

One of the areas where the application of metabolomics may become a reality soon is the evaluation of response to pharmacologic treatment. Although this is one of the first areas were metabolomics were applied, in the case of cardiovascular diseases so far it has only been reported in animal studies (see above). Still, it has been show that drugs do influence the metabolic pattern in human studies of plasma [Kirschenlohr et al., 2006] and that altering metabolism could be a therapeutic target [Lee et al., 2005] thus paharmacogenomics application may not be far away in the area of cardiovascular disease.

Work has started in the integration of various 'omics' technologies in global systems biology approaches [Mayr et al., 2007, 2008, 2009a, 2009b. Wheelock et al., 2009, De Souza et al., 2010]. Systems biology should provide with a complete and definitive view of a biomedical problem [Barabasi et al., 2011] but there are some problems associated that need to be solved. For example, just to integrate all the data it has to be considered that response time after a stimulus is not the same in transcripts, proteins or metabolites. Also, fold change in metabolite levels does not have to mimic changes in mRNA or protein levels.

4. Conclusion

In conclusion, the future of metabolomics is now. It is clear that metabolomics can be applied to various cardiovascular related diseases, although its clinical value in different settings remains to be determined; this is the next big challenge in the field.

Metabolomics, being a high throughput methodology is very well suited for biomarker discovery. The detection of biomolecules is an established methodology in the everyday clinical practice thus once a new biomarker has been found its application to the clinic should be straight forward. In our opinion, this approach will be successful in the sort term if it is able to address specific and relevant clinical situations.

Also, efforts should focus on the integration of metabolomics with systems biology analysis as in the long term, for the success of personalized medicine, the treatment of diseases will give way to the treatment of patients each with individual co-morbidities and environment. How well the integration of systems biology is archived will define the future not only of metabolomics but of all the 'omics' approaches.

5. Acknowledgment

This work has been founded by the Spanish ministry of Science SAF-2008-03067 and Instituto de Salud Carlos III, RECAVA DR06/0014/0025. I Barba is recipient of a Ramón y Cajal Fellowship.

6. References

Abozguia K, Clarke K, Lee L, Frenneaux M. (2006) Modification of myocardial substrate use as a therapy for heart failure. Nat Clin Pract Cardiovasc Med. Sep;3(9):490-8

Albert R, Jeong H, Barabasi AL. (2000) Error and attack tolerance of complex networks. Nature. Jul 27;406(6794):378-82.

Andreadou I, Papaefthimiou M, Zira A, Constantinou M, Sigala F, Skaltsounis AL, Tsantili-Kakoulidou A, Iliodromitis EK, Kremastinos DT, Mikros E. (2009) Metabonomic identification of novel biomarkers in doxorubicin cardiotoxicity and protective effect of the natural antioxidant oleuropein. NMR Biomed. Jul;22(6):585-92.

Ardenkjaer-Larsen JH, Fridlund B, Gram A, Hansson G, Hansson L, Lerche MH, Servin R, Thaning M, Golman K. (2003) Increase in signal-to-noise ratio of > 10,000 times in liquid-state NMR. Proc Natl Acad Sci U S A. Sep 2;100(18):10158-63.

Ashrafian H, Docherty L, Leo V, Towlson C, Neilan M, Steeples V, Lygate CA, Hough T, Townsend S, Williams D, Wells S, Norris D, Glyn-Jones S, Land J, Barbaric I, Lalanne Z, Denny P, Szumska D, Bhattacharya S, Griffin JL, Hargreaves I, Fernandez-Fuentes N, Cheeseman M, Watkins H, Dear TN. (2010) A mutation in the mitochondrial fission gene Dnm1l leads to cardiomyopathy. PLoS Genet. Jun 24;6(6):e1001000

Atherton HJ, Gulston MK, Bailey NJ, Cheng KK, Zhang W, Clarke K, Griffin JL. (2009) Metabolomics of the interaction between PPAR-alpha and age in the PPAR-alpha-null mouse. Mol Syst Biol. 5:259.

Barabási AL, Gulbahce N, Loscalzo J. (2011) Network medicine: a network-based approach to human disease. Nat Rev Genet. Jan;12(1):56-68.

Barba I, Jaimez-Auguets E, Rodriguez-Sinovas A, Garcia-Dorado D. (2007) 1H NMR-based metabolomic identification of at-risk areas after myocardial infarction in swine. MAGMA. Dec;20(5-6):265-71

Barba I, de León G, Martín E, Cuevas A, Aguade S, Candell-Riera J, Barrabés JA, Garcia-Dorado D. (2008) Nuclear magnetic resonance-based metabolomics predicts exercise-induced ischemia in patients with suspected coronary artery disease. Magn Reson Med. Jul;60(1):27-32.

Bollard ME, Stanley EG, Lindon JC, Nicholson JK, Holmes E. (2005) NMR-based metabonomic approaches for evaluating physiological influences on biofluid composition. NMR Biomed. 18:143–162

Bothwell JH, Griffin JL. (2011) An introduction to biological nuclear magnetic resonance spectroscopy. Biol Rev Camb Philos Soc. May;86(2):493-510.

Brindle JT, Antti H, Holmes E, Tranter G, Nicholson JK, Bethell HW, Clarke S, Schofield PM, McKilligin E, Mosedale DE, Grainger DJ. (2002) Rapid and noninvasive diagnosis of the presence and severity of coronary heart disease using 1H-NMR-based metabonomics. Nat Med. Dec;8(12):1439-44.

Brindle KM. (2003) Metabolomics. Pandora's box or Aladdin's cave? The biochemist. February.

Cascante M, Boros LG, Comin-Anduix B, de Atauri P, Centelles JJ, Lee PW. (2002) Metabolic control analysis in drug discovery and disease. Nat Biotechnol. Mar;20(3):243-9.

Clark AL, Poole-Wilson PA, Coats AJ. (1996) Exercise limitation in chronic heart failure: central role of the periphery. J Am Coll Cardiol. Nov 1;28(5):1092-10

Clayton TA, Lindon JC, Cloarec O, Antti H, Charuel C, Hanton G, Provost JP, Le Net JL, Baker D, Walley RJ, Everett JR, Nicholson JK. (2006) Pharmaco-metabonomic phenotyping and personalized drug treatment. Nature. Apr 20;440(7087):1073-7.

Constantinou MA, Tsantili-Kakoulidou A, Andreadou I, Iliodromitis EK, Kremastinos DT, Mikros E. (2007) Application of NMR-based metabonomics in the investigation of myocardial ischemia-reperfusion, ischemic preconditioning and antioxidant intervention in rabbits. Eur J Pharm Sci. Mar;30(3-4):303-14.

De Souza AI, Cardin S, Wait R, Chung YL, Vijayakumar M, Maguy A, Camm AJ, Nattel S. (2010) Proteomic and metabolomic analysis of atrial profibrillatory remodelling in congestive heart failure. J Mol Cell Cardiol. Nov;49(5):851-63.

Duarte NC, Becker SA, Jamshidi N, Thiele I, Mo ML, Vo TD, Srivas R, Palsson BØ. (2007) Global reconstruction of the human metabolic network based on genomic and bibliomic data. Proc Natl Acad Sci U S A. Feb 6;104(6):1777-82.

Dunn WB, Broadhurst DI, Atherton HJ, Goodacre R, Griffin JL. (2011) Systems level studies of mammalian metabolomes: the roles of mass spectrometry and nuclear magnetic resonance spectroscopy. Chem Soc Rev. Jan;40(1):387-426.

Ellis DI, Dunn WB, Griffin JL, Allwood JW, Goodacre R. (2007) Metabolic fingerprinting as a diagnostic tool Pharmacogenomics. Sep;8(9):1243-66.

Fiehn O. (2002) Metabolomics--the link between genotypes and phenotypes. Plant Mol Biol. Jan;48(1-2):155-71

Freedman DS, Otvos JD, Jeyarajah EJ, Shalaurova I, Cupples LA, Parise H, D'Agostino RB, Wilson PW, Schaefer EJ. (2004) Sex and age differences in lipoprotein subclasses measured by nuclear magnetic resonance spectroscopy: the Framingham Study. Clin Chem. Jul;50(7):1189-200.

Gallagher FA, Kettunen MI, Day SE, Hu DE, Ardenkjaer-Larsen JH, Zandt R, Jensen PR, Karlsson M, Golman K, Lerche MH, Brindle KM (2008) Magnetic resonance imaging of pH in vivo using hyperpolarized 13C-labelled bicarbonate. Nature. Jun 12;453(7197):940-3.

Golman K, Petersson JS, Magnusson P, Johansson E, Akeson P, Chai CM, Hansson G, Månsson S. (2008) Cardiac metabolism measured noninvasively by hyperpolarized 13C MRI. Magn Reson Med. May;59(5):1005-13.

Goodacre R. (2007) Metabolomics of a superorganism. J Nutr. Jan;137(1 Suppl):259S-266S.

Griffin JL, Sang E, Evens T, Davies K, Clarke K. (2002) Metabolic profiles of dystropyn and utrophyn expressuion in mouse models of Duchenne muscular dystrophy. FEBS Letters, 26618 1-8.

Griffin JL. (2003) Metabonomics: NMR spectroscopy and pattern recognition analysis of body fluids and tissues for characterisation of xenobiotic toxicity and disease diagnosis. Curr Opin Chem Biol. Oct;7(5):648-54

Griffin JL, Nicholls AW. (2006) Metabolomicsas a functional genomic tool for understanding lipid dysfunction in diabetes, obesity and related disorders. Pharmacogenomics. Oct;7(7):1095-107

Griffin JL, Des Rosiers C. (2009) Applications of metabolomics and proteomics to the mdx mouse model of Duchenne muscular dystrophy: lessons from downstream of the transcriptome. Genome Med. Mar 25;1(3):32.

Hotelling, H. Analysis of a complex of statistical variables into principal components. Journal of Educational Psychology, Vol 24(6), 1933, 417-441

Inserte J, Molla B, Aguilar R, Través PG, Barba I, Martín-Sanz P, Boscá L, Casado M, Garcia-Dorado D. (2009) Constitutive COX-2 activity in cardiomyocytes confers permanent cardioprotection Constitutive COX-2 expression and cardioprotection. J Mol Cell Cardiol. Feb;46(2):160-8.

Jeong H, Tombor B, Albert R, Oltvai ZN, Barabási AL. (2000) The large-scale organization of metabolic networks. Nature. Oct 5;407(6804):651-4.

Jones GL, Sang E, Goddard C, Mortishire-Smith RJ, Sweatman BC, Haselden JN, Davies K, Grace AA, Clarke K, Griffin JL. (2005) A functional analysis of mouse models of cardiac disease through metabolic profiling. J Biol Chem. Mar 4;280(9): 7530-9.

Kang SM, Park JC, Shin MJ, Lee H, Oh J, Ryu do H, Hwang GS, Chung JH. (2011) H nuclear magnetic resonance based metabolic urinary profiling of patients with ischemic heart failure. Clin Biochem. Mar;44(4):293-9

Kell DB. (2004) Metabolomics and systems biology: making sense of the soup. Curr Opin Microbiol. Jun;7(3):296-307.

Kirschenlohr HL, Griffin JL, Clarke SC, Rhydwen R, Grace AA, Schofield PM, Brindle KM, Metcalfe JC. (2006) Proton NMR analysis of plasma is a weak predictor of coronary artery disease. Nat Med. Jun;12(6):705-10.

Lee L, Campbell R, Scheuermann-Freestone M, Taylor R, Gunaruwan P, Williams L, Ashrafian H, Horowitz J, Fraser AG, Clarke K, Frenneaux M. (2005) Metabolic modulation with perhexiline in chronic heart failure: a randomized, controlled trial of short-term use of a novel treatment. Circulation. Nov 22;112(21):3280-8

Lewis GD, Wei R, Liu E, Yang E, Shi X, Martinovic M, Farrell L, Asnani A, Cyrille M, Ramanathan A, Shaham O, Berriz G, Lowry PA, Palacios IF, Taşan M, Roth FP, Min J, Baumgartner C, Keshishian H, Addona T, Mootha VK, Rosenzweig A, Carr SA, Fifer MA, Sabatine MS, Gerszten RE. (2008) Metabolite profiling of blood from individuals undergoing planned myocardial infarction reveals early markers of myocardial injury. J Clin Invest. Oct;118(10):3503-12.

Loscalzo J, Kohane I, Barabasi AL. (2007) Human disease classification in the postgenomic era: a complex systems approach to human pathobiology. Mol Syst Biol. 3:124.

Mayr M, Madhu B, Xu Q. (2007) Proteomics and metabolomics combined in cardiovascular research. Trends Cardiovasc Med. Feb;17(2):43-8.

Mayr M, Grainger D, Mayr U, Leroyer AS, Leseche G, Sidibe A, Herbin O, Yin X, Gomes A, Madhu B, Griffiths JR, Xu Q, Tedgui A, Boulanger CM. (2009a) Proteomics, metabolomics, and immunomics on microparticles derived from human atherosclerotic plaques. Circ Cardiovasc Genet. Aug;2(4):379-88

Mayr M, Liem D, Zhang J, Li X, Avliyakulov NK, Yang JI, Young G, Vondriska TM, Ladroue C, Madhu B, Griffiths JR, Gomes A, Xu Q, Ping P. (2009b) Proteomic and metabolomic analysis of cardioprotection: Interplay between protein kinase C epsilon and delta in regulating glucose metabolism of murine hearts. J Mol Cell Cardiol. Feb;46(2):268-77.

Mendes P, Kell DB, Westerhoff HW. (1996) Why and when channelling can decrease pool size at constant net flux in a simple dynamic channel. BBA 1289, 2, 175-186

Müller G. (2010) Personalized prognosis and diagnosis of type 2 diabetes--vision or fiction? Pharmacology. 85(3):168-87.

Nicholson JK, Lindon JC, Holmes E. (1999) 'Metabonomics': understanding the metabolic responses of living systems to pathophysiological stimuli via multivariate statistical analysis of biological NMR spectroscopic data. Xenobiotica. Nov;29(11):1181-9

Nicholson JK, Lindon JC. (2008) Systems biology: Metabonomics. Nature. Oct 23;455(7216):1054-6.

Nicholson JK, Wilson ID, Lindon JC. (2011) Pharmacometabonomics as an effector for personalized medicine. Pharmacogenomics. Jan;12(1):103-11

Oh JE, Krapfenbauer K, Fountoulakis M, Frischer T, Lubec G. (2004) Evidence for the existence of hypothetical proteins in human bronchial epithelial, fibroblast, amnion, lymphocyte, mesothelial and kidney cell lines. Amino Acids. Feb;26(1):9-18.

Perrine SA, Michaels MS, Ghoddoussi F, Hyde EM, Tancer ME, Galloway MP. (2009) Cardiac effects of MDMA on the metabolic profile determined with 1H-magnetic resonance spectroscopy in the rat. NMR Biomed. May;22(4):419-25.

Raamsdonk LM, Teusink B, Broadhurst D, Zhang N, Hayes A, Walsh MC, Berden JA, Brindle KM, Kell DB, Rowland JJ,Westerhoff HV, van Dam K, Oliver SG. (2001) A functional genomics strategy that uses metabolome data to reveal the phenotype of silent mutations. Nat Biotechnol. Jan;19(1):45-50.

Rodriguez-Sinovas A, Sanchez JA, Gonzalez-Loyola A, Barba I, Morente M, Aguilar R, Agullo E, Miro-Casas E, Esquerda E, Ruiz-Meana M, Garcia-Dorado D. (2010) Effects of substitution of Cx43 by Cx32 on myocardial energy metabolism tolerance to ischemia and preconditioning protection. J Physiol. Apr 1;588(Pt 7):1139-51

Sabatine MS, Liu E, Morrow DA, Heller E, McCarroll R, Wiegand R, Berriz GF, Roth FP, Gerszten RE. (2005) Metabolomic identification of novel biomarkers of myocardial ischemia. Circulation. Dec 20;112(25):3868-75.

Sauer U, Heinemann M, Zamboni N. (2007) Genetics. Getting closer to the whole picture. Science. Apr 27;316(5824):550-1.

Schroeder MA, Atherton HJ, Ball DR, Cole MA, Heather LC, Griffin JL, Clarke K, Radda GK, Tyler DJ. (2009) Real-time assessment of Krebs cycle metabolism using hyperpolarized 13C magnetic resonance spectroscopy. FASEB J. Aug;23(8):2529-38.

Schroeder MA, Swietach P, Atherton HJ, Gallagher FA, Lee P, Radda GK, Clarke K, Tyler DJ. (2010) Measuring intracellular pH in the heart using hyperpolarized carbon dioxide and bicarbonate: a 13C and 31P magnetic resonance spectroscopy study. Cardiovasc Res. Apr 1;86(1):82-91.

Schroeder MA, Atherton HJ, Heather LC, Griffin JL, Clarke K, Radda GK, Tyler DJ (2011) Determining the in vivo regulation of cardiac pyruvate dehydrogenase based on label flux from hyperpolarised [1-(13) C]pyruvate. NMR Biomed. Mar 8. doi: 10.1002/nbm.1668.

Spratlin JL, Serkova NJ, Eckhardt SG. (2009) Clinical Applications of Metabolomics in Oncology: A Review Clin Cancer Res; 15, 2009

Sreekumar A, Poisson LM, Rajendiran TM, Khan AP, Cao Q, Yu J, Laxman B, Mehra R, Lonigro RJ, Li Y, Nyati MK, Ahsan A, Kalyana-Sundaram S, Han B, Cao X, Byun J, Omenn GS, Ghosh D, Pennathur S, Alexander DC, Berger A, Shuster JR, Wei JT, Varambally S, Beecher C, Chinnaiyan AM. (2009) Metabolomic profiles delineate potential role for sarcosine in prostate cancer progression. Nature. Feb 12;457(7231):910-4.

Sundgren PC, Nagesh V, Elias A, Tsien C, Junck L, Gomez Hassan DM, Lawrence TS, Chenevert TL, Rogers L, McKeever P, Cao Y. (2009) Metabolic alterations: a biomarker for radiation-induced normal brain injury-an MR spectroscopy study. J Magn Reson Imaging. Feb;29(2):291-7.

van de Woestijne AP, Monajemi H, Kalkhoven E, Visseren FL. (2011) Adipose tissue dysfunction and hypertriglyceridemia: mechanisms and management. Obes Rev. Jul 12. doi: 10.1111/j.1467-789X.2011.00900.x

Wang TJ, Larson MG, Vasan RS, Cheng S, Rhee EP, McCabe E, Lewis GD, Fox CS, Jacques PF, Fernandez C, O'Donnell CJ, Carr SA, Mootha VK, Florez JC, Souza A, Melander O, Clish CB, Gerszten RE. (2011) Metabolite profiles and the risk of developing diabetes. Nat Med. Apr;17(4):448-53

Weckwerth W, Morgenthal K. (2005) Metabolomics: from pattern recognition to biological interpretation. Drug Discov Today. Nov 15;10(22):1551-8

Wheelock CE, Wheelock AM, Kawashima S, Diez D, Kanehisa M, van Erk M, Kleemann R, Haeggström JZ, Goto S. (2009) Systems biology approaches and pathway tools for investigating cardiovascular disease. Mol Biosyst. Jun;5(6):588-602.

Xia J, Psychogios N, Young N, Wishart DS. (2009) "MetaboAnalyst: a web server for metabolomic data analysis and interpretation" Nucleic Acids Research 37(Web Server issue):W652-W660

11

Novel Regulators of Low-Density Lipoprotein Receptor and Circulating LDL-C for the Prevention and Treatment of Coronary Artery Disease

Guoqing Cao, Robert J. Konrad,
Mark C. Kowala and Jian Wang
Lilly Research Laboratories, Indianapolis, Indiana, USA

1. Introduction

Low-density lipoprotein cholesterol (LDL-C) is a major risk factor for atherosclerosis and coronary artery disease (CAD). The role of LDL-C in CAD has been established through experimental studies, epidemiological and genetic studies and the elucidation of the low-density lipoprotein receptor (LDLR) pathway (Brown and Goldstein, 1986). LDLR deficient mice develop frank hypercholesterolemia and atherosclerosis on western diet (Ishibashi et al., 1994). In humans, people with low LDL-C have very low risk of developing CAD and plasma LDL-C is positively associated with CAD (Stamler et al., 2000). Mutations in LDLR in humans form the molecular basis for familial hypercholesterolemia and patients with this disease develop premature CAD (Hobbs et al., 1990). Statins are a class of small molecule compounds that inhibit HMG-CoA reductase, a rate-limiting enzyme in cholesterol biosynthesis, thereby reducing LDL-C in humans. Statins effectively reduce LDL-C and the associated cardiovascular disease risk by about 30%, but residual risks for developing cardiovascular disease remain. In recent years, clinical studies have suggested that further lower circulating LDL-C is closely associated with additional reduction of cardiovascular risk. The majority of the high risk patients often fail to reach their LDL-C goal, and thus, novel targets and medications are highly desirable for the prevention and treatment of cardiovascular disorders. In the last few years, novel regulators of LDLR and/or circulating LDL-C have emerged that suggest potentially more therapeutic opportunities. These include proprotein convertase subtilisin/kexin type 9 (PCSK9) and the inducible degrader of LDLR (Idol) that regulate LDLR and LDL-C levels. Novel therapeutic modalities thus may provide additional clinical options to further reduce LDL-C and cardiovascular disease risk.

2. Cholesterol homeostasis and the management of cholesterol

While cholesterol is an essential component of cellular membranes, excessive cholesterol is detrimental to cells. Accordingly, the cellular cholesterol level is tightly controlled through intricate regulatory mechanisms. The steady state cholesterol level is dictated by cholesterol biosynthesis, cellular cholesterol uptake, and cholesterol efflux. The cholesterol biosynthetic pathway involves more than 30 enzymes to make cholesterol from acetyl-CoA, while cholesterol uptake is primarily mediated by the receptor-mediated endocytosis. Cholesterol carried in LDL particles is readily taken up by its cognitive plasma membrane receptor, LDLR. Cholesterol is delivered eventually to the lysosomal compartment, and LDLRs either recycle back to plasma membrane or are degraded in lysosomes. Cholesterol efflux is mediated by ATP-binding cassette transporters (ABC proteins). ABCA1 primarily mediates apolipoprotein AI dependent cholesterol efflux while ABCG1 is largely responsible for apolipoprotein E/high-density lipoprotein (HDL) particle mediated cholesterol efflux. Cholesterol biosynthesis and LDLR levels are feedback-regulated by sterol-responsive element binding protein 2 (SREBP2) (Goldstein et al., 2006), while ABCA1/ABCG1 are both regulated through liver X receptors (LXRs) (Cao et al., 2004).

Physiologically, the circulating LDL-C concentration is determined by the rate of LDL-C production and its clearance. Very low-density lipoprotein (VLDL) particles are assembled and secreted from liver and are converted to LDL particles in circulation through triglyceride lipolysis by lipoprotein lipase (LPL). Proteins involved in this process are intimately related to the rate of VLDL secretion and contribute to circulating LDL-C levels. For instance, apolipoprotein B (apoB) deficiency leads to impaired VLDL assembly and secretion, and accordingly very low levels of plasma cholesterol. LDL particle clearance is primarily mediated through hepatic LDLR, and thus proteins or other agents that affect liver LDLR levels greatly impact LDL-C. In hypercholesterolemic patients, dysfunctional LDLR results in increased circulating LDL-C and premature coronary artery disease.

LDL-C is a major cardiovascular risk factor that has been established through epidemiological, genetic, and pharmacological studies. Statins are small molecule inhibitors of the rate-limiting enzyme HMG-CoA reductase in the cholesterol biosynthetic pathway. Statins reduce intracellular cholesterol and increase hepatic LDLR levels through the feedback mechanism of SREBP2 activation. Statins decrease circulating LDL-C by 20-50% in humans and effectively reduce cardiovascular risk by approximately 30%. Additionally, the cholesterol absorption inhibitor ezetimibe inhibits an intestinal epithelial membrane protein Niemann-Pick C1-Like 1 (NPC1L1) to reduce cholesterol absorption and accordingly lowers LDL-C by about 20% in humans. The cardiovascular risk reduction from ezetimibe, however, is yet to be proven in clinical studies.

In recent years, it has been found that additional reduction of LDL-C has been associated with further reduced cardiovascular risk, suggesting a strategy of "the lower, the better" for cardiovascular disease prevention and treatment (O'Keefe et al., 2004). However, LDL-C lowering efficacy is limited by statins, since doubling the dose of statins typically results in only an additional 6% reduction in LDL-C, a so-called "6% rule". As a result, many patients cannot achieve their cholesterol goal. Additionally, in high risk patients, an LDL-C of 50-70 mg/dl is recommended, which poses more challenges for patients and physicians to achieve this goal. Novel therapeutic modalities are thus highly desirable. The recent discoveries of novel regulators of LDL-C therefore provide new opportunities for such development and will be reviewed in this chapter.

3. PCSK9

3.1 Cell biology, biochemistry, and physiology of PCSK9

Proprotein subtilisin kexin type 9 (PCSK9) was originally named NARC-1 for neural apoptosis-regulated convertase 1 and was found expressed in hepatocytes, kidney mesenchymal cells, intestinal and colon epithelial cells and brain telencephalen neurons (Seidah et al., 2003). PCSK9 belongs to and is the ninth member of the proprotein convertase family that also includes S1P/SKI-1, an essential serine protease that cleaves SREBPs within the luminal region of the endoplasmic reticulum (ER). PCSK9 encodes a protein of 692 amino acids whose structure includes a signal peptide at its amino terminus, followed by a prodomain, catalytic domain, and carboxyl terminal cysteine and histidine rich domain of unknown function (Horton et al., 2009) (Figure 1). PCSK9 is synthesized as a proprotein/zymogen, and the prodomain of PCSK9 is self-cleaved between glutamine 152 and serine 153 producing a prodomain fragment of 14 kD. After self-cleavage, the prodomain remains associated with the catalytic domain to form a non-covalent protein complex. The protein complex is about 74 kD, and in a denaturing polyacrylamide gel electrophoresis (PAGE) system, two fragments of 60 kD (mature protein) and 14 kD (prodomain) are observed. The association of the prodomain with the rest of the catalytic domain is fairly tight, and as a result, catalytic activity is completely inhibited by the presence of the prodomain (Horton et al., 2009). The details of the molecular basis of the protein complex have been described in recent reports that elaborated the crystal structure of the protein complex (Kwon et al., 2008). PCSK9 is glycosylated at Asn 533 and Tyr-sulfated at Tyr 38, but mutants without glycosylation and sulfation retain their secretion and function in degrading LDLR. PCSK9 is also phosphorylated at Ser 47 and 688. Loss of phosphorylation at Ser 47 leads to increased degradation of PCSK9, suggesting its potential role in regulating PCSK9 protein levels and function (Dewpura et al., 2008).

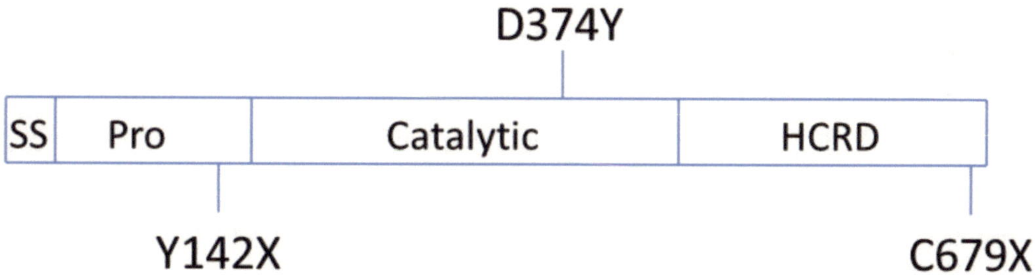

Fig. 1. Domain structure of PCSK9. SS, signal sequence; Pro, prodomain; catalytic, catalytic domain; CHRD, Cys/His rich domain. The gain-of-function mutation D374Y and the two loss-of-function mutations were highlighted.

The amino terminal signal sequence serves to lead the protein into the endoplasmic reticulum and the secretory pathway. The prodomain serves in general as an inhibitor of the mature, catalytic domain before it is cleaved. In PCSK9, however, the prodomain continues to serve as an inhibitory factor even after its auto-processing from the catalytic domain in a non-covalent fashion. This implies that the catalytic activity is either regulated and activated at some specific physiological condition or is not essential for the function. Indeed, in an important paper, Horton and colleagues reported making a secreted form of catalytically inactive mutant PCSK9 through transexpression of both the prodomain and the catalytic domain and showed that the catalytically inactive mutants were able to degrade cellular LDLR proteins (McNutt et al., 2007). This elegant work along with the reports from other laboratories indicates that the protease activity of PCSK9 is not essential for its physiological function. In addition, it was observed recently that the acidic stretch within the prodomain functions to inhibit PCSK9 degradation of LDLR. Deletion of these acidic residues further increases PCSK9 protein binding to LDLR (Benjannet et al., 2010).

The carboxyl terminus of PCSK9 contains a Cys and His rich domain, the function of which is not well understood. This domain is speculated to be important for protein interaction, and it was recently reported that the carboxyl terminus of PCSK9 binds annexin A2, but not closely related annexin A1. Annexin A2 co-localizes with PCSK9 at the cellular surface and serves to inhibit PCSK9 function in degrading LDLR (Mayer et al., 2008). This speculated role of annexin A2 is consistent with the observation that some monoclonal antibodies with epitopes against the carboxyl terminus of PCSK9 inhibit PCSK9 function (Ni et al., 2010), possibly through mimicking annexin A2 function.

PCSK9 binds to the EGFA domain of the extracellular portion of LDLR, and the binding affinity increases by more than 50-fold when the pH is reduced to 5.5 (Zhang et al., 2007). Upon binding to LDLR, the PCSK9/LDLR complex undergoes receptor mediated endocytosis and traffics to the endosomal compartment, where an acidic environment facilitates tighter binding of the two proteins. This increased affinity between the two proteins presumably results in the escorting of LDLR to lysosomal degradation instead of recycling back to plasma membrane (Lagace et al., 2006; Qian et al., 2007). LDLR and PCSK9 co-localize to endosomal/lysosomal compartments, and the binding of two proteins have been studied in detail with the resolution of co-crystal structure of PCSK9 and the EGFA domain (Kwon et al., 2008). EGFA binds to the catalytic domain of PCSK9 (Figure 2).

While its potential physiological role was initially speculated in neuronal cell differentiation and development, it was found later through primarily human genetic studies that PCSK9 plays a major role in regulating hepatic LDLR protein levels and thus circulating LDL-C in humans (Abifadel et al., 2009; Abifadel et al., 2003). In addition to the potential role of degrading LDLR intracellularly, secreted PCSK9 protein is functional in degrading cellular and hepatic LDLR and thus elevates LDL-C *in vivo*. Recombinant PCSK9 protein, when added to cell cultures, dose dependently reduces total cellular LDLR protein and cell surface LDLR levels. This results in reduced LDL particle uptake into the cells as evaluated by a fluorescent labeled LDL particle uptake assay. The half-maximum effective concentration (EC_{50}) is achieved at 0.8 μg/ml. When injected into wild type mice intravenously, PCSK9 decreased primarily hepatic LDLR protein levels and increased circulating LDL-C, as evaluated by fast protein liquid chromatography (FPLC) (Qian et al., 2007). When used at the pharmacological levels, PCSK9 appears to degrade LDLR in other tissues as well (Schmidt et al., 2008). When grossly over expressed in mouse liver through adenovirus, PCSK9 dramatically reduces hepatic LDLR protein levels. Circulating LDL-C is thus elevated to a level similar to that seen in LDLR deficient mice (Maxwell and Breslow, 2004). Conversely, PCSK9 deficient mice have a significant increase in hepatic LDLR protein levels.

Importantly, statin treatment of PCSK9 deficient mice further augmented the liver LDLR protein levels, demonstrating the additive effects of PCSK9 deficiency and statin treatment on LDLR protein expression (Rashid et al., 2005).

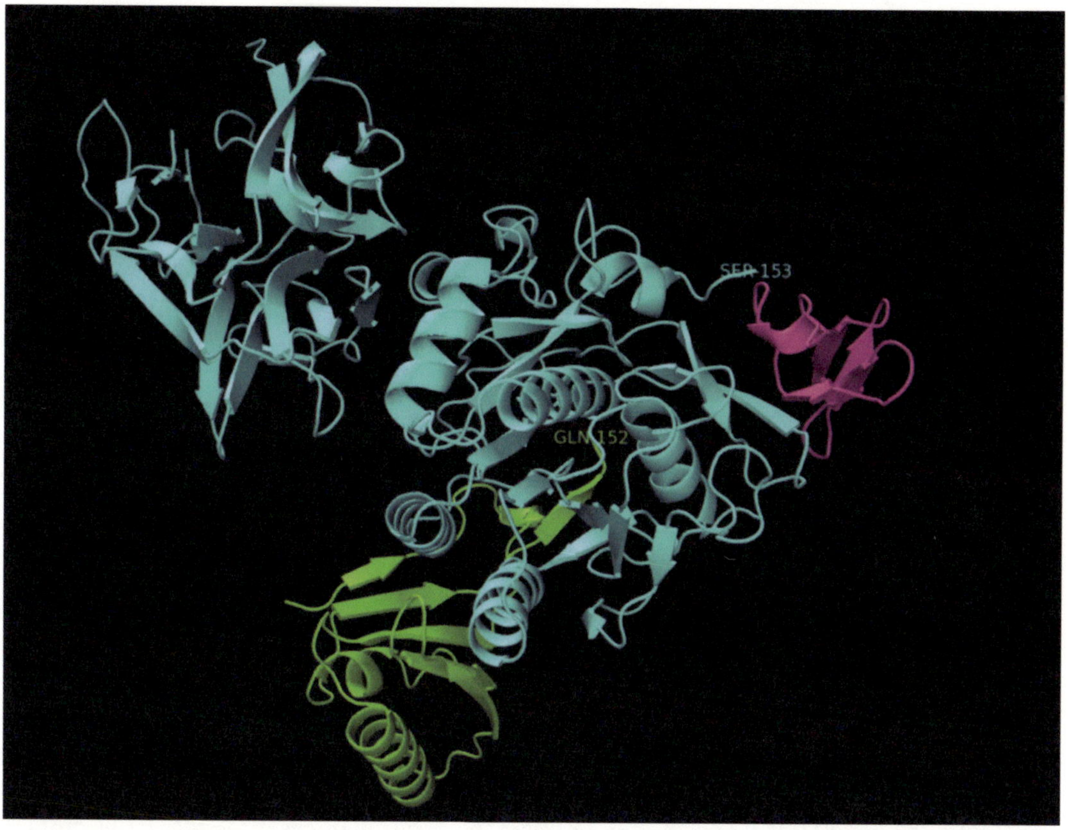

Fig. 2. Co-crystal structure of PCSK9 and EGFA domain of LDLR. Green, prodomain. Blue catalytic and CHRD. Purple, EGFA. Gln152 and Ser153 were labeled (Courtesy of Dr. Yong Wang and Dr. Yue-Wei Qian).

Besides the well-documented role of PCSK9 in regulating circulating LDL-C primarily through LDLR, a proposed role for PCSK9 in VLDL secretion has been suggested. It appears that increased PCSK9 levels through adenoviral expression in mice accelerates the VLDL secretion rate while PCSK9 deficiency in mice reduces postprandial hypertriglyceridemia. These observations, however, were not substantiated by reports from other labs and remain controversial. Beyond LDLR as the substrate for PCSK9, some *in vitro* data indicate that very low-density lipoprotein receptor (VLDLR) and apolipoprotein E receptor 2 (apoER2), two proteins that share about 60% homology with LDLR, can be substrates for PCSK9 as well (Poirier et al., 2008). VLDLR is primarily expressed in heart, muscle, and adipose tissue and possibly plays a role in mobilizing triglyceride (TG) from VLDL to these tissues as the energy source. The role of PCSK9 in regulating VLDLR implies a role in regulating energy homeostasis in muscle, heart, and fat. Indeed, a recent study reported increased fat mass in

PCSK9 deficient mice and increased cell surface VLDLR receptor expression in adipose tissue. Conversely, hepatic PCSK9 expression dramatically reduced VLDLR in adipose tissue (Roubtsova et al., 2011). ApoER2 is primarily expressed in brain and is speculated to play a major role in neuronal differentiation and brain development. Regulation of apoER2 by PCSK9 suggests its potential role in brain development and function. In zebra fish, PCSK9 deficiency leads to impaired brain development. In mice, PCSK9 reduces LDLR during brain development and ischemic stroke, whereas in adult mice, LDLR protein levels in the brain are similar in wild type and PCSK9 deficient mice (Liu et al., 2010; Rousselet et al., 2011).

3.2 Human genetics, physiology, and regulation of PCSK9

PCSK9 was cloned as the ninth member of the proprotein convertase family. Its potential role in cholesterol homeostasis was discovered through human genetic studies. In 2003, through extensive genetic mapping studies, mutations in PCSK9 were discovered and reported as the third locus for autosomal dominant familial hypercholesterolemia (ADH) in addition to the well-established loci of apoB and LDLR in this disease (Abifadel et al., 2003). Following the original study, many mutations or polymorphisms within PCSK9 have been reported. These have been categorized into gain-of-function (GOF) mutations, loss-of-function (LOF) mutations, or polymorphisms that result in either elevated or reduced circulating LDL-C levels in humans (Abifadel et al., 2009).

The molecular basis for most GOF mutants is not clear at the moment. However, a D374Y mutation, which was originally described in an Anglo-Saxon family, led to a more severe clinical hypercholesterolemic phenotype than other heterozygous GOF mutations of PCSK9 or LDLR mutations, and is associated with a very early onset of coronary artery disease. Asp374 of PCSK9 is intimately involved in EGFA domain binding as was revealed by the co-crystal structure of PCSK9 and the EGFA domain. The D374Y mutation results in a conformational change that enables PCSK9 to bind LDLR more tightly (Kwon et al., 2008). In cultured cells, the D374Y mutant demonstrated a more than a 10-fold increase in potency in degrading cellular LDLR proteins, highlighting the molecular basis for this GOF mutant (McNutt et al., 2007). Even the plasma level of PCSK9 is decreased in patients carrying this mutation, which probably reflects its tight binding to LDLR and faster clearance through receptor-mediated endocytosis. It is conceivable that such an increase in affinity towards LDLR would dramatically increase LDLR degradation. Indeed, in heterozygous carriers of this mutation, statin use actually worsens the hypercholesterolemia. This occurs presumably as a result of statins inducing more D374Y mutant PCSK9, which significantly reduces hepatic LDLR proteins. In a transgenic mouse model, PCSK9 D374Y mutant significantly elevated plasma LDL-C and led to a more accelerated development of atherosclerosis under hypercholesterolemic conditions (Herbert et al., 2010).

Contrary to the GOF mutations, LOF mutants were found at a relatively high frequency in humans. The combined incidence of LOF mutations of a Y142X mutant, which encodes a truncated protein and a C679X mutant, that leads to lack of protein secretion, was 2.6% in blacks in the ARIC (Atherosclerosis Risk In Communities) study. The two heterozygous LOF mutants in blacks resulted in a 28% lower plasma LDL-C and an 88% reduction in CAD risk. The R46L mutation, which results in reduced secretory efficiency and lower plasma protein levels, was present in 3.2% whites in the ARIC study and was associated with a 47% reduction in CAD risk (Cohen et al., 2006). These data suggest that the life-long reduction in LDL-C appears to have greater benefit in CAD risk reduction than drug therapy, thus highlighting the potential benefit of reducing LDL-C at an early stage of the disease progression for CAD prevention.

Circulating PCSK9 is largely produced hepatically based on the liver-specific PCSK9 knockout mouse studies, although it is also expressed in intestines and kidney. Circulating PCSK9 exists either in the form of the 74 kD complex or can be further cleaved by furin at Arg 218 to result in a truncated, inactive form of PCSK9 (Benjannet et al., 2006; Konrad et al., 2011). The ELISA method our labs have been using detects both the wild type and the furin cleaved forms. The circulating PCSK9 levels in humans vary significantly and the average level is estimated around 100-500 ng/ml. Not surprisingly, circulating PCSK9 levels are significantly associated with total cholesterol and LDL-C, but not high-density lipoprotein cholesterol (Konrad et al., 2011). Although PCSK9 plays a critical role in regulating hepatic LDLR protein levels and plasma LDL-C, PCSK9 only explains about 7% of the variability in circulating LDL-C levels (Lakoski et al., 2009). In large population studies, PCSK9 is also associated with plasma TG, implying its possible role in VLDL metabolism as suggested by some of the studies in animal models. PCSK9 is positively associated with body mass index in these studies, which is not entirely consistent with the observation in PCSK9 deficient mice that increased visceral adipose mass was observed. Plasma PCSK9 is associated with plasma glucose levels, although the role of PCSK9 in glucose homeostasis has been controversial. Contradicting results have been reported from two different labs, suggesting that in PCSK9 deficient mice, there was either compromised or unchanged insulin sensitivity, as evaluated by an oral glucose tolerant test (Cui et al., 2010; Lakoski et al., 2009; Langhi et al., 2009; Mbikay et al., 2010).

PCSK9 is regulated by many physiological processes and pharmacological agents. The most prominent regulating factor is SREBP2. PCSK9 is a direct target gene of SREBP2, with a sterol-responsive element residing in its proximal region of its promoter. In cultured cells, statins inhibit cholesterol biosynthesis, reduce intracellular cholesterol levels, and activate SREBP2 and its target genes, including PCSK9. The parallel regulation of cholesterol biosynthesis, LDLR, and PCSK9 represents a complicated and intricate regulatory system to fine tune cholesterol homeostasis. In humans, statins significantly increase plasma PCSK9 levels, which attenuates statin efficacy (Careskey et al., 2007; Konrad et al., 2011). In this regard, therapeutic agents that inhibit PCSK9 expression or function will additively reduce LDL-C with statin therapy. The bile acid binding resin cholestyramine, expectedly increased circulating PCSK9 levels through accelerating the conversion of cholesterol to bile acid in liver and depleting hepatic cholesterol (Persson et al., 2010). Conversely, cholesterol or sterols in cultured cells repress SREBP2 activity and accordingly PCSK9 expression (Schmidt et al., 2006).

Circulating PCSK9 has a very distinct diurnal rhythm that peaks around 4:00 am and has a nadir from 4-9 pm with a fluctuation of 15% of its plasma levels. This diurnal rhythm is completely paralleled by the cholesterol biosynthesis surrogate lathosterol, suggesting that circulating PCSK9 is tightly controlled together with hepatic cholesterol biosynthesis (Persson et al., 2010). Although cholesterol biosynthesis fluctuates during the 24 hour shift, plasma cholesterol levels remain constant, and this may be achieved through paralleled expression of PCSK9, which implies a physiological role of PCSK9 in maintaining a constant plasma cholesterol level during the daily fluctuation of cholesterol biosynthesis (Persson et al., 2010). In animal models and humans, fasting reduces SREBP2 activity, and the plasma PCSK9 level is reduced accordingly. Re-feeding results in recovery of PCSK9 expression and circulating PCSK9 levels (Browning and Horton, 2010; Persson et al., 2010). PCSK9 is also reported to be regulated by insulin, LXRs, and the SREBP1c axis in cultured cells. Bile acids, on the other hand, reduce PCSK9 expression presumably through the farnesoid X receptor (Langhi et al., 2008). Fenofibrate reduces PCSK9 expression in cultured cells and in animal models. In the clinic, however, the majority of available data point to the fact that fibrates significantly elevate PCSK9 levels in both diabetic and non-diabetic subjects, which possibly attenuates fibrate effects in reducing LDL-C levels (Konrad et al., 2011). Berberine, a compound that reduces LDL-C in humans and is derived from a Chinese herb (Coptis sinensis), dramatically reduces PCSK9 mRNA and protein expression in cultured hepatoma cells (Cameron et al., 2008). PCSK9 is regulated by several hormones. In humans, females have higher circulating PCSK9 levels than males, and post-menopausal women have higher PCSK9 levels than premenopausal women (Cui et al., 2010; Lakoski et al., 2009). Estradiol reduces PCSK9 in rats but not in humans, while growth hormone significantly reduces PCSK9 levels in humans (Persson et al., 2010).

3.3 Therapeutic approaches to modulate PCSK9 expression and function

An effective therapy is based on a solid hypothesis and human validation. LDL-C as a major risk factor for CAD is firmly established, and in addition, genetic data from PCSK9 mutations in humans have provided the strongest validation to pursue PCSK9 modulators to either suppress its expression or inhibit its function. Furthermore, data collected in recent years indicate that the lower the LDL-C, the more CAD protection, thus PCSK9 also provides a unique opportunity for LDL-C lowering since statins increase PCSK9 in humans, which attenuates their efficacy. Thus, novel agents targeting PCSK9 that function in an additive fashion to statins are highly desirable and will be a valuable addition for physicians to effectively manage circulating LDL-C.

Anti-sense oligonucleotides (ASO) have been explored as a potential therapeutic agent for years, and recently an ASO against apoB has proven successful in phase III clinical studies that effectively reduced LDL-C. In mice, an ASO effectively reduced liver PCSK9 mRNA and thus its production, leading to significantly elevated hepatic LDLR levels (Graham et al., 2007). Recently, a new generation of ASO called locked nucleic acid (LNA) modified gap-mer antisense oligonucleotides has been developed. These LNA oligonucleotides are short in length, single stranded, and have high affinity towards mRNA and microRNA. LNAs are readily delivered in saline and have been shown to safely and potently inhibit mRNA targets in mice and humans. LNA against PCSK9 effectively reduced PCSK9 expression in cultured cells. In mice, LNA reduced PCSK9 expression by 60%, and the effect lasted more than two weeks. Hepatic LDLR levels were elevated by more than 2-fold (Gupta et al., 2010). These studies suggest that ASO or LNA have potential to reduce circulating LDL-C in humans through inhibiting PCSK9 expression. An LNA against PCSK9 is currently in phase I clinical studies.

A similar approach involves inhibiting PCSK9 expression through RNA interference. A small interfering RNA (siRNA) was delivered to animals through lipidoid nanoparticles.

Liver specific knockdown of PCSK9 in mice and rats reduced PCSK9 mRNA by 50-70% and reduced circulating cholesterol concentrations by 60%. In non-human primates, a single dose of siRNA targeting PCSK9 reduced plasma PCSK9 by more than 70% and caused an accompanying reduction of LDL-C by more than 50%. The reduced LDL-C only returned to baseline 21 days following the siRNA delivery (Frank-Kamenetsky et al., 2008). These data suggest that siRNA targeting of PCSK9 to reduce LDL-C is technically feasible and support the possibility of LDL-C lowering through suppressing PCSK9 expression. A clinical trial application for ALN-PCS, an RNAi therapeutic targeting PCSK9 for the treatment of severe hypercholesterolemia was filed recently.

An alternative approach is to inhibit PCSK9 function through developing monoclonal antibodies against PCSK9. PCSK9 functions through binding to EGFA domain of LDLR. Blocking the interaction of PCSK9 and LDLR is thus a promising approach. Indeed, a monoclonal antibody that blocks the interaction of PCSK9 and EGFA domain of LDLR blocked PCSK9 function and increased cellular LDLR protein levels in cultured cells. Notably, the effect of preserving LDLR protein level was further enhanced when cultured cells were treated with statins, suggesting the additive effect with statins (Chan et al., 2009). In a mouse model over expressing human PCSK9, this antibody reduced LDL-C significantly (Chan et al., 2009). In non-human primates, a single injection of the antibody at 3 mg/kg reduced LDL-C by 80% within one week of treatment, and the significant reduction of LDL-C was maintained more than 10 days after antibody administration (Chan et al., 2009). In humans, single dose administration through either intravenous or subcutaneous injection of a PCSK9 monoclonal antibody developed by Regeneron dose-dependently reduced LDL-C up to 60% (2011 The Deuel Conference on Lipids). This antibody is currently in phase II clinical trials.

A small molecule approach to inhibit PCSK9 function or its auto-catalytic processing has proven very challenging. However, it was reported that berberine, a natural product, dramatically reduced PCSK9 expression through transcriptional repression (Cameron et al., 2008; Li et al., 2009). While the mechanism is not entirely understood, this observation suggests the possibility that developing small molecule modulators to mediate PCSK9 expression is potentially viable.

PCSK9 appears to be a very safe target. While it was shown in zebra fish that PCSK9 is essential for brain development, PCSK9 deficient mice have appeared normal. In humans, compound heterozygous carriers for LOF mutations for PCSK9 who lack circulating PCSK9 have been reported. These individuals have very low levels of serum PCSK9 levels (below 20 mg/dl) but otherwise appear completely healthy. Thus, PCSK9 is a well validated target in humans for LDL-C reduction and CAD prevention and treatment.

4. The role of Idol in regulating LDLR

The inducible degrader of LDLR (Idol) was recently identified as another post-translational regulator of LDLR. Idol was originally cloned from neuronal cells as a myosin regulatory light chain (MRLC) interacting protein (Olsson et al., 1999), and named Mylip (or MIR). Mylip has a FERM (4.1 band, ezrin, radixin and moesin) at its amino terminal end and a RING zinc finger ubiquitin ligase domain at its carboxy terminal end. The FERM domain is thought to mediate protein-protein or protein-membrane interactions. Proteins containing a

FERM domain provide a link between the cell membrane and cytoskeleton. The RING domain is the active site of a large number of E3 ubiquitin ligases which catalyze the transfer of activated ubiquitin to substrate proteins leading to their degradation in the proteasome or lysosome. Mylip is the only FERM-containing protein that also has a RING domain. It has been shown that the RING domain of Mylip can mediate its self-ubiquitination and degradation in the proteasome (Bornhauser et al., 2003). Over expression of Mylip can inhibit nerve growth factor-stimulated neurite outgrowth in PC12 neuronal cells, presumably due to the ubiquitination and degradation of myosin regulatory light chain (Bornhauser and Lindholm, 2005). In the rat, Mylip expression is localized especially to neurons in the hippocampus and cerebellum, both during development and in adult brain (Olsson et al., 2000). Mylip expression can also be detected in many other tissues, suggesting additional functions and targets for this protein.

The Liver X receptors (LXRs) are important transcriptional factors regulating cellular cholesterol content. LXRs. LXR-α and LXR-β are sterol-response nuclear receptors activated by excess cellular cholesterols. Activated LXRs stimulate expression of ATP-binding cassette transporters A1 and G1 (ABCA1 and ABCG1) to promote efflux of cellular cholesterol, resulting in hepatic secretion of cholesterol into the bile and enhancement of reverse cholesterol transport in peripheral tissues. In mouse models of atherosclerosis, LXR agonists suppressed the development of atherosclerosis lesions. However, LXR agonists also stimulate hepatic fatty acid and triglyceride synthesis. This is due to the fact that sterol responsive element-binding protein 1c (SREBP1c) is a down-stream target of LXR. Activation of SREBP1c would lead to increased expression of genes involved in fatty acids and triglyceride synthesis.

In a recent publication, Zecler and co-workers investigated the effect of LXR agonists on cholesterol uptake in cultured liver cells (Zelcer et al., 2009). They found that LXR agonists suppressed LDL-C uptake by these cells. Further investigation revealed that LXR agonist GW3956 did not change LDLR mRNA level. Instead, the compound reduced LDLR protein level and redistributed LDLR from the plasma membrane to intracellular compartments. To explore the mechanism by which LXR agonists reduced LDLR protein, Zecler and colleagues also performed transcription profiling in cells treated with LXR agonists. Mylip is one of the genes whose mRNA is stimulated by LXR agonists. Treatment of primary hepatocytes with the LXR agonist GW3956 resulted in a 4-fold increase in Mylip mRNA level. GW3956 also stimulated Mylip transcription in multiple tissues in mice, including spleen, adrenal gland, intestine, and liver. The fact that Mylip is an ubiquitin E3 ligase capable of self-ubiquitination promoted Zecler and co-workers to investigate if Mylip can also mediate LDLR ubiquitination. Immunoprecipitation coupled with immunoblotting analysis revealed LDLR ubiquitination and subsequent degradation in HEK293 cells co-transfected with LDLR and Mylip. Additionally, Mylip carrying a mutation in the RING domain failed to induce LDLR ubiquitination and degradation when co-transfected into HEK293 cells. MG132, a proteasome inhibitor, did not block Idol-induced LDLR degradation. This observation is consistent with studies of PCSK9-mediated LDLR degradation in which the degradation occurs in the lysosome and not the proteasome. These data suggested that Mylip functions as an E3 ligase to trigger LDLR ubiquitination and degradation. Therefore, Mylip was renamed as inducible degrader of LDLR (Idol).

Amino acid sequence alignment revealed a conserved lysine residue in the C-terminal portion of LDLR, immediately following the NPVY endocytotic motif. Mutation of this lysine residue was not able to block Idol-stimulated LDLR ubiquitination and degradation. However, double mutation containing lysine 20 and cysteine 29 (K20R/C29A) rendered LDLR resistant to Idol-modulated ubiquitination and degradation in HEK293 cells (Zelcer et al., 2009). LDLR belongs to the LDLR family of receptors that share sequence and structure homology. The very-low-density lipoprotein receptor (VLDLR) and lipoprotein E receptor 2 (ApoER2) are two members of this receptor family that share a high degree of homology with LDLR. In co-transfection assays, Idol was able to stimulate ubiquitination and degradation of both VLDLR and apoER2. The C-terminal lysine residue (K20) is conserved in both VLDLR and ApoER2, while the cysteine (C29) is not conserved. Single mutation at K20 of VLDLR was able to block Idol-mediated ubiquitination and degradation (Hong et al., 2010). However, other members of this receptor family that also contain this conserved lysine residue, such as LPR1b, are not targets of Idol. It has been reported that PCSK9 can also reduce the protein levels of VLDLR and ApoER2. Thus it appears that the substrate specificities of Idol and PCSK9 overlap.

Using a floxed gene trap cassette system, Idol-deficient embryonic stem (ES) cells were generated (Scotti et al., 2011). LDLR protein level was much higher in Idol$^{-/-}$ ES cells than in wild type ES cells. When the cells were switched to medium containing 10% lipoprotein-deficient serum (LPDS), LDLR protein level increased in both types of ES cells. In Idol$^{-/-}$ ES cells, membrane-bound and intracellular LDLR protein levels both increased, suggesting that Idol can mediate degradation of LDLR before and after it reaches the cell membrane. Remarkably, treatment with the LXR agonist GW3965 reduced LDLR protein levels in wild type, but not in Idol$^{-/-}$ ES cells. This observation confirmed the previous finding that LXR-induced LDLR reduction was mediated through Idol. While PCSK9 binds to the extracellular EGFA domain of LDLR, Idol interacts with the C-terminal region of LDLR. Yet both pathways resulted in LDLR degradation in the lysosome. In Idol-deficient ES cells, recombinant PCSK9 is still able to induce LDLR degradation. This suggests that the Idol and PCSK9 pathways acted independently of each other. It could be speculated that owing to the importance of tightly controlling cellular cholesterol levels and circulating LDL-C levels, mammalian cells evolved two independent post-transcriptional pathways to regulate LDLR protein levels, and hence LDL-cholesterol uptake. These two pathways could complement each other or counterbalance each other depending on the specific situation. As discussed above, statins increase hepatic cholesterol uptake largely due to activation of LDLR transcription through SREBP-2. However, activation of SREBP-2 also increases expression of PCSK9, which in turn functions to reduce LDLR protein level. In a recent report, Dong and colleagues observed that statins suppressed Idol expression in HepG2 cells (Dong B et al., 2011). More interestingly, the ability of statins to increase LDLR protein level in these cells was compromised if the cells were transfected with Idol siRNA. The authors proposed that suppressing Idol expression is one of the mechanisms through which statins increase LDLR expression. This notion, however, was not confirmed by studies in Idol-deficient ES cells. Statins maintain their ability to increase LDLR protein level in Idol$^{-/-}$ ES cells (Scotti et al., 2011). In fact, LDLR levels in Idol$^{-/-}$ ES cells are much higher than wild type cells, even after statin treatment. Thus the exact relationship between these different LDLR regulatory pathways remains to be elucidated.

Studies in rodent models of hypercholesterolemia show that Idol can affect LDLR protein levels and cholesterol metabolism *in vivo*. In mice treated with the LXR agonist GW3965, LDLR protein levels were reduced in multiple tissues, including macrophages, small intestine, and to a lesser degree, liver. Conversely, the LDLR protein level was increased in these tissues in mice deficient for both LXR genes. More direct evidence was provided with studies using adenoviral construct harboring mouse Idol (Ad-Idol). Mice infected with Ad-Idol displayed dramatically reduced hepatic LDLR protein expression and a significantly increased plasma cholesterol levels compared to mice infected with control viral construct. Size fractionation of plasma lipoproteins revealed that the increased plasma cholesterol was largely due to increases in LDL cholesterol (Zelcer et al., 2009).

Idol has also been shown to play a role in impaired cholesterol metabolism in the Niemann-Pick type C and ApoE double knockout mice (NPC$^{-/-}$ApoE$^{-/-}$) (Ishibashi et al., 2010). The plasma cholesterol level is significantly higher in NPC$^{-/-}$ApoE$^{-/-}$ mice than in ApoE$^{-/-}$ mice. A large portion of this elevated plasma cholesterol is in the form of VLDL-C, due to reduced clearance of VLDL-C in the double knock-out mice. The double knock-out mice have significantly less LDLR protein in the liver, despite increased mRNA levels. Further analysis revealed that the expression of both Idol and PCSK9 is increased in livers of NPC$^{-/-}$ApoE$^{-/-}$ mice. In fact, all LXR and SREBP-2 target genes were stimulated in the livers, including LDLR at the transcriptional level. However, increased expression of Idol and PCSK9 resulted in accelerated degradation of hepatic LDLR protein, leading to reduced VLDL-cholesterol clearance in the NPC$^{-/-}$ApoE$^{-/-}$ mice. In this situation, Idol and PCSK9 worked in a complementary fashion to reduce hepatic LDLR levels, which resulted in significant hypercholesterolemia.

Recent genome-wide association studies (GWAS) provided some clues that Idol might be involved in the regulation of LDL-cholesterol in humans. The Women's Genome Health Study (WGHS) included 17,296 North American women with self-reported European ancestry who were non-diabetic and not on lipid lowering therapy at baseline (Chasman et al., 2009). Plasma lipid profiles and genotyping analysis were performed in these subjects. A total of forty-three loci displayed significant association with at least one lipid marker, including LDL-C, HDL-C, triglycerides, ApoA1, and ApoB100 levels, as well as lipoprotein size. The majority of these loci correspond to genes known to affect plasma lipid levels, such as PCSK9, LDLR, CETP, and HMG-CoA reductase. However, three novel loci were identified that showed significant association with at least one of the lipids measured, and one of the loci (rs2480) associated with LDL-cholesterol resides on chromosome 6q22.3, near the Mylip gene. In a separate report, Waterworth and co-workers performed a meta-analysis of 8 independent GWAS studies with a total of 17,723 participants of Caucasian European descent (Waterworth et al., 2010). This analysis confirmed most of the known genes affecting lipid metabolism as well as new loci identified from other GWAS. Additionally, six new loci were identified that reached genome-wide statistical association with circulating lipids. These are SBPs at Mylip/GMPR and PPP1R3B loci with LDL-C; at SLC39A8, TTC39B and FADS1 loci with HDL-C; and FADS1 loci with triglycerides. SNP rs2142672 lies in a distinct block of high linkage disequilibrium (LD) between 2 genes; Mylip and guanosine monophosphate reductase (GMPR) on chromosome 6q23. The C allele, with a frequency of 74%, is associated with relatively high levels of circulating LDL-C. These studies demonstrated the potential association between Idol gene polymorphisms and circulating

LDL-cholesterol levels, although there have been no reports on gain-of-function or loss-of-function of Idol so far. Therefore, a causal relationship between Idol gene function and LDL-C levels in humans is yet to be established.

To summarize, biochemical studies have demonstrated that Idol functions as an ubiquitin ligase for LDLR leading to its degradation in the lysosome. *In vivo* studies provided evidence that increased Idol expression in the liver could lead to reduced LDL-C clearance and elevated plasma cholesterol levels. GWAS data suggested associations between Idol gene polymorphisms and circulating LDL-cholesterol levels. It is conceivable that compounds capable of inhibiting Idol-mediated LDLR degradation could lead to increased hepatic cholesterol clearance and reduce circulating LDL-C. Idol is an intracellular protein that interacts with the intracellular domain of LDLR. Thus, unlike the situation with PCSK9, small molecular inhibitors that can penetrate cell membrane will have to be developed. Ubiquitin ligases represent one of the largest protein families in mammalian cells. It is estimated that over six hundred ubiquitin ligases exist in humans with each one targeting only a few specific substrates. Dysfunction of the ubiquitin proteasome system (UPS) has been shown to be involved in multiple diseases (Cohen and Tcherpakov, 2010). The development of small molecule inhibitors targeting UPS represents one of the exciting new frontiers in drug discovery (Ceccarelli et al., 2011). A small molecule inhibitor of Idol would be useful as an additional LDL-C lowering agent for those patients who cannot tolerate statins, or those unable to reach an aggressive LDL-C lowering goal with statins.

5. Concluding remarks

In summary, recent evidence has emerged that supports further reducing LDL-C for CAD prevention and treatment. It is expected that the new guidelines for LDL-C will be even lower. Existing therapies to reduce LDL-C, however, do not appear to be sufficient to meet these new guidelines, and therefore, there are significant unmet medical needs in this area. The identification of PCSK9 and Idol as novel regulators of LDLR has provided novel opportunities to develop additional therapeutics to further reduce LDL-C. New experimential drugs particularly targeting PCSK9 are already in clinical development. We anticipate that one or more of these agents will be able to demonstrate significant efficacy in reducing LDL-C and additional benefit in CAD prevention and treatment. Such compounds may likely become the next generation of medicines for managing cardiovascular disease.

6. Abbreviations

- apoER2 ApoE receptor 2
- ApoB Apolipoprotein B
- CAD Coronary artery disease
- EGFA Epidermal growth factor domain A
- Idol Inducible degrader of LDLR
- LDL-C Low-density lipoprotein cholesterol
- LDLR Low-density lipoprotein receptor
- LXR Liver X receptor
- PCSK9 Proprotein convertase subtilisin/kexin type 9
- SREBP2 Sterol-responsive element binding protein 2
- VLDLR Very low-density lipoprotein receptor

7. References

Abifadel, M., Rabes, J.P., Devillers, M., Munnich, A., Erlich, D., Junien, C., Varret, M., and Boileau, C. (2009). Mutations and polymorphisms in the proprotein convertase subtilisin kexin 9 (PCSK9) gene in cholesterol metabolism and disease. Hum Mutat 30, 520-529.

Abifadel, M., Varret, M., Rabes, J.P., Allard, D., Ouguerram, K., Devillers, M., Cruaud, C., Benjannet, S., Wickham, L., Erlich, D., Derre, A., Villeger, L., Farnier, M., Beucler, I., Bruckert, E., Chambaz, J., Chanu, B., Lecerf, J.M., Luc, G., Moulin, P., Weissenbach, J., Prat, A., Krempf, M., Junien, C., Seidah, N.G., and Boileau, C. (2003). Mutations in PCSK9 cause autosomal dominant hypercholesterolemia. Nat Genet 34, 154-156.

Benjannet, S., Rhainds, D., Hamelin, J., Nassoury, N., and Seidah, N.G. (2006). The proprotein convertase (PC) PCSK9 is inactivated by furin and/or PC5/6A: functional consequences of natural mutations and post-translational modifications. J Biol Chem 281, 30561-30572.

Benjannet, S., Saavedra, Y.G., Hamelin, J., Asselin, M.C., Essalmani, R., Pasquato, A., Lemaire, P., Duke, G., Miao, B., Duclos, F., Parker, R., Mayer, G., and Seidah, N.G. (2010). Effects of the prosegment and pH on the activity of PCSK9: evidence for additional processing events. J Biol Chem 285, 40965-40978.

Bornhauser, B.C., Johansson, C., and Lindholm, D. (2003). Functional activities and cellular localization of the ezrin, radixin, moesin (ERM) and RING zinc finger domains in MIR. FEBS Letters 553, 195-199.

Bornhauser, B.C., and Lindholm, D. (2005). MSAP enhances migration of C6 glioma cells through phosphorylation of the myosin regulatory light chain. Cellular and Molecular Life Sciences 62, 1260-1266.

Brown, M.S., and Goldstein, J.L. (1986). A receptor-mediated pathway for cholesterol homeostasis. Science 232, 34-47.

Browning, J.D., and Horton, J.D. (2010). Fasting reduces plasma proprotein convertase, subtilisin/kexin type 9 and cholesterol biosynthesis in humans. J Lipid Res 51, 3359-3363.

Cameron, J., Ranheim, T., Kulseth, M.A., Leren, T.P., and Berge, K.E. (2008). Berberine decreases PCSK9 expression in HepG2 cells. Atherosclerosis 201, 266-273.

Cao, G., Liang, Y., Jiang, X.C., and Eacho, P.I. (2004). Liver X receptors as potential therapeutic targets for multiple diseases. Drug News Perspect 17, 35-41.

Careskey, H.E., Davis, R.A., Alborn, W.E., Troutt, J.S., Cao, G., and Konrad, R.J. (2007). Atorvastatin increases human serum levels of proprotein convertase subtilisin kexin type 9 (PCSK9). J Lipid Res 21, 21.

Ceccarelli, Derek F., Tang, X., Pelletier, B., Orlicky, S., Xie, W., Plantevin, V., Neculai, D., Chou, Y.-C., Ogunjimi, A., Al-Hakim, A., Varelas, X., Koszela, J., Wasney, Gregory A., Vedadi, M., Dhe-Paganon, S., Cox, S., Xu, S., Lopez-Girona, A., Mercurio, F., Wrana, J., Durocher, D., Meloche, S., Webb, David R., Tyers, M., and Sicheri, F. (2011). An Allosteric Inhibitor of the Human Cdc34 Ubiquitin-Conjugating Enzyme. Cell 145, 1075-1087.

Chan, J.C., Piper, D.E., Cao, Q., Liu, D., King, C., Wang, W., Tang, J., Liu, Q., Higbee, J., Xia, Z., Di, Y., Shetterly, S., Arimura, Z., Salomonis, H., Romanow, W.G., Thibault, S.T., Zhang, R., Cao, P., Yang, X.P., Yu, T., Lu, M., Retter, M.W., Kwon, G., Henne, K., Pan, O., Tsai, M.M., Fuchslocher, B., Yang, E., Zhou, L., Lee, K.J., Daris, M., Sheng, J., Wang, Y., Shen, W.D., Yeh, W.C., Emery, M., Walker, N.P., Shan, B., Schwarz, M., and Jackson, S.M. (2009). A proprotein convertase subtilisin/kexin type 9 neutralizing antibody reduces serum cholesterol in mice and nonhuman primates. Proc Natl Acad Sci U S A 106, 9820-9825.

Chasman, D.I., ParÃ©, G., Mora, S., Hopewell, J.C., Peloso, G., Clarke, R., Cupples, L.A., Hamsten, A., Kathiresan, S., MÃ¤larstig, A., Ordovas, J.M., Ripatti, S., Parker, A.N., Miletich, J.P., and Ridker, P.M. (2009). Forty-Three Loci Associated with Plasma Lipoprotein Size, Concentration, and Cholesterol Content in Genome-Wide Analysis. PLoS Genet 5, e1000730.

Cohen, J.C., Boerwinkle, E., Mosley, T.H., Jr., and Hobbs, H.H. (2006). Sequence variations in PCSK9, low LDL, and protection against coronary heart disease. N Engl J Med 354, 1264-1272.

Cohen, P., and Tcherpakov, M. (2010). Will the Ubiquitin System Furnish as Many Drug Targets as Protein Kinases? Cell 143, 686-693.

Cui, Q., Ju, X., Yang, T., Zhang, M., Tang, W., Chen, Q., Hu, Y., Haas, J.V., Troutt, J.S., Pickard, R.T., Darling, R., Konrad, R.J., Zhou, H., and Cao, G. (2010). Serum PCSK9 is associated with multiple metabolic factors in a large Han Chinese population. Atherosclerosis 213, 632-636.

Dewpura, T., Raymond, A., Hamelin, J., Seidah, N.G., Mbikay, M., Chretien, M., and Mayne, J. (2008). PCSK9 is phosphorylated by a Golgi casein kinase-like kinase ex vivo and circulates as a phosphoprotein in humans. Febs J 275, 3480-3493.

Dong B, Wu M, Cao A, Li H, and J., L. (2011). Suppression of Idol expression is an additional mechanism underlying statin-induced up-regulation of hepatic LDL receptor expression. Int J Mol Med. 27, 103-110.

Frank-Kamenetsky, M., Grefhorst, A., Anderson, N.N., Racie, T.S., Bramlage, B., Akinc, A., Butler, D., Charisse, K., Dorkin, R., Fan, Y., Gamba-Vitalo, C., Hadwiger, P., Jayaraman, M., John, M., Jayaprakash, K.N., Maier, M., Nechev, L., Rajeev, K.G., Read, T., Rohl, I., Soutschek, J., Tan, P., Wong, J., Wang, G., Zimmermann, T., de Fougerolles, A., Vornlocher, H.P., Langer, R., Anderson, D.G., Manoharan, M., Koteliansky, V., Horton, J.D., and Fitzgerald, K. (2008). Therapeutic RNAi targeting PCSK9 acutely lowers plasma cholesterol in rodents and LDL cholesterol in nonhuman primates. Proc Natl Acad Sci U S A 105, 11915-11920.

Goldstein, J.L., DeBose-Boyd, R.A., and Brown, M.S. (2006). Protein sensors for membrane sterols. Cell. 124, 35-46.

Graham, M.J., Lemonidis, K.M., Whipple, C.P., Subramaniam, A., Monia, B.P., Crooke, S.T., and Crooke, R.M. (2007). Antisense inhibition of proprotein convertase subtilisin/kexin type 9 reduces serum LDL in hyperlipidemic mice. J Lipid Res. 48, 763-767. Epub 2007 Jan 2022.

Gupta, N., Fisker, N., Asselin, M.C., Lindholm, M., Rosenbohm, C., Orum, H., Elmen, J., Seidah, N.G., and Straarup, E.M. (2010). A locked nucleic acid antisense oligonucleotide (LNA) silences PCSK9 and enhances LDLR expression in vitro and in vivo. PLoS One 5, e10682.

Herbert, B., Patel, D., Waddington, S.N., Eden, E.R., McAleenan, A., Sun, X.M., and Soutar, A.K. (2010). Increased secretion of lipoproteins in transgenic mice expressing human D374Y PCSK9 under physiological genetic control. Arterioscler Thromb Vasc Biol 30, 1333-1339.

Hobbs, H.H., Russell, D.W., Brown, M.S., and Goldstein, J.L. (1990). The LDL receptor locus in familial hypercholesterolemia: mutational analysis of a membrane protein. Annu Rev Genet 24, 133-170.

Hong, C., Duit, S., Jalonen, P., Out, R., Scheer, L., Sorrentino, V., Boyadjian, R., Rodenburg, K.W., Foley, E., Korhonen, L., Lindholm, D., Nimpf, J., van Berkel, T.J.C., Tontonoz, P., and Zelcer, N. (2010). The E3 Ubiquitin Ligase IDOL Induces the Degradation of the Low Density Lipoprotein Receptor Family Members VLDLR and ApoER2. J. Biol. Chem. 285, 19720-19726.

Horton, J.D., Cohen, J.C., and Hobbs, H.H. (2009). PCSK9: a convertase that coordinates LDL catabolism. J Lipid Res 50 Suppl, S172-177.

Ishibashi, M., Masson, D., Westerterp, M., Wang, N., Sayers, S., Li, R., Welch, C.L., and Tall, A.R. (2010). Reduced VLDL clearance in Apoe−/−Npc1−/− mice is associated with increased Pcsk9 and Idol expression and decreased hepatic LDL-receptor levels J. Lipid Res. 51, 2655-2663.

Ishibashi, S., Goldstein, J.L., Brown, M.S., Herz, J., and Burns, D.K. (1994). Massive xanthomatosis and atherosclerosis in cholesterol-fed low density lipoprotein receptor-negative mice. J Clin Invest 93, 1885-1893.

Konrad, R.J., Troutt, J.S., and Cao, G. (2011). Effects of currently prescribed LDL-C-lowering drugs on PCSK9 and implications for the next generation of LDL-C-lowering agents. Lipids Health Dis 10, 38.

Kwon, H.J., Lagace, T.A., McNutt, M.C., Horton, J.D., and Deisenhofer, J. (2008). Molecular basis for LDL receptor recognition by PCSK9. Proc Natl Acad Sci U S A. 105, 1820-1825. Epub 2008 Feb 1824.

Lagace, T.A., Curtis, D.E., Garuti, R., McNutt, M.C., Park, S.W., Prather, H.B., Anderson, N.N., Ho, Y.K., Hammer, R.E., and Horton, J.D. (2006). Secreted PCSK9 decreases the number of LDL receptors in hepatocytes and inlivers of parabiotic mice. J Clin Invest 116, 2995-3005.

Lakoski, S.G., Lagace, T.A., Cohen, J.C., Horton, J.D., and Hobbs, H.H. (2009). Genetic and metabolic determinants of plasma PCSK9 levels. J Clin Endocrinol Metab 94, 2537-2543.

Langhi, C., Le May, C., Gmyr, V., Vandewalle, B., Kerr-Conte, J., Krempf, M., Pattou, F., Costet, P., and Cariou, B. (2009). PCSK9 is expressed in pancreatic delta-cells and does not alter insulin secretion. Biochem Biophys Res Commun 390, 1288-1293.

Langhi, C., Le May, C., Kourimate, S., Caron, S., Staels, B., Krempf, M., Costet, P., and Cariou, B. (2008). Activation of the farnesoid X receptor represses PCSK9 expression in human hepatocytes. FEBS Lett 582, 949-955.

Li, H., Dong, B., Park, S.W., Lee, H.S., Chen, W., and Liu, J. (2009). Hepatocyte nuclear factor 1alpha plays a critical role in PCSK9 gene transcription and regulation by the natural hypocholesterolemic compound berberine. J Biol Chem 284, 28885-28895.

Liu, M., Wu, G., Baysarowich, J., Kavana, M., Addona, G.H., Bierilo, K.K., Mudgett, J.S., Pavlovic, G., Sitlani, A., Renger, J.J., Hubbard, B.K., Fisher, T.S., and Zerbinatti, C.V. (2010). PCSK9 is not involved in the degradation of LDL receptors and BACE1 in the adult mouse brain. J Lipid Res 51, 2611-2618.

Maxwell, K.N., and Breslow, J.L. (2004). Adenoviral-mediated expression of Pcsk9 in mice results in a low-density lipoprotein receptor knockout phenotype. Proc Natl Acad Sci U S A 101, 7100-7105. Epub 2004 Apr 7126.

Mayer, G., Poirier, S., and Seidah, N.G. (2008). Annexin A2 is a C-terminal PCSK9-binding protein that regulates endogenous low density lipoprotein receptor levels. J Biol Chem 283, 31791-31801.

Mbikay, M., Sirois, F., Mayne, J., Wang, G.S., Chen, A., Dewpura, T., Prat, A., Seidah, N.G., Chretien, M., and Scott, F.W. (2010). PCSK9-deficient mice exhibit impaired glucose tolerance and pancreatic islet abnormalities. FEBS Lett 584, 701-706.

McNutt, M.C., Lagace, T.A., and Horton, J.D. (2007). Catalytic activity is not required for secreted PCSK9 to reduce LDL receptors in HepG2 cells. J Biol Chem 29, 29.

Ni, Y.G., Condra, J.H., Orsatti, L., Shen, X., Di Marco, S., Pandit, S., Bottomley, M.J., Ruggeri, L., Cummings, R.T., Cubbon, R.M., Santoro, J.C., Ehrhardt, A., Lewis, D., Fisher, T.S., Ha, S., Njimoluh, L., Wood, D.D., Hammond, H.A., Wisniewski, D., Volpari, C., Noto, A., Lo Surdo, P., Hubbard, B., Carfi, A., and Sitlani, A. (2010). A proprotein convertase subtilisin-like/kexin type 9 (PCSK9) C-terminal domain antibody antigen-binding fragment inhibits PCSK9 internalization and restores low density lipoprotein uptake. J Biol Chem 285, 12882-12891.

O'Keefe, J.H., Jr., Cordain, L., Harris, W.H., Moe, R.M., and Vogel, R. (2004). Optimal low-density lipoprotein is 50 to 70 mg/dl: lower is better and physiologically normal. J Am Coll Cardiol 43, 2142-2146.

Olsson, P.-A., Bornhauser, B.C., Korhonen, L., and Lindholm, D. (2000). Neuronal Expression of the ERM-like Protein MIR in Rat Brain and Its Localization to Human Chromosome 6. Biochemical and Biophysical Research Communications 279, 879-883.

Olsson, P.-A., Korhonen, L., Mercer, E.A., and Lindholm, D. (1999). MIR Is a Novel ERM-like Protein That Interacts with Myosin Regulatory Light Chain and Inhibits Neurite Outgrowth. J Biol Chem. 274, 36288-36292.

Persson, L., Cao, G., Stahle, L., Sjoberg, B.G., Troutt, J.S., Konrad, R.J., Galman, C., Wallen, H., Eriksson, M., Hafstrom, I., Lind, S., Dahlin, M., Amark, P., Angelin, B., and Rudling, M. (2010). Circulating proprotein convertase subtilisin kexin type 9 has a diurnal rhythm synchronous with cholesterol synthesis and is reduced by fasting in humans. Arterioscler Thromb Vasc Biol 30, 2666-2672.

Poirier, S., Mayer, G., Benjannet, S., Bergeron, E., Marcinkiewicz, J., Nassoury, N., Mayer, H., Nimpf, J., Prat, A., and Seidah, N.G. (2008). The proprotein convertase PCSK9 induces the degradation of low density lipoprotein receptor (LDLR) and its closest family members VLDLR and ApoER2. J Biol Chem. 283, 2363-2372. Epub 2007 Nov 2326.

Qian, Y.W., Schmidt, R.J., Zhang, Y., Chu, S., Lin, A., Wang, H., Wang, X., Beyer, T.P., Bensch, W.R., Li, W., Ehsani, M.E., Lu, D., Konrad, R.J., Eacho, P.I., Moller, D.E., Karathanasis, S.K., and Cao, G. (2007). Secreted proprotein convertase subtilisin/kexin-type 9 downregulates low-density lipoprotein receptor through receptor-mediated endocytosis. J Lipid Res 20, 20.

Rashid, S., Curtis, D.E., Garuti, R., Anderson, N.N., Bashmakov, Y., Ho, Y.K., Hammer, R.E., Moon, Y.A., and Horton, J.D. (2005). Decreased plasma cholesterol and hypersensitivity to statins in mice lacking Pcsk9. Proc Natl Acad Sci U S A 102, 5374-5379. Epub 2005 Apr 5371.

Roubtsova, A., Munkonda, M.N., Awan, Z., Marcinkiewicz, J., Chamberland, A., Lazure, C., Cianflone, K., Seidah, N.G., and Prat, A. (2011). Circulating proprotein convertase subtilisin/kexin 9 (PCSK9) regulates VLDLR protein and triglyceride accumulation in visceral adipose tissue. Arterioscler Thromb Vasc Biol 31, 785-791.

Rousselet, E., Marcinkiewicz, J., Kriz, J., Zhou, A., Hatten, M.E., Prat, A., and Seidah, N.G. (2011). PCSK9 reduces the protein levels of the LDL receptor in mouse brain during development and after ischemic stroke. J Lipid Res 52, 1383-1391.

Schmidt, R.J., Beyer, T.P., Bensch, W.R., Qian, Y.W., Lin, A., Kowala, M., Alborn, W.E., Konrad, R.J., and Cao, G. (2008). Secreted proprotein convertase subtilisin/kexin type 9 reduces both hepatic and extrahepatic low-density lipoprotein receptors in vivo. Biochem Biophys Res Commun. 370, 634-640. Epub 2008 Apr 2010.

Schmidt, R.J., Ficorilli, J.V., Zhang, Y., Bramlett, K.S., Beyer, T.P., Borchert, K., Dowless, M.S., Houck, K.A., Burris, T.P., Eacho, P.I., Liang, G., Guo, L.W., Wilson, W.K., Michael, L.F., and Cao, G. (2006). A 15-ketosterol is a liver X receptor ligand that suppresses sterol-responsive element binding protein-2 activity. J Lipid Res 47, 1037-1044.

Scotti, E., Hong, C., Yoshinaga, Y., Tu, Y., Hu, Y., Zelcer, N., Boyadjian, R., de Jong, P.J., Young, S.G., Fong, L.G., and Tontonoz, P. (2011). Targeted Disruption of the Idol Gene Alters Cellular Regulation of the Low-Density Lipoprotein Receptor by Sterols and Liver X Receptor Agonists. Mol Cell Biol. 31, 1885-1893.

Seidah, N.G., Benjannet, S., Wickham, L., Marcinkiewicz, J., Jasmin, S.B., Stifani, S., Basak, A., Prat, A., and Chretien, M. (2003). The secretory proprotein convertase neural apoptosis-regulated convertase 1 (NARC-1): liver regeneration and neuronal differentiation. Proc Natl Acad Sci U S A 100, 928-933. Epub 2003 Jan 2027.

Stamler, J., Daviglus, M.L., Garside, D.B., Dyer, A.R., Greenland, P., and Neaton, J.D. (2000). Relationship of baseline serum cholesterol levels in 3 large cohorts of younger men to long-term coronary, cardiovascular, and all-cause mortality and to longevity. JAMA 284, 311-318.

Waterworth, D.M., Ricketts, S.L., Song, K., Chen, L., Zhao, J.H., Ripatti, S., Aulchenko, Y.S., Zhang, W., Yuan, X., Lim, N., Luan, J.a., Ashford, S., Wheeler, E., Young, E.H., Hadley, D., Thompson, J.R., Braund, P.S., Johnson, T., Struchalin, M., Surakka, I., Luben, R., Khaw, K.-T., Rodwell, S.A., Loos, R.J.F., Boekholdt, S.M., Inouye, M., Deloukas, P., Elliott, P., Schlessinger, D., Sanna, S., Scuteri, A., Jackson, A., Mohlke, K.L., Tuomilehto, J., Roberts, R., Stewart, A., Kesaniemi, Y.A., Mahley, R.W., Grundy, S.M., Wellcome Trust Case Control, C., McArdle, W., Cardon, L., Waeber, G., Vollenweider, P., Chambers, J.C., Boehnke, M., Abecasis, G.R., Salomaa, V., Jarvelin, M.-R., Ruokonen, A., Barroso, I., Epstein, S.E., Hakonarson, H.H., Rader, D.J., Reilly, M.P., Witteman, J.C.M., Hall, A.S., Samani, N.J., Strachan, D.P., Barter, P., van Duijn, C.M., Kooner, J.S., Peltonen, L., Wareham, N.J., McPherson, R., Mooser, V., and Sandhu, M.S. (2010). Genetic Variants Influencing Circulating Lipid Levels and Risk of Coronary Artery Disease. Arterioscler Thromb Vasc Biol 30, 2264-2276.

Zelcer, N., Hong, C., Boyadjian, R., and Tontonoz, P. (2009). LXR Regulates Cholesterol Uptake Through Idol-Dependent Ubiquitination of the LDL Receptor. Science 325, 100-104.

Zhang, D.W., Lagace, T.A., Garuti, R., Zhao, Z., McDonald, M., Horton, J.D., Cohen, J.C., and Hobbs, H.H. (2007). Binding of PCSK9 to EGF-A repeat of LDL receptor decreases receptor recycling and increases degradation. J Biol Chem 23, 23.

12

Serum Choline Plasmalogen is a Reliable Biomarker for Atherogenic Status

Ryouta Maeba[1] and Hiroshi Hara[2]
[1]*Department of Biochemistry, Teikyo University School of Medicine*
[2]*Division of Applied Bioscience, Research Faculty of Agriculture, Hokkaido University*
Japan

1. Introduction

Plasmalogens (Pls) belong to a subclass of glycerophospholipids, and widely distributed in human and animal tissues (Nagan & Zoeller, 2001). Although the clinical significance of these phospholipids is recognized in relation to peroxisomal disorders (Wanders & Waterham, 2006), the physiopathological roles of Pls are not fully understood. Recently, serum (or plasma) Pls have gained interest in several clinical symptoms of life-style related disease possibly because of their antioxidant properties (Brites et al., 2004). We have developed a highly sensitive and simple method to determine the serum concentrations of choline (PlsCho) and ethanolamine plasmalogen (PlsEtn) separately, using a radioactive iodine and high-performance liquid chromatography (^{125}I-HPLC method) (Maeba & Ueta, 2004; Maeba et al, 2012). The method has improved as auto-analytical system by introducing online detection with flow γ-counter. We have applied the system to the determination of serum Pls from normal subjects and CAD patients, and investigated the clinical significance of serum Pls as a biomarker for metabolic syndrome and atherosclerosis. This chapter briefly describes Pls structure, distribution, functions, and biosynthesis, and describes in detail the methods for measurement of Pls and clinical significance of serum Pls.

2. Plasmalogens (Pls)

Pls are one of the three subclasses of glycerophospholipids, and characterized by a vinyl-ether bond (-O-CH=CH-) in *sn*-1 and an ester bond in *sn*-2 position of the glycerol backbone (**Fig.1**).

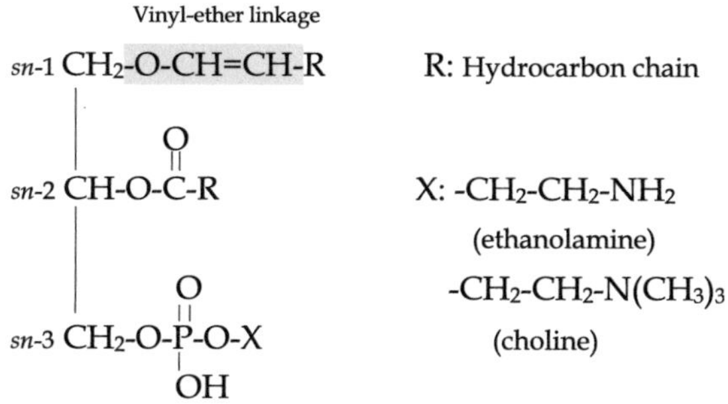

Fig. 1. Chemical structure of Pls

Pls constitute 18% of the total phospholipids mass in humans, mostly as membrane structure component. The polar head group of Pls mainly consists of choline or ethanolamine. Ethanolamine plasmalogens (PlsEtn) are predominantly distributed in almost organs, tissues and cells except heart and blood plasma, in which PlsEtn and choline plasmalogens (PlsCho) are equally contained. Pls are abundantly distributed in brain, heart, kidney, lung, testis, skeletal muscle, erythrocyte, macrophage, and lymphocytes in human body. These organs, tissues, and cells are characterized by the frequent occurrence of cell membrane fusion or oxidative stress.

2.1 Functions and biosynthesis of Pls

Major functions of Pls are shown in **Fig.2**. 1) Modulating membrane fluidity is essential for regulating membrane protein functions, as well as cell fusion, exocytosis, and endocytosis. This function is derived from high propensity of PlsEtn to form locally inverse hexagonal phase in phospholipid bilayer membranes (Glaser & Gross, 1994). 2) Endogenous antioxidant function of Pls is derived from the presence of vinyl ether double bond, which is capable of scavenging free radicals (Zoeller et al., 1988). In addition, we have recently found a novel antioxidant function of PlsEtn to lower the susceptibility of cholesterol in phospholipid bilayer and membranes to oxidation, probably through modulating the physical property of membranes (Maeba & Ueta, 2003a, 2003b). 3) The function of storage of bioactive lipid source comes from the fact that the lipid mediator producing fatty acids such as arachidonic acid, eicosapentaenoic acid (EPA), and docosahexaenoic acid (DHA) are preferentially located at *sn*-2 position of Pls.

1. Membrane modulator

membrane fluidity, membrane fusion

2. Endogenous antioxidant

radical scavenger

lower susceptibility of cholesterol and membranes to oxidation

3. Storage of bioactive lipid source

arachidonic acid, DHA, EPA

Fig. 2. Major functions of Pls

Next, dihydroxyacetone phosphate (DHAP) is a starting material for biosynthesis of Pls. DHAP-acyltransferase (DHAP-AT) and alkyl DHAP synthase (ADHAP-S) are responsible for the 1st and 2nd steps of Pls biosynthesis, respectively, and are localized in peroxisome (**Fig.3**). Therefore, peroxisomal disorders often show Pls deficiency (Wanders & Waterham, 2006). Mental retardation represents a phenotype of peroxisomal disorders, suggesting the essential role of Pls in the normal function of central nervous system (CNS). This is supported by Pls-deficient mouse, which revealed severe phenotypic alterations, including defects in CNS myelination (Gorgas et al., 2006). In addition to peroxisomal disorders, decreased brain Pls content has been reported in a number of neurological disorders such as spinal cord injury, Alzheimer's disease, Down syndrome, and multiple sclerosis (Lessig & Fuchs, 2009). The final step of PlsEtn biosynthesis is the desaturation of 1-alkyl-2-acyl-GPE via the action of $\Delta 1$ desaturase, whereas PlsCho is primarily formed from PlsEtn via polar-head group modification, by which mechanism remains still obscure (Lee, 1998). Facilitation of PlsCho biosynthesis is presumably important to prevent from atherogenic status, as described later, therefore elucidation of the regulatory mechanism of transfer from PlsEtn to PlsCho must become important.

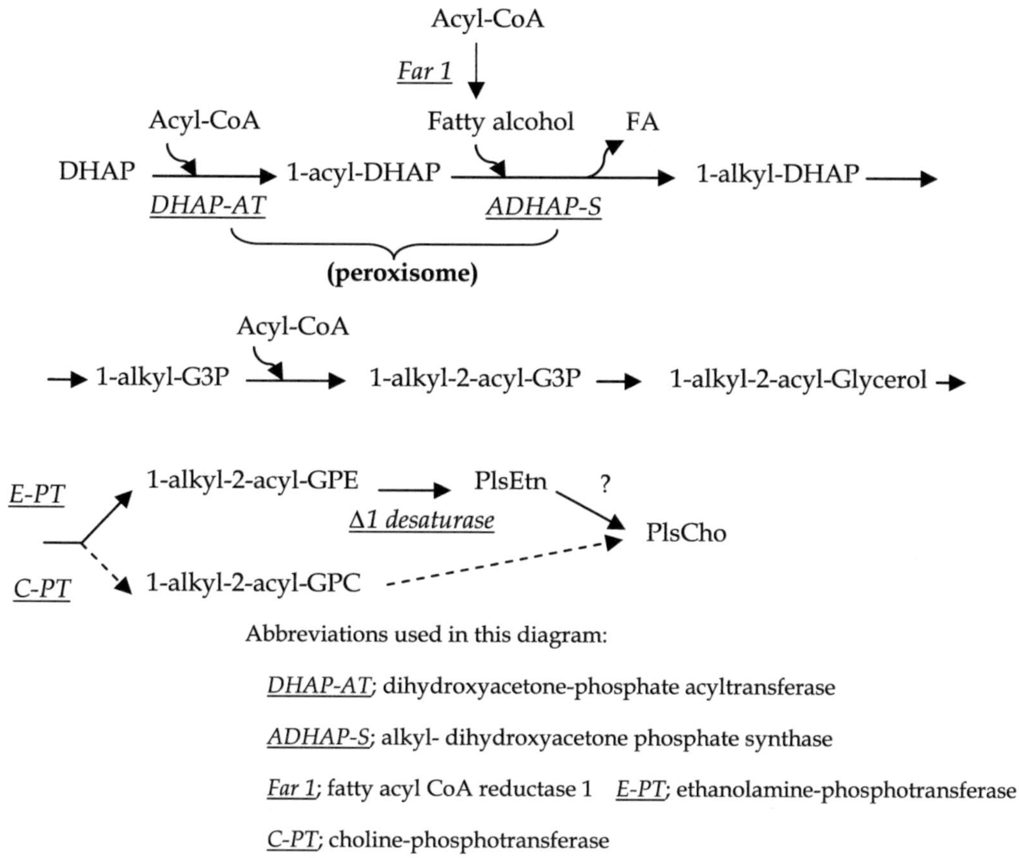

Fig. 3. Biosynthetic pathway of Pls

2.2 Quantification of Pls

Analytical methods for Pls have been developed principally based on acid labile property of the vinyl-ether linkage of Pls, which leads to the sequential decomposition into fatty aldehydes and 1-lysophospholipids. The resultant fatty aldehydes are usually measured as dimethyl acetal derivatives using gas chromatography/mass spectrometry (GC/MS) (Ingrand et al., 2000), and 1-lysophospholipids are measured by two-dimensional thin layer chromatography (TLC) (Horrocks, 1968). However, these methods are laborious and insufficient to accurately quantify Pls in a small amount of serum (or plasma).

2.2.1 LC/MS analysis of Pls

Recently, LC/MS has been applied to the analysis of Pls at the molecular species levels (Zemski & Murphy, 2004). We also have established the analytical method for Pls molecular species with UPLC-MS/MS (**Fig.4**).

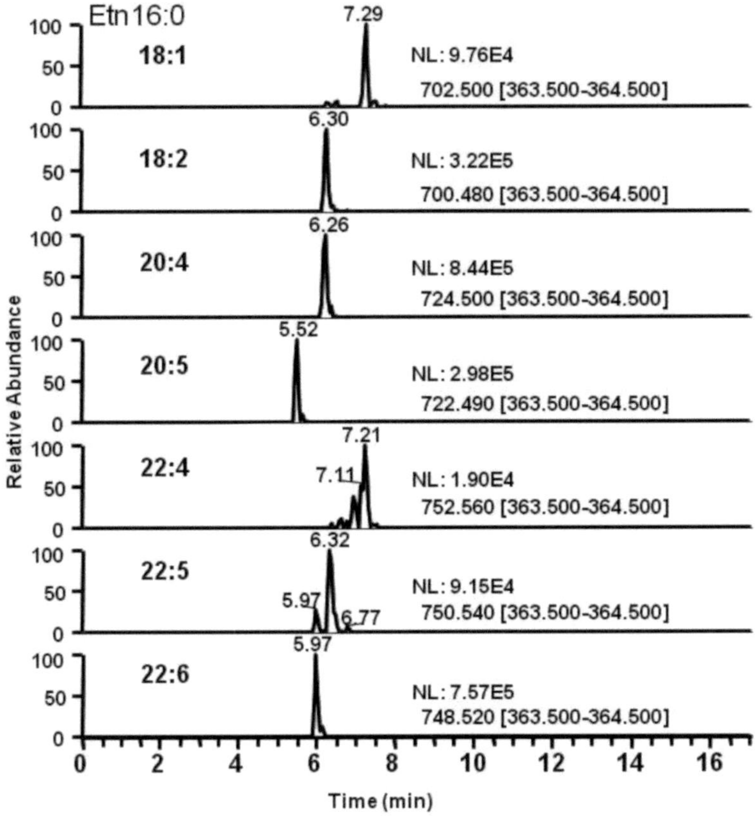

Fig. 4. UPLC-MS/MS analysis of PlsEtn 16:0 molecular species

The long chain fatty alcohol in *sn*-1 position consists almost exclusively of 16:0, 18:0, and 18:1 alkenyl groups, while *sn*-2 position is esterified predominantly with n-6 or n-3 series polyunsaturated fatty acids. LC/MS analysis is powerful method to provide substantial useful information, but the excess data is unlikely suitable for a routine diagnostic test, except for specific diagnostic molecular species for particular disorders such as Alzheimer's disease (Goodenowe et al, 2007).

2.2.2 ^{125}I-HPLC method for determination of Pls

We have originally developed a unique method to determine total amounts of PlsCho and PlsEtn separately, using radioactive iodine (^{125}I) and high-performance liquid chromatography (^{125}I-HPLC method) (Maeba & Ueta, 2004; Maeba et al, 2012). The method is based on the binding specificity of iodine to Pls. Triiodide (1-) ion (I_3^-) specifically reacts with a vinyl-ether double bond of Pls at molar ratio 1:1 in methanol solution. Pls assay based on this principle had already been established (Williams et al., 1962). However, the "cold" iodine method has some problems of low detectable Pls and interfering substances in the extracted lipids from biomaterials like serum. ^{125}I-HPLC method permitted the highly sensitive and accurate determination of serum (or plasma) Pls by using a radioactive iodine (^{125}I), and removing interfering substances with HPLC. The primary advantage of this method enabled to measure PlsCho and PlsEtn separately. ^{125}I-HPLC method has been markedly improved by introducing a quantitative standard (Q.S.) and online detection with flow γ-counter. 1-Alkenyl 2,3-cyclic glycerophosphate was decided as Q.S. in view of both the same quantitative property of Pls and the proper retention time in the HPLC elution profile (**Fig.5, 6**).

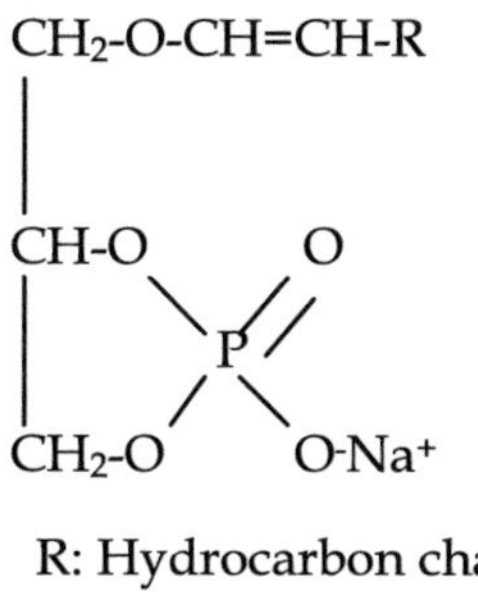

Fig. 5. Chemical structure of 1-Alkenyl 2,3-cyclic glycerophosphate (Q.S.)

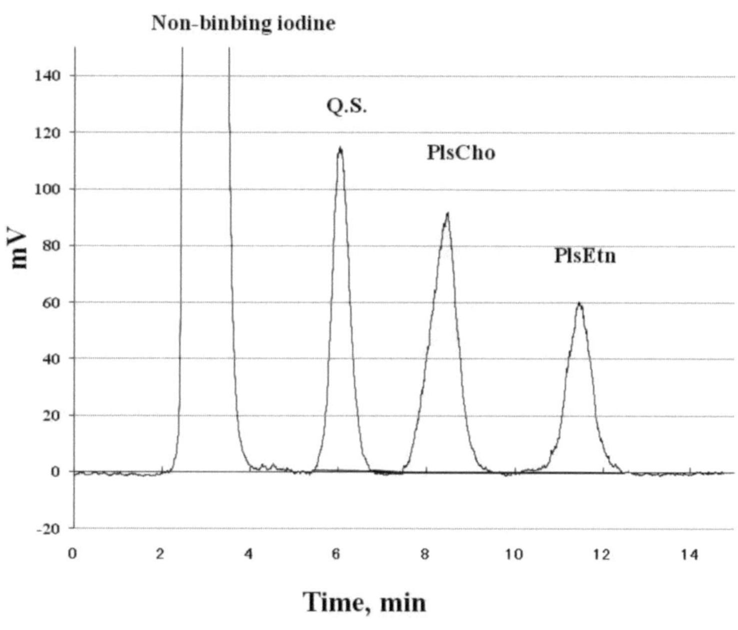

Fig. 6. A typical HPLC elusion profile of Pls and Q.S. detected with flow γ-counter

Online detection with flow γ-counter permitted more precise and safe measurement of Pls-related radio activity. The improved method has been fully validated in terms of selectivity, sensitivity, linearity, precision, accuracy, and has applied to the determination of human serum Pls. To minimize diffusion of radioactive contamination, the treatment column for HPLC waste fluid was prepared. The radioactive iodine adsorbents column reduced the radioactivity in waste fluid less than 500cpm/ml, even when 100 times sample injections. ^{125}I-HPLC method is useful as a continious auto-analytical system for a routine diagnostic test of human serum (or plasma) Pls.

2.3 Pls as a serum (plasma) biomarker

We have focused on the antioxidant property of Pls, and the potential utility of serum Pls as a biomarker for oxidative stress and aging (Brosche, 1997). It is well known that the number and the capability of peroxisome reduce with aging (Poynter & Davnes, 1998), which may induce the reduction of Pls biosynthesis. Decreased antioxidant Pls level may lead to predominant oxidative status in redox balance, which may cause the diseases associated with aging or oxidative stress such as atherosclerosis, metabolic syndrome (MetS) and Alzheimer's disease (**Fig.7**).

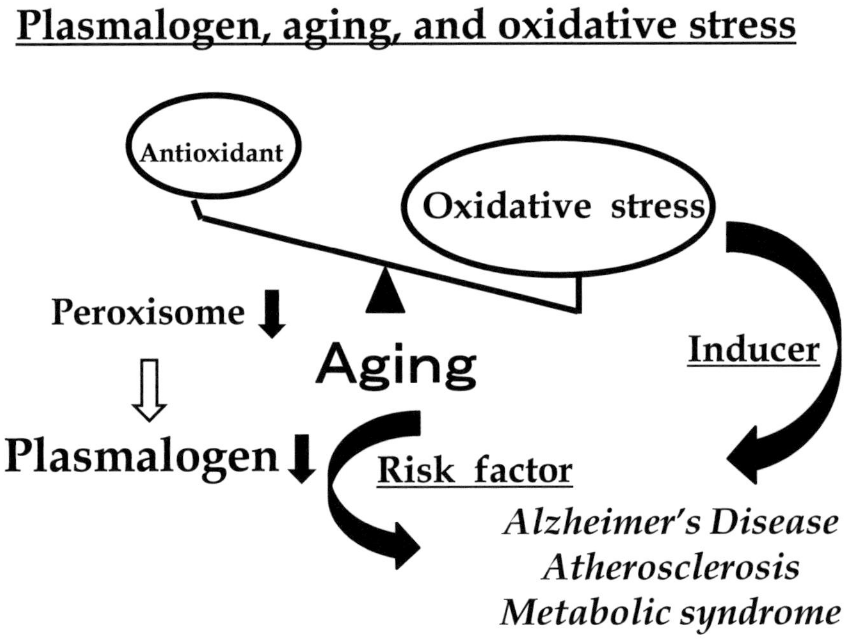

Fig. 7. Hypothesis for Pls deficiency causing life-style related disease

2.3.1 Serum (plasma) Pls

Serum (plasma) Pls are mainly synthesized in and secreted by liver as a structural component of lipoproteins (Vance, 1990), and potentially prevent lipoprotein oxidation relevant to atherosclerosis probably due to the radical scavenging ability of vinyl-ether double bond (Engelmann et al., 1994; Zoeller et al, 1999). The profile of human serum (plasma) Pls is as follows. Pls concentration is 100-300 µM with the content ratio of PlsCho/PlsEtn ranging from 0.5 to 1.5. PlsCho represent approximately 5% of choline glycerophospholipid, while PlsEtn represent 50~60% of ethanolamine glycerophospholipid. Total phospholipids concentration is 2-4 mM in serum (plasma), including 60~75% choline glycerophospholipid and 2~5% ethanolamine glycerophospholipid. The distribution of Pls on lipoprotein classes shows higher proportion of HDL, LDL, and VLDL in the order (Wiesner et al., 2009).

2.3.2 Pls in serum (plasma) or red blood cells of normal subjects

Pls levels in serum (plasma) or red blood cells of normal subjects have been determined with ^{125}I-HPLC method in each generation (**Table 1**).

	Blood serum or plasma						Red blood cells	
	Young		Middle-age		Elderly		Young	
	M	F	M	F	M	F	M	F
n	74	27	383	69	8	65	74	27
Age	23.9	22.7	40.4	34.8***	77.6	72.3*	23.9	22.7
	±3.7	±3.9	±10.7	±10.3	±5.0	±5.1	±3.7	±3.9
PlsCho	98.5	115.2**	62.5	69.8***	54.9	54.7		
μM	±23.0	±24.5	±12.2	±13.0	±10.2	±11.2		
PlsEtn	133.8	142.9	73.3	71.0	68.8	68.5		
μM	±33.3	±38.7	±19.4	±20.5	±13.0	±16.6		
PlsCho+PlsEtn	232.4	258.1	135.8	140.7	123.6	123.2		
μM	±53.3	±61.2	±29.0	±29.8	±21.7	±25.5		
PlsCho/PlsEtn	0.75	0.83*	0.88	1.04***	0.80	0.82	0.29	0.29
ratio	±0.12	±0.14	±0.17	±0.28	±0.11	±0.15	±0.04	±0.03
PL	2.17	2.14	2.99	2.94	3.28	3.44		
mM	±0.34	±0.41	±0.49	±0.33	±0.40	±0.38		
PlsCho/PL	4.6	5.6*	2.2	2.4***	1.7	1.6	5.7	6.5*
mol %	±1.1	±1.6	±0.4	±0.5	±0.3	±0.3	±1.6	±1.6
PlsEtn/PL	6.3	6.9	2.5	2.5	2.1	2.0	19.2	22.3*
mol %	±1.8	±2.2	±0.6	±0.7	±0.5	±0.5	±4.6	±4.8
(PlsCho+PlsEtn)/PL	10.9	12.5	4.6	4.8	3.8	3.6	24.9	28.8*
mol %	±2.7	±3.7	±0.9	±1.1	±0.8	±0.8	±6.0	±6.3

Mean ±S.D., *t*-test between Male and Female in each generation, * $p<0.05$, ** $p<0.01$, *** $p<0.001$

Table 1. Pls levels in serum (plasma) or red blood cells of normal subjects

There were significant differences in almost all Pls parameters as well as age and total phospholipids (PL) among generations, except for PlsEtn level between middle-age and elderly. Pls in serum (plasma) is decreased with aging, especially substantial reduction was observed between young and middle-age. Interestingly, there were significant differences in PlsCho, PlsCho/PlsEtn ratio, and PlsCho/PL mol% between male (M) and female (F) of young and middle-aged normal subjects. However, the sex differences in PlsCho-related parameters disappeared in elderly normal subjects, suggesting that PlsCho biosynthesis may be partly affected by sex hormone like estrogen. Analysis of serum Pls of middle-aged normal subjects (n=452) showed a strong correlation between PlsCho and PlsEtn. Correlative analysis of PlsCho/PlsEtn ratio with PlsCho or PlsEtn suggested that the ratio is highly influenced by the variation of PlsEtn (**Fig.8**). PlsCho/PlsEtn ratio in red blood cells considerably differs from that in serum (plasma), indicating predominance of PlsEtn similarly to other many organs, tissues and cells. Both PlsCho/PL and PlsEtn/PL mol% in red blood cells of young female were significantly higher than those of young male, whereas only PlsCho/PL mol% in plasma of young female was significantly higher than that of young male. Analysis of Pls in plasma and red blood cells of young normal subjects (n=101) showed a strong correlation between PlsCho and PlsEtn in both specimens. Correlative analysis of PlsCho/PlsEtn ratio with PlsCho or

PlsEtn suggested that the ratio is highly influenced by the variation of PlsCho in the case of red blood cells (n.d.). There were no strong correlations (coefficient >0.3) in all Pls-related parameters between plasma and red blood cells (n.d.).

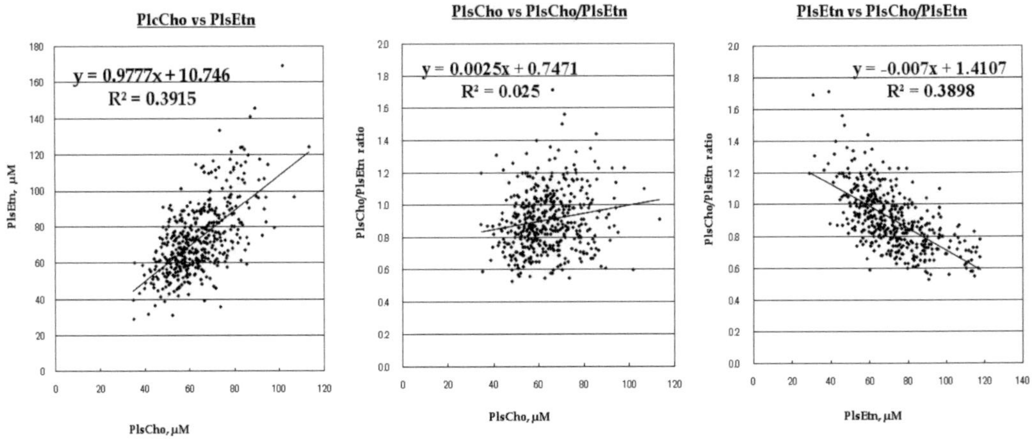

Fig. 8. Relationship between PlsCho and PlsEtn

Next, to investigate the clinical significance of serum Pls, correlative analyses were made of over 40 years old in middle-aged normal subjects (n=216). Their clinical and serum biochemical data are shown in **Table 2**. Almost all data showed in the normal range. Total Pls level was 137.0±29.6, and PlsCho/PlsEtn ratio was 0.87±0.19.

n (M/F)	216 (195/21)	γ-GTP (U/l)	58±58	Adiponectin (μg/mg)	6.9±4.8
Age	48.9±7.1	HDL-C (mg/dl)	65±18	PlsCho (μM)	62.7±12.9
Body weight (kg)	68.5±11.3	LDL-C (mg/dl)	124±27	PlsEtn (μM)	74.2±19.6
BMI (kg/m²)	24.6±6.0	TG (mg/dl)	121±88	PlsCho+PlsEtn (μM)	137.0±29.6
Waist circumstance (cm)	83.0±8.9	sdLDL (mg/dl)	33.0±12.9	PlsCho/PlsEtn ratio	0.87±0.19
Systolic pressure (mmHg)	126±14	Glu (mg/dl)	96±13	PL (mM)	3.13±0.47
Diastolic pressure (mmHg)	81±11	UA (mg/dl)	6.2±1.5	PlsCho/PL (mol %)	2.0±0.4
GOT (U/l)	25±10	Hcy (μmol/l)	11.0±5.0	PlsEtn/PL (mol %)	2.4±0.6
GPT (U/l)	28±18	hsCRP (μg/dl)	78±67	(PlsCho+PlsEtn)/PL (mol %)	4.4±1.0

Mean±S.D.

Table 2. Clinical and biochemical data of middle-aged (≧40 years old) normal subjects

Correlative analyses revealed significant positive correlations between PlsCho and HDL-C (r = 0.714) or adiponectin (r = 0.314), and negative correlations between PlsCho and body weight (r = -0.334), waist circumference (r = -0.375), TG (r = -0.327), hsCRP (r = -0.250), respectively. Furthermore, PlsCho/PL mol% correlated with age (r = -0.266), systolic (r = -0.292) and diastolic pressure (r = -0.283), sdLDL-C (r = -0.458), UA (r = -0.255), as well as atherogenic index of plasma, calculated as log (TG/HDL-C) (r = -0.674) (**Table 3**).

n=216 correlation coefficient >0.25, p< 0.001

Correlation coefficient	age	Body weight	Waist size	Systolic pressure	Diastolic pressure	HDL-C	LDL-C	sdLDL-C
PlsCho	-0.194	**-0.334**	**-0.375**	-0.134	-0.092	**0.714**	0.036	-0.224
PlsEtn	-0.023	-0.098	-0.118	0.020	0.125	**0.408**	0.120	0.016
PlsCho+PlsEtn	-0.100	-0.210	-0.240	-0.045	0.043	**0.580**	0.096	-0.086
PlsCho/PlsEtn	-0.140	-0.185	-0.196	-0.152	-0.241	0.167	-0.127	-0.242
PL	0.052	0.066	0.068	**0.252**	**0.293**	**0.285**	**0.301**	**0.367**
PlsCho/PL	**-0.266**	**-0.374**	**-0.408**	**-0.292**	**-0.283**	**0.506**	-0.162	**-0.458**
PlsEtn/PL	-0.109	-0.157	-0.162	-0.128	-0.050	**0.307**	-0.033	-0.200
(PlsCho+PlsEtn)/PL	-0.191	**-0.271**	**-0.290**	-0.215	-0.162	**0.427**	-0.095	**-0.337**

Correlation coefficient	TG	AIP	Glu	UA	hsCRP	Adipo-nectin	Hcy
PlsCho	**-0.327**	**-0.576**	-0.168	-0.151	**-0.250**	**0.314**	-0.233
PlsEtn	-0.038	-0.248	0.107	-0.012	-0.105	0.103	-0.194
PlsCho+PlsEtn	-0.166	**-0.414**	-0.001	-0.073	-0.178	0.205	-0.230
PlsCho/PlsEtn	**-0.265**	-0.241	**-0.265**	-0.119	-0.032	0.172	0.031
PL	**0.382**	0.188	0.101	**0.253**	-0.068	-0.024	-0.063
PlsCho/PL	**-0.542**	**-0.674**	-0.236	**-0.318**	-0.226	**0.319**	-0.179
PlsEtn/PL	-0.271	**-0.396**	0.042	-0.172	-0.054	0.125	-0.158
(PlsCho+PlsEtn)/PL	**-0.421**	**-0.561**	-0.081	**-0.255**	-0.138	0.226	-0.183

AIP; atherogenic index of plasma, calculated as log (TG/HDL-C)

Table 3. Correlations between Pls and clinical or serum parameters of middle-aged (≧40) normal subjects

Surprisingly, the correlation between PlsCho and HDL-C was stronger rather than that between PlsCho and PlsEtn (**Fig.8, 9**). Indeed, PlsCho preferentially distribute in HDL class compared to other lipoprotein fractions, but this fact cannot explain the strong correlation of PlsCho with HDL-C, because PlsEtn as well as PlsCho also show preferential distribution in HDL compartment.

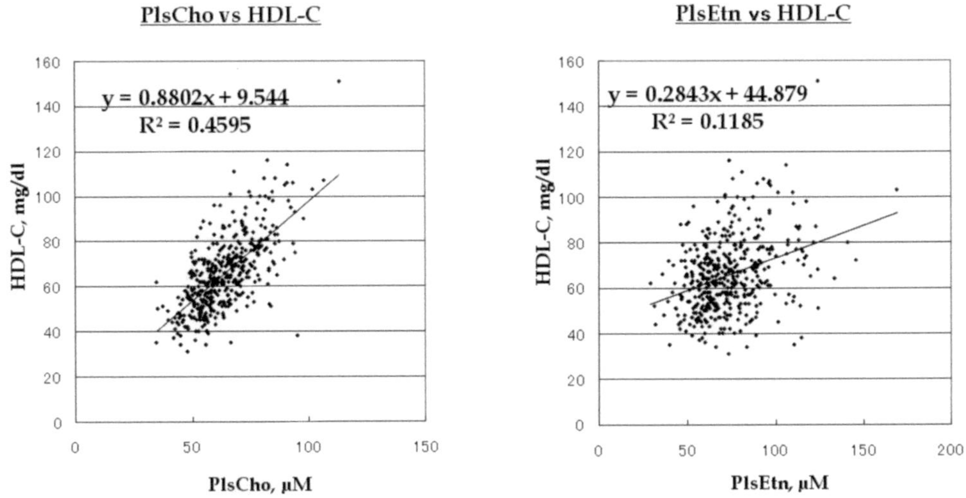

Fig. 9. Relationship between Pls and HDL

2.3.3 Pls in serum of CAD patients

Pls levels in serum and lipoproteins were determined for the CAD patients referred for coronary angiography (*n*=50), and compared with those of patients with (≧75%) and without (<50%) significant stenosis (**Table 4-1**). Serum PlsCho was significantly decreased in CAD patients with ≧75% stenosis compared to patients without significant stenosis (<50%). Total phospholipids (PL), cholesterol (CH), triglyceride (TG), and protein content as well as Pls were determined in HDL and LDL fractions from patients' serum. The ratios of Pls to each lipid (mol %) or protein (μmol/g) in lipoprotein particles were compared between patients with and without significant stenosis. The CAD patients with ≧75% stenosis showed significant reduction in PlsCho/protein ratio in both HDL and LDL, indicating that PlsCho content of each lipoprotein particle is entirely decreased. Concomitantly, tocopherols (V.E.), lipid-soluble antioxidant vitamin, levels in serum were determined, and compared with those of patients with (≧75%) and without (<50%) significant stenosis (**Table 4-2**). There were no significant differences in all tocopherol homolog between them. These results demonstrate the specific reduction in serum PlsCho in CAD patients, and show clinical utility of PlsCho as a serum biomarker for atherogenic status.

Next, to investigate the relationship between Pls and other serum lipids or lipoproteins, correlative analyses were made of another CAD patients referred for coronary angiography (*n*=148). Their serum lipids and lipoproteins data including Pls are shown in **Table 5**.

Interestingly, in addition to the strong correlation of PlsCho with HDL (Maeba et al., 2007), LDL particle size significantly correlated with PlsCho/PlsEtn ratio as well as TG and HDL-C (**Table 6**). Small dense LDL (sdLDL) is well-known risk factor for atherosclerosis, and frequently observed in dyslipidemia of type-2 diabetes or MetS, which is characterized by low HDL and high TG (Nozue et al, 2007). As PlsEtn is presumably a precursor of PlsCho in biosynthetic pathway, PlsCho/PlsEtn ratio can be regarded as an indicator of transfer rate from PlsEtn to PlsCho. Therefore, the cause or effect of declining transfer rate is assumed to be potentially related to the appearance of atherogenic sdLDL, but it is obscure how Pls are involved in the alteration of lipoprotein metabolism.

Serum

stenosis	*n* (M/F)	Age	PlsCho μM	PlsEtn μM	PlsCho+PlsEtn μM
≧75%	30 (20/10)	67.8±10.3	39.2±10.5**	63.0±14.5	102.2±21.6
<50%	20 (11/9)	61.0±17.7	49.0±12.4	66.9±18.8	115.9±25.7

stenosis	PlsCho/PlsEtn ratio	PL mM	PlsCho/PL mol %	PlsEtn/PL mol %	(PlsCho+PlsEtn)/PL mol %
≧75%	0.64±0.16	2.34±0.39	1.7±0.5	2.8±0.7	4.5±1.1
<50%	0.78±0.28	2.59±0.54	1.9±0.4	2.6±0.7	4.5±0.9

HDL

stenosis	PlsCho/PlsEtn ratio	PlsCho/PL mol %	PlsEtn/PL mol %	PlsCho/CH mol %	PlsEtn/CH mol %
≧75%	0.72±0.20	1.7±0.4	2.5±0.8	1.5±0.4	2.1±0.7
<50%	0.86±0.34	1.7±0.4	2.2±0.6	1.5±0.3	1.9±0.6

stenosis	PlsCho/TG mol %	PlsEtn/TG mol %	PlsCho/protein μmol/g	PlsEtn/protein μmol/g
≧75%	14.6±8.2	21.4±13.8	11.3±3.5*	16.3±6.1
<50%	12.7±4.8	16.1±7.1	14.2±4.9	17.7±6.4

LDL

stenosis	PlsCho/PlsEtn ratio	PlsCho/PL mol %	PlsEtn/PL mol %	PlsCho/CH mol %	PlsEtn/CH mol %
≧75%	0.80±0.19	1.4±0.3	1.8±0.3	0.6±0.1	0.7±0.2
<50%	0.94±0.30	1.6±0.4	1.8±0.4	0.7±0.2	0.7±0.2

stenosis	PlsCho/TG mol %	PlsEtn/TG mol %	PlsCho/protein μmol/g	PlsEtn/protein μmol/g
≧75%	3.3±1.4	4.2±1.8	24.9±6.0*	31.6±6.5
<50%	4.3±1.9	4.8±2.2	29.8±7.3	32.8±7.4

Mean±S.D. t-test between patients with and without significant stenosis, * $p < 0.05$ ** $p < 0.01$

Table 4-1. Comparison of Pls levels in serum and lipoproteins between CAD patients with and without significant stenosis

stenosis	α-Toc. μM	β-Toc. μM	γ-Toc. μM	δ-Toc. μM
≧75%	29.6±5.8	0.6±0.2	1.9±0.7	0.1±0.1
<50%	30.4±8.5	0.6±0.2	2.1±0.8	0.1±0.1

Table 4-2. Comparison of V.E levels in serum between patients with and without significant stenosis

n (M/F)	148 (110/38)	LDL size, nm	25.5 ± 0.5
Age	65.2±12.2	MDA-LDL, U/l	105 ± 40
CAD ≥75% stenosis	63.5%	LP (a), mg/dl	26 ± 21
PlsCho, μM	65 ± 18	TG, mg/dl	123 ± 80
PlsEtn, μM	83 ± 33	LPL mass, ng/ml	42.7 ±13.3
PlsCho +PlsEtn, μM	148 ± 50	apo A-I, mg/dl	119 ± 22
PlsCho/PlsEtn ratio	0.83 ± 0.17	apo A-II, mg/dl	24 ± 6
PL, mM	2.2 ± 0.4	apo B, mg/dl	102 ± 26
TC, mg/dl	189 ± 40	apo B-48, mg/dl	6.9 ± 3.2
LDL-C, mg/dl	119 ± 45	apo C-II, mg/dl	4 ± 2
HDL-C, mg/dl	47 ± 11	apo C-III, mg/dl	9 ± 3
RLP-C, mg/dl	5 ± 2	apo E, mg/dl	4.3 ± 1.3

Mean±S.D.

Table 5. Serum lipids and lipoproteins data of CAD patients

Correlation coefficient	RLP-C	TG	apo C-II	HDL-C	PlsCho/PlsEtn ratio
LDL particle size	-0.452	-0.442	-0.431	0.415	0.402

RLP-C; remnant-like particle-cholesterol

Table 6. Parameters indicating significant strong correlation (coefficient > 0.4, p<0.001) with LDL particle size

Most of the PlsCho in the plasma membrane are considered to be probably made by *N*-methylation of PlsEtn in three steps by reaction with *S*-adenosylmethionine (AdoMet), rather than base exchange via exchange of choline (Cho) for ethanolamine (Etn) or serine (Ser), or the Kennedy pathway by reaction of cytidine monophosphate with PlsEtn (Horrocks et al, 1986). Serum PlsCho is also possibly derived from *N*-methylation of PlsEtn, catalyzed by a hepatocyte-specific enzyme, phosphatidylethanolamine *N*-methyltransferase (PEMT) (Fig.10). Interestingly, PEMT knockout mice reveal that PEMT is required for hepatic secretion of triacylglycerol (TG) in very low density lipoproteins (VLDL) (Noga et al, 2002). This finding suggests that PlsCho may have an essential role in lipoprotein metabolism, because PEMT is responsible for ~30% of phosphatidylcholine (PC), major Cho-containing glycerophospholipid, formed in liver, while PlsCho is primarily made from PlsEtn probably via PEMT pathway. Furthermore, a polymorphism of the human *PEMT* gene is associated with diminished activity and may confer susceptibility to nonalcoholic fatty liver disease (NAFLD) (Song et al, 2005). This observation also suggests the importance of PlsCho in the transport of TG from liver, and the participation of the lack of PlsCho in the onset of metabolic syndrome (MetS), because NAFLD shares many features of the MetS, such as abdominal obesity, type 2 diabetes, dyslipidemia, and insulin resistance (Pacifico et al, 2011). Human *PEMT* gene is regulated by estrogen (Resseguie et al, 2007), which may explain the sex difference in serum levels of PlsCho, despite no significant sex difference in serum levels of PC, and provide an evidence supporting the involvement of PEMT pathway in the synthesis of PlsCho. Moreover, a nutritional insufficiency in the methyl donor such as methionine or choline also causes lack of PlsCho and elevated homocysteine (Hcy), a risk factor for cardiovascular disease. These reports may provide the physiopathological basis for the validity of PlsCho as a biomarker for atherogenic status.

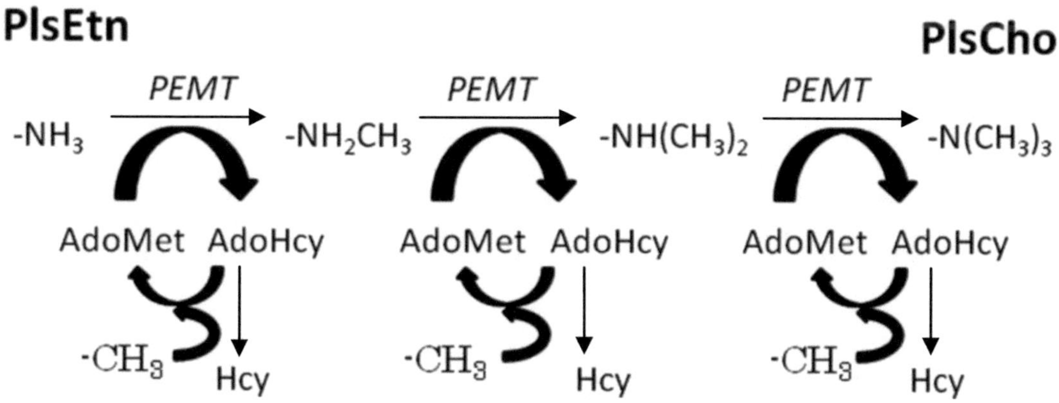

Fig. 10. PEMT pathway for conversion of PlsEtn to PlsCho

2.3.4 Intervention study of increasing serum Pls

Myo-inositol (MI) is one of 9 isomers of inositol, and is the most abundant in nature including human body. Besides dietary intake, MI is synthesized from glucose in vivo. MI contributes to numerous functions as a precursor molecule, such as signal transduction through biosynthesis of inositol phospholipids, or ca^{2+} homeostasis through biosynthesis of inositol phosphates (Vanhaesebroeck et al., 2001). Moreover, MI itself plays an important role in normal functions of CNS as an organic osmolyte (Gullans & Verbalis, 1993), and also possibly involves in myelin formation (Berry et al., 2003). Pls are major component of myelin membranes, and essential for myelin formation and functions. In animal studies, oral administration of MI showed to increase Pls level in rat brain (Hoffman-Kuczynski & Reo, 2004). Therefore, we have undertaken MI intervention study to investigate whether MI administration improves the dyslipidemia of MetS through facilitating Pls biosynthesis, and to explore the relationship between serum Pls and sdLDL. Clinical background of study subjects is shown in **Table 7**. Almost all subjects (n=17) were hyperlipidemia, and half of the subjects were diagnosed as MetS. Treatment of MI 5g daily for 1 week, followed by MI 10g daily for 1 week markedly reduced sdLDL, and significantly increased PlsCho as well as PlsCho/PL and blood glucose particularly for MetS subjects, without alteration in the levels of TG and HDL-C (**Table 8**). This result suggests that facilitating PlsCho biosynthesis potentially prevents from atherogenic status trough reducing sdLDL. The increase in Pls levels after MI treatment tended to be inversely proportional to the serum Pls levels before treatment (Fig.11). Serum Pls reached a plateau level of around 150 μM with MI treatment, which corresponds to the average level observed in normal subjects (Maeba et al., 2008). Pls biosynthesis is strictly regulated and the Pls levels in cells or tissues are physiologically kept constant (Liu et al., 2005). Our result appears to support these facts.

n (M/F)	17 (15/2)
Age	43.6 ± 6.6
Rate of obesity (BMI≧25)	65%
Rate of hyperlipidemia	94%
Rate of diabetes mellitus	18%
Rate of hypertension	29%
Rate of metabolic syndrome (MetS) (according to Japanese guideline*)	47%
Rate of current cigarette smoking	71%

* Japanese criteria for MetS
MetS is diagnosed when 1) plus more than two of the risk determinants among 2) – 4).
1) Waist circumstance: M≧85 cm, F≧90 cm
2) TG≧150 mg/dl and/or HDL-C<40 mg/dl
3) Systolic pressure≧130mmHg and/or Diastolic pressure≧85 mmHg
4) Fasting glucose≧110 mg/dl

Table 7. Clinical background of study subjects

	MetS (*n* = 8)		non- MetS (*n* = 9)	
	before	after	before	after
BMI, kg/m2	29.3±3.0	29.7±3.7 (101.4)	25.3±2.3	25.2±2.6 (99.6)
Waist circumstance, cm	99.6±6.3	99.9±9.1 (100.3)	85.0±4.6	82.9±4.0 (97.5)
Systolic pressure, mmHg	136±13	140±26 (102.9)	132±11	125±9 (94.7)
Diastolic pressure, mmHg	85±12	93±16 (109.4)	78±7	81±5 (103.8)
Blood glucose, mg/dl	104.1±16.6	87.5±11.6 (84.1)*	96.2±18.6	97.7±17.4 (101.6)
hsCRP, mg/dl	0.316±0.315	0.171±0.137 (54.1)	0.056±0.029	0.453±0.995 (808.9)
apo A-I, mg/dl	121.3±21.6	122.5±15.2 (101.0)	147.6±14.7	146.0±16.4 (98.9)
apo B, mg/dl	142.6±43.4	130.6±40.4 (91.6)	123.9±41.2	119.8±48.9 (96.7)
apo E, mg/dl	6.0±1.2	5.8±1.3 (96.7)	4.3±1.5	4.2±2.0 (97.7)
TG, mg/dl	230.1±89.9	239.5±142.4 (104.1)	151.8±87.4	135.3±100.8 (89.1)
TC, mg/dl	261.9±69.7	246.1±62.6 (94.0)	256.3±66.1	249.3±85.2 (97.3)
HDL-C, mg/dl	44.9±11.1	45.5±11.3 (100.9)	58.2±7.1	58.6±6.7 (100.7)
LDL-C, mg/dl	185.5±71.4	166.1±68.0 (89.5)	174.4±58.0	164.4±70.8 (94.3)
sdLDL-C, mg/dl	56.4±25.0	39.2±19.7 (69.5)	37.5±21.4	32.5±23.3 (86.7)
PL, mM	2.8±0.5	2.8±0.5 (100.0)	2.9±0.5	2.8±0.8 (96.6)
PlsCho, μM	40.9±9.0	51.5±3.6 (125.9)*	50.7±12.5	57.3±18.5 (113.0)
PlsEtn, μM	44.9±13.1	53.9±6.7 (120.0)	56.6±20.6	60.0±20.3 (106.0)
PlsCho+ PlsEtn, μM	85.8±20.3	105.4±8.6 (122.8)*	107.2±30.3	117.3±37.4 (109.4)
PlsCho/PL, mol%	1.5±0.2	1.9±0.2 (130.3)***	1.7±0.4.	2.1±0.5.(115.8)
PlsEtn/PL, mol%	1.6±0.4	2.0±0.4 (124.4)	2.0±0.9	2.2±0.8 (106.4)
(PlsCho+PlsEtn)/PL, mol%	3.1±0.5	3.9±0.6 (127.2)**	3.8±1.3	4.2±1.2 (111.0)
PlsCho/PlsEtn ratio	0.94±0.23	0.97±0.12 (103.2)	0.94±0.21	0.98±0.17 (104.3)

Values are mean±S.D., and values in parentheses are relative percentage to each value before treatment.
t-test between before and after treatment, * $p < 0.05$, ** $p < 0.01$, *** $p < 0.001$

Table 8. Effect of *myo*-inositol treatment on clinical and serum biochemical parameters of the hyperlipidemic subjects with (MetS) and without metabolic syndrome (non-MetS)

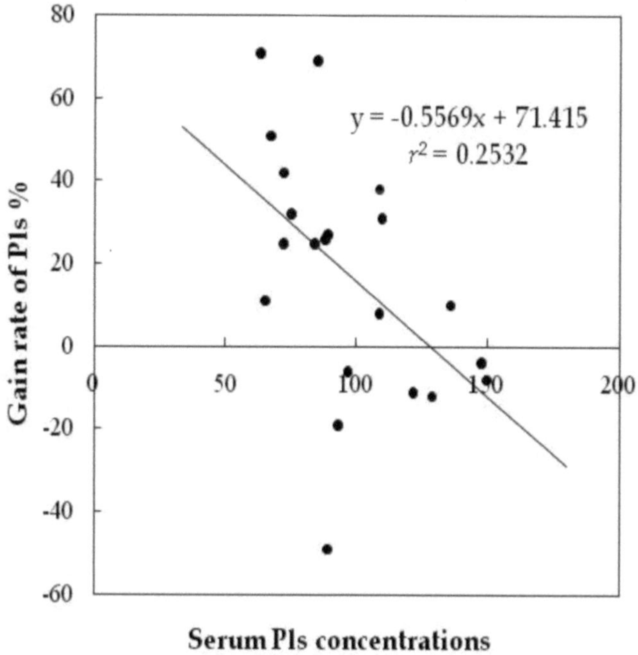

Fig. 11. Relationship between the gain rate of Pls after MI treatment and serum Pls levels before treatment

3. Conclusion

We have established auto-analytical ^{125}I-HPLC system for a routine diagnostic test of human serum (or plasma) Pls. We have applied the system to the determination of serum (or plasma) Pls from normal subjects and CAD patients, and found that serum (or plasma) PlsCho is a novel and reliable biomarker for MetS and atherosclerosis. Intervention study of increasing PlsCho by MI treatment demonstrated clinical utility of PlsCho as a serum (or plasma) biomarker for atherogenic status. Improvement of PlsCho deficiency is important for preventing from life-style related disease associated with aging and oxidative stress. MI intake is one of the effective ways to enhance Pls biosynthesis.

4. Acknowledgement

We especially thank the subjects who participated in these studies. We thank Mr. Yuya Yamazaki of the Life Science Department, Advanced Materials R&D Laboratory, ADEKA Co., for developing ^{125}I-HPLC method. These works were supported by "Knowledge Cluster Initiative" (2nd stage, "Sapporo Bio-cluster Bio-S") of the Ministry of Education, Science, Sports and Culture of Japan. Part of these works was enabled by a Grant-in-Aid for the Technology Development Project for the Creation of Collective Private Agribusiness (H15-7) from the Ministry of Agriculture, Forestry and Fisheries, Japan.

5. References

Berry, G.; Wu, S.; Buccafusca, R.; Ren, J.; Gonzales, L.; Ballard, P.; Golden, J.; Stevens, M. & Greer, J. (2003). Loss of murine Na^+/myo-inositol cotransporter leads to brain myo-inositol depletion and central apnea, *J Biol Chem,* Vol.278, pp. 18297-18302

Brites, P; Waterham, H. & Wanders, R. (2004). Functions and biosynthesis of plasmalogens in heath and disease, *Biochim Biophys Acta,* Vol.1636, pp. 219-231

Brosche, T. (1997). Plasmalogen phospholipids - facts and theses to their antioxidative qualities, *Arch Gerontol Geriatr,* Vol.25, pp. 73-81

Engelmann, B.; Brautigam, C. & Thiery, J. (1994). Plasmalogen phospholipids as potential protectors against lipid peroxidation of low density lipoproteins, *Biochem Biophys Res Commun,* Vol.204, pp.1235-1242

Glaser, P. & Gross, R. (1994). Plasmenylethanolamine facilitates rapid membrane fusion: a stopped-flow kinetic investigation correlating the propensity of a major plasma membrane constituent to adapt an H_{II} phase with its ability to promote membrane fusion, *Biochemistry,* Vol.33, pp. 5805-5812

Goodenow, D.; Cook, L.; Liu, J.; Lu, Y.; Jayasinghe, D.; Ahiahonu, P.; Heath, D.; Yamazaki, Y.; Flax, J.; Krenitsky, K.; Sparks D.; Lerner, A.; Friedland, R.; Kudo, T.; Kamino, K.; Morihara, T.; Takeda, M. & Wood, P. (2007). Peripheral ethanolamine plasmalogen deficiency: A logical causative factor in alzheimer's disease and dementia, J Lipid Res, Vol.48, pp. 2485-2498

Gorgas, K.; Teigler, A.; Komljenovic, D. & Just, W. (2006). The ether lipid-deficient mouse: Tracking down plasmalogen functions, *Biochim Biophys Acta,* Vol.1763, pp. 1511-1526

Gullans, S. & Verbalis, J. (1993). Control of brain volume during hyperosmolar and hypoosmolar conditions, *Annu Rev Med,* Vol.44, pp. 289-301

Hoffman-Kuczynski, B. & Reo, N. (2004). Studies of myo-inositol and plasmalogen metabolism in rat brain, *Neurochem Re,s* Vol.29, pp. 843-855

Horrocks, L. (1968). The alk-1-enyl group content of mammalian myelin phosphoglycerides by quantitative two-dimensional thin-layer chromatography, *J Lipid Res,* Vol.9, pp. 469-472

Horrocks, L.; Yeo, Y.; Harder, H.; Mozzi, R. & Goracci, G. (1986). Choline plasmalogen, glycerophospholipid methylation, and receptor-mediated activation of adenylate cyclase, In: *Advances in cyclic nucleotide and protein phsophorylation research,* Greengard, P. & Robison, G., pp.263-291, Raven Press, New York

Ingrand, S.; Wahl, A.; Favreliere, S.; Barbot, F. & Tallineau, C. (2000). Quantification of long-chain aldehydes by gas chromatography coupled to mass spectrometry as a tool for simultaneous measurement of plasmalogens and their aldehydic breakdown products, *Anal Biochem,*Vol.280, pp. 65-72

Lee, T. (1998). Biosynthesis and possible biological functions of plasmalogens, *Biochim Biophys Acta,* Vol.1394, pp. 129-145

Lessig, J. & Fuchs, B. (2009). Plasmalogens in biological systems: Their role in oxidative processes in biological membranes, their contribution to pathological processes and aging and plasmalogen analysis, *Curr Med Chem,* Vol.16, pp. 2021-2041

Liu, D.; Nagan, N.; Just, W.; Rodemer, C.; Thai, T. & Zoeller, R. (2005). Roles of dihydroxyacetonephosphate acyltransferase in the biosynthesis of plasmalogens and nonether glycerolipids, *J Lipid Res*, Vol.46, pp.727-735

Maeba, R. & Ueta, N. (2003a). Ethanolamine plasmalogen prevent the oxidation of cholesterol by reducing the oxidizability of cholesterol in phospholipids bilayers, *J Lipid Res*, Vol.44, pp. 164-171

Maeba, R. & Ueta, N. (2003b). Ethanolamine plasmalogen and cholesterol reduce the total membrane oxidizability measured by the oxygen uptake method, *Biochem Biophys Res Commun*, Vol.302, pp. 265-270

Maeba, R. & Ueta, N. (2004). Determination of choline and ethanolamine plasmalogens in human plasma by HPLC using radioactive triiodide (1-) ion ($^{125}I_3^-$), *Anal Biochem*, Vol.331, pp. 169-176

Maeba, R.; Maeda, T.; Kinoshita, M.; Takao, K.; Takenaka, H.; Kusana, J.; Yoshimura, N.; Takeoka, Y.; Yasuda, D.; Okazaki, T. & Teramoto, T. (2007). Plasmalogens in human serum positively correlate with high-density lipoprotein and decrease with aging, *J Atheroscler Thromb*, Vol.14, pp. 12-18

Maeba, R.; Hara, H.; Ishikawa, H.; Hayashi, S.; Yoshimura, N.; Kusano, J.; Takeoka, Y.; Yasuda, D.; Okazaki, T.; Kinoshita, M. & Teramoto, T. (2008). *Myo*-inositol treatment increases serum plasmalogens and decreases small dense LDL, particularly in the hyperlipidemic subjects with metabolic syndrome, *J Nutr Sci Vitaminol*, Vol.54, pp. 196-202

Maeba, R.; Yamazaki, Y.; Nezu, T. & Okazaki, T. (2012). Improvement and validation of ^{125}I-high-performance liquid chromatography method for determination of total human serum choline and ethanolamine plasmalogens, *Ann Clin Biochem*, Vol.49, pp. 86-93

Nagan, N. & Zoeller, R. (2001). Plasmalogens: biosynthesis and functions, *Prog Lipid Res*, Vol.40, pp. 199-229

Noga, A.; Zhao, Y. & Vance, D. (2002). An unexpected requirement for phosphatidylethanolamine *N*-methyltransferase in the secretion of very low density lipoproteins, *J Biol Chem*, Vol.277, pp. 42358-42365

Nozue, T.; Michishita, I.; Ishibashi, Y.; Ito, S.; Iwaki, T.; Mizuguchi, I.; Miura, M.; Ito, Y. & Hirano, T. (2007). Small dense low-density lipoprotein cholesterol is a useful marker of metabolic syndrome in patients with coronary artery disease, *J Atheroscler Thromb*, Vol.14, pp. 202-207

Pacifico, L.; Nobili, V.; Anania, C.; Verdecchia, P. & Chiesa, C. (2011). Pediatric nonalcoholic fatty liver disease, metabolic syndrome and cardiovascular risk, *World J Gastroenterol*, Vol.17, pp. 3082-3091

Poynter, M. & Davnes, R. (1998). Peroxisome proliferators-activated receptor α activation modulates cellular redox status, represses nuclear factor-κB signaling, and reduces inflammatory cytokine production in aging, *J Biol Chem*, Vol.273, pp. 32833-32841

Resseguie, M.; Song, J.; Niculescu, M.; Costa, K.; Randall, T. & Zeisel S. (2007). Phosphatidylethanolamine *N*-methyltransferase (*PEMT*) gene expression is induced by estrogen in human and mouse primary hepatocytes, *FASEB J*, Vol.21, pp. 2622-2632

Song, J.; Costa, K.; Fischer, L.; Kohlmeier, M.; Kwock, L.; Wang, S. & Zeisel S. (2005). Polymorphism of the *PEMT* gene and susceptibility to nonalcoholic fatty liver disease (NAFLD), *FASEB J*, Vol.19, pp. 1266-1271

Vance, J. (1990). Lipoproteins secreted by cultured rat hepatocytes contain the antioxidant 1-alk-1-enyl-2-acylglycerophosphoethanolamine, *Biochim Biophys Acta,* Vol.1045, pp. 128-134

Vanhaesebroeck, B.; Leevers, S.; Ahmadi, K.; Timms, J.; Katso, R.; Driscoll, P.; Woscholski, R.; Parker, P. & Waterfield, M. (2001). Synthesis and function of 3-phosphorylated inositol lipids, *Annu Rev Biochem*, Vol.70, pp. 535-602

Wanders, R. & Waterham H. (2006). Peroxisomal disorders: The single peroxisomal enzyme deficiencies, *Biochim Biophys Acta,* Vol.1763, pp. 1707-172 169-176

Wiesner, P.; Leidl, K.; Boettcher, A.; Schmitz, G. & Liebisch, G. (2009). Lipid profiling of FPLC-separated lipoprotein fractions by electrospray ionization tandem mass spectrometry, *J Lipid Res,* Vol.50, pp. 574-585

Williams, J.; Anderson, C. & Jasik, A. (1962). A sensitive and specific method for plasmalogens and other enol ethers, *J Lipid Res,* Vol.3, pp. 378-381

Zemski, B. & Murphy, R. (2004). Electrospray ionization tandem mass spectrometry of glycerophosphoethanolamine plasmalogen phospholipids, *J Am Soc Mass Spectrom,* Vol.15, pp. 1499-1508

Zoeller, R.; Morand, O. & Raetz, C. (1988). A possible role for plasmalogens in protecting animal cells against photosensitized killing, *J Biol Chem*, Vol.263, pp. 11590-11596

Zoeller, R.; Lake, A.; Nagan. N.; Gaposchkin, D.; Legner, M. & Lieberthal, W. (1999). Plasmalogens as endogenous antioxidants: somatic cell mutants reveal the importance of the vinyl ether, *Biochem J,* Vol.338, pp.769-776